Statistics for Biology and Health

Series Editors:
M. Gail
K. Krickeberg
J. Samet
A. Tsiatis
W. Wong

T0255165

For other titles published in this series, go to
http://www.springer.com/series/2848

Mark Chang

Modern Issues and Methods in Biostatistics

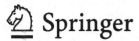 Springer

M. Chang
AMAG Pharmaceuticals, Inc.
Biometrics
Hayden Ave. 100
02421 Lexington Massachusetts
USA

Statistics for Biology and Health Series Editors

M. Gail
National Cancer Institute
Bethesda, MD 20892
USA

A. Tsiatis
Department of Statistics
North Carolina State University
Raleigh, NC 27695
USA

Klaus Krickeberg
Le Châtelet
F-63270 Manglieu
France

W. Wong
Department of Statistics
Stanford University
Stanford, CA 94305-4065
USA

Jonathan M. Samet
Department of Preventive Medicine
Keck School of Medicine
University of Southern California
1441 Eastlake Ave. Room 4436, MC 9175
Los Angles, CA 90089

ISSN 1431-8776
ISBN 978-1-4614-2945-6   ISBN 978-1-4419-9842-2 (eBook)
DOI 10.1007/978-1-4419-9842-2
Springer New York Dordrecht Heidelberg London

Springer is part of Springer Science+Business Media (www.springer.com)

Preface

Classic biostatistics, a branch of statistical science, has as its main focus the applications of statistics in public health, the life sciences, and the pharmaceutical industry. Modern biostatistics, beyond just a simple application of statistics, is a confluence of statistics and knowledge of multiple intertwined fields. Biostatistics often requires innovations across disciplines. Over the years, biostatistics has gradually shaped its own unique characteristics and approaches. Indeed, the application demands, the advancements in computer technology, and the rapid growth of life science data (e.g., genomics data) have promoted the formation of modern biostatistics.

There are at least three characteristics of modern biostatistics: (1) in-depth engagement in the application fields that require penetration of knowledge across several fields, (2) high-level complexity of data because they are longitudinal, incomplete, or latent because they are heterogeneous due to a mixture of data or experiment types, because of high-dimensionality, which may make meaningful reduction impossible, or because of extremely small or large size; and (3) dynamics, the speed of development in methodology and analyses, has to match the fast growth of data with a constantly changing face.

This book is written for researchers, biostatisticians/statisticians, and scientists who are interested in quantitative analyses. The goal is to introduce modern issues and methods in biostatistics and help researchers and students quickly grasp key concepts and methods. Bear in mind that many methods can solve the same problem and many problems can be solved by the same method, which becomes apparent when those topics are discussed in a single volume. Modern biostatistics requires researchers to possess diverse knowledge. However, given the vast number of publications in the research area, it requires a huge investment of time to gain insight into modern biostatistics. Therefore, I hope this book can serve as a vehicle to achieve this objective, though by no means do I want or am I able to cover this fast-growing field completely. I would also like to warn readers that, inevitably, the book will often reflect the author's opinions, especially in discussing controversial matters. Nevertheless, it displays broad coverage and can be used as a textbook or as a reference text.

The book consists of ten chapters: Multiple-Hypothesis Testing Strategy, Pharmaceutical Decision and Game Theory, Noninferiority Trial Design, Adaptive Trial Design, Missing Data Imputation and Analysis, Multivariate and Multistage Survival Data Modeling, Meta-analysis, Data Mining and Signal Detection, Monte Carlo Simulation, and Bayesian Methods and Applications. Some of these titles are new; others are not that new but include novel ingredients or developments in methodology, computation algorithms, or applications. These areas have a common reason for their popularity in that they are in high demand by the real world and especially from the pharmaceutical industry.

Each chapter includes an introduction to the concepts, discussions of methodology, and examples of applications. Controversies and challenges are also included. Each chapter is limited to about 30 pages. Given the limit in length, materials are selected to focus on the key concepts and methods that have been used in practice; lengthy mathematical derivations are generally omitted, but references to them are provided. At the end of each chapter, exercises are provided as well as a list of references for further reading.

I point out that, due to the nature of each of the ten topics, the mathematical complexity varies from chapter to chapter. Some are more theoretical, whereas others are more scientifically involved and require thinking rather beyond straight mathematics. I have fully realized the importance of consistency in presentation across chapters but will not over-emphasize it. The book is organized as follows.

Chapter 1, Multiple – Hypothesis Testing Strategy, introduces commonly used methods for multiplicity adjustment in the frequentist paradigm, including commonly used single-step and stepwise procedures such as gatekeeping and tree-structured test procedures. Discussions of applications will focus on clinical trials. The controversies surrounding multiplicity issues particularly are addressed.

Chapter 2, Pharmaceutical Decision and Game Theory, addresses decision and game theory, which has a long history in economics. However, recently the need for more cost-effective R & D programs has demanded a shift in the pharmaceutical decision-making process from the qualitative decision paradigm to the quantitative decision approaches that are based on formal decision and game theory. For this reason, this chapter first introduces decision and game theory in general and then discusses how to apply it to the pharmaceutical decision process by using models, such as the Markov decision process and implementations using computer simulations. Applications presented include clinical development program and R & D portfolio optimizations, and prescription drug commercialization among others.

Chapter 3, Noninferiority Trial Design, discusses the needs of noninferiority (NI) trials and summarizes three common methods for NI trial designs, including the fixed-margin, lamda, and synthetic methods. Comparisons are made among the different methods, and the controversies surrounding such trials are discussed. The materials covered in this chapter should meet the basic needs for designing an NI trial.

Chapter 4, Adaptive Trial Design, deals with adaptive trials, a coming storm in the pharmaceutical industry thanks to the leadership of biostatistics. This chapter introduces the adaptive design concept and provides a uniform formulation for hypothesis-based adaptive trial designs. The evaluation matrix and various applications are studied. Controversies and challenges are considered.

Chapter 5, Missing Data Imputation and Analysis, discusses the problem of imperfect or incomplete information. Traditional methods such as the general linear model, which ignore subjects with incomplete observations, often cause bias and often are not applicable in practice. Statistical models that effectively deal with missing observations are becoming increasingly important, and research in this area is developing rapidly. This chapter discusses different types of missing data and various models for analyses with ignorable and nonignorable missing patterns. Implementations using software such as SAS are presented as well.

Chapter 6, Multivariate and Multistage Survival Data Modeling, addresses the fact that the survival data model we are dealing with today in the life sciences is more complicated than ever, involving multivariates and many covariates. Multistage models provide powerful tools for solving various problems with survival data such as competing risks, adaptive treatment switching, informative dropouts, progressive disease, and longitudinal data modeling. This chapter starts with a review of various survival models, including Cox's proportional hazard model, the frailty model, the copula model, the first-hitting-time model, and nonparametric approaches. The frailty, copula, and first-hitting-time models are discussed in detail and expanded to multivariate and multistage models. We discuss step-by-step model building using various examples.

Chapter 7, Meta-analysis, discusses what is in a sense an art, with many controversies, especially for post hoc meta-analysis. Meta-analysis methods are classified into three categories based on data type: subject-based data, study-based data, and mixed-data models. Fixed-effect and random-effect models and sequential methods are at the center of the discussion. Graphical presentations and interpretations of the results are also made.

Chapter 8, Data Mining and Signal Detection, introduces supervised, unsupervised, and reinforcement learning mechanics in data mining methods, including link analysis, the nearest-neighbor method, kernel and tree methods, the support vector machine, artificial neural networks, the k-means algorithm, genetic programming, cellular automata, and agent-based methods. Applications in the life sciences and drug development are discussed. Signal detection with various sequential likelihood ratio tests and other data mining methods is studied.

Chapter 9, Monte Carlo Simulation, notes that computer simulations have become a very powerful and cost-effective approach in the life sciences and in the pharmaceutical industry. This chapter discusses several random sampling methods, clinical trial simulations, molecular designs, biological pathway simulations, and pharmacokinetic and pharmacodynamic simulations.

Chapter 10, Bayesian Methods and Applications, introduces Bayesian inferences, hierarchical models, decision models, model selection, Bayesian multiplicity, and computational methods. It also provides application examples for clinical trials, signal detection, missing data-imputation, meta-analysis, disease mapping, and other areas.

The draft manuscripts were reviewed by nine statisticians. Their constructive comments have greatly improved the manuscript. In the big picture, they consistently suggested reducing the mathematical complexity and adding more motivating examples. As a result, I have added about 20 examples and 40 pages. I have also removed some mathematical content; but I found it difficult to cut math too much and at the same time cover a reasonable scope in depth of topic within 30 pages – I wanted it to be concise.

My little daughter, Monica, a middle school student, reviewed an early draft manuscript of all ten chapters and corrected many of my grammatical errors (she very much enjoyed doing that for me!). I want to thank her a lot! Dr. Robert Pierce carefully reviewed parts of the manuscript before I submitted it to the publisher. Without his review, the quality of the book would not be as good as you have right now. Finally, I would like to thank Mr. John Kimmel and Mr. Marc Strauss at Springer for providing me with the opportunity to work on this project.

Mark Chang (张扬)

Contents

Chapter 1
Multiple-Hypothesis Testing Strategy

1.1 Multiple-Testing Problems

1.1.1 Statistical Hypothesis Testing

In this chapter, we will discuss multiple hypothesis-testing issues from a frequentist perspective. The Bayesian approaches for multiple-testing problems will be discussed briefly in Chap. 10. As we all know, a typical hypothesis test in the frequentist paradigm can be written as

$$H_o : \delta \in \Omega_0 \text{ or } H_a : \delta \in \Omega_1, \tag{1.1}$$

where δ is a parameter such as treatment effect, the domain Ω_0 can be, for example, a set of nonpositive values, and the domain Ω_1 can be the negation of Ω_0. In this case, (1.1) becomes

$$H_o : \delta \leq 0 \text{ or } H_a : \delta > 0. \tag{1.2}$$

The probability of erroneously rejecting H_o when it is true is called the type-I error rate, α. Similarly, the probability of erroneously rejecting H_a when it is true is called the type-II error rate, β. The probability of rejecting H_o is the power of the hypothesis test, which is dependent on the particular value of δ. The power is numerically equal to $1 - \beta$ when H_a is true. When H_o is true, the power is numerically equal to the type-I error rate, α.

1.1.2 Sources of Multiplicity

It is well known that multiple-hypothesis testing (multiple-testing) can inflate the type-I error dramatically without proper adjustments for the p-values or significance level. This is referred to as a multiplicity issue. The multiplicity

M. Chang, *Modern Issues and Methods in Biostatistics*, Statistics for Biology and Health, DOI 10.1007/978-1-4419-9842-2_1, © Springer Science+Business Media, LLC 2011

can come from different sources, for example, in clinical trials, it can come from (1) multiple-treatment comparisons, (2) multiple tests performed at different times, (3) multiple tests for several endpoints, (4) multiple tests conducted for multiple populations using the same treatment within a single experiment, and (5) a combination of some or all of the sources above.

Multiple-treatment comparisons are often conducted in dose-finding studies. Multiple time-point analyses are often conducted in longitudinal studies with repeated measures, or in trials with group sequential or adaptive designs.

Why are multiple-endpoint analyses required? Lemuel Moyé points out (2003, p. 76) that there are three primary reasons why we conduct a multiple-endpoint study: (1) a disease has an unknown aetiology or no clinical consensus on the single most important clinical efficacy endpoint exists; (2) a disease manifests itself in multidimensional ways; and (3) a therapeutic area for which the prevailing methods for assessment of treatment efficacy dictate a multifaceted approach both for selection of the efficacy endpoints and for their evaluation.

The statistical analyses of multiple-endpoint problems can be categorized as (1) a single primary efficacy endpoint with one or more secondary endpoints, (2) coprimary endpoints (more than one primary endpoint) with secondary endpoints, (3) composite primary efficacy endpoints with interest in each individual endpoint, or (4) a surrogate primary endpoint with supportive secondary endpoints. A surrogate endpoint is a biological or clinical marker that can replace a gold standard endpoint such as survival.

In the case of diseases of unknown etiology, where no clinical consensus has been reached on the single most important clinical efficacy endpoint, coprimary endpoints may be used. When diseases manifest themselves in multidimensional ways, drug effectiveness is often characterized by the use of composite endpoints, global disease scores, or the disease activity index (DAI). When a composite primary efficacy endpoint is used, we are often interested in the particular aspect or endpoint where the drug has demonstrated benefits. An ICH guideline (European Medicines Agency 1998) suggests: "If a single primary variable cannot be selected from multiple measurements associated with the primary objective, another useful strategy is to integrate or combine the multiple measurements into a single or 'composite' variable, using a predefined algorithm... This approach addresses the multiplicity problem without requiring adjustment to the type-I error." For some indications, such as oncology, it is difficult to use a gold standard endpoint, such as survival, as the primary endpoint because it requires a longer follow-up time and because patients switch treatments after disease progression. Instead, a surrogate endpoint, such as time-to-progression, might be chosen as the primary endpoint with other supporting efficacy evidence, such as infection rate. Huque and Röhmel (2010) provide an excellent overview of multiplicity problems in clinical trials from the regulatory perspective. Following are some motivating examples.

(1) A trial compares two doses of a new treatment to a control with respect to the primary efficacy endpoint. (2) In a clinical trial, there are two endpoints; at least one needs to be statistically significant or all need to be statistically significant. (3) Given three specified primary endpoints E1, E2 and E3, either E1 needs to

be statistically significant or both E2, and E3 need to be statistically significant. (4) One of the two specified endpoints must be statistically significant and the other one needs to show noninferiority. (5) A trial tests for treatment effects for multiple primary and secondary endpoints at low, medium and high doses of a new treatment compared with a placebo with the restriction that tests for the secondary endpoints for a specific dose can be carried out only when certain primary endpoints show meaningful treatment efficacy for that dose. (6) A clinical trial uses a surrogate endpoint S for an accelerated approval and a clinically important endpoint T for a full approval. (7) In a multiple-group oncology trial, each treatment group represents a single drug or combination of drugs. The goal is to identify the most effective drug or combination of drugs, if any. (8) In pharmacovigilance or sequential drug safety monitoring in postmarketing, how can we effectively control the false signals? (9) In adaptive sequential design, multiple tests are performed at different time points. How can we control the type-I error rate?

In this chapter, we will discuss various multiplicity issues and methods. However, multiplicity due to sequential analyses or adaptive designs will be discussed in Chap. 4. The multiplicity in data mining and pharmacovigilance will be discussed in Chap. 8.

1.1.3 Multiple-Testing Taxonomy

Let H_{oi} $(i = 1, \ldots, K)$ be the null hypotheses of interest in an experiment. There are at least three different types of global multiple-hypothesis testing that can be performed.

1.1.3.1 Union-Intersection Testing

$$H_o : \cap_{i=1}^{K} H_{oi} \text{ versus } H_a : \bar{H}_o. \tag{1.3}$$

In this setting, if any H_{oi} is rejected, the global null hypothesis H_o is rejected. For union-intersection testing, if the global testing has a size of α, then this has to be adjusted to a smaller value for testing each individual H_{io}, called the local significance level.

Example 1.1. In a typical dose-finding trial, patients are randomly assigned to one of several (K) parallel dose levels or a placebo. The goal is to find out if there is a drug effect and which dose(s) has the effect. In such a trial, H_{oi} will represent the null hypothesis that the ith dose level has no effect in comparison with the placebo. The goal of the dose-finding trial can be formulated in terms of hypothesis testing (1.3).

1.1.3.2 Intersection-Union Testing

$$H_o : \cup_{i=1}^{K} H_{oi} \text{ versus } H_a : \bar{H}_o. \tag{1.4}$$

In this setting, if and only if all H_{0i} $(i = 1, \ldots, K)$ are rejected is the global null hypothesis H_o rejected. For intersection-union testing, the global α will apply to each individual H_{io} testing.

Example 1.2. Alzheimer's trials in mild to moderate disease generally include ADAS Cog and CIBIC (Clinician's Interview Based Impression of Change) endpoints as coprimaries. The ADAS Cog endpoint measures patients' cognitive functions, while the CIBIC endpoint measures patients' deficit in activities of daily living. For proving a claim of a clinically meaningful treatment benefit for this disease, it is generally required to demonstrate statistically significant treatment benefit on each of these two primary endpoints (called coprimary endpoints). If we denote H_{o1} as the null hypothesis of no effect in terms of the ADAS Cog and H_{o2} as the null hypothesis of no effect in terms of CIBIC, then the hypothesis testing for the efficacy claim in the clinical trial can be expressed as (1.4).

1.1.3.3 Union-Intersection Mixture Testing

This is a mixture of (1) and (2), for example,

$$H_o : \cap_{i=1}^{K} H_{oi}^* \text{ versus } H_a : \bar{H}_o, \tag{1.5}$$

where $H_{oi}^* = \cup_{j=1}^{K_i} H_{oij}$.

Example 1.3. This example is a combination of Examples 1.1 and 1.2, Suppose this dose-finding trial has $K = 2$ dose levels and a placebo. For each dose level, the efficacy claim is based on the coprimary endpoints, ADAS Cog and CIBIC. Let H_{oi1} and H_{oi2} be the null hypotheses for the two primary endpoints for the ith dose level. Rejection of H_{oi}^* will lead to an efficacy claim for the ith dose in terms of the two coprimary endpoints. Then, the efficacy claim in this trial can be postulated in terms of hypothesis test (1.5).

Familywise Error Rate

Familywise Error Rate (FWER) is the maximum (sup) probability of falsely rejecting H_o under all possible null hypothesis configurations:

$$FWER = \sup_{H_o} P \text{ (rejecting } H_o). \tag{1.6}$$

In intersection-union testing, a null hypothesis configuration can be just a combination of some H_{oi} $(i = 1, \ldots, K)$.

Table 1.1 Error inflation due to correlations between endpoints

Level α_A	Level α_B	Correlation R_{AB}	FWER
		0	0.098
		0.25	0.097
0.05	0.05	0.50	0.093
		0.75	0.083
		1.00	0.050

Note: $\alpha_A = \alpha$ for endpoint A, $\alpha_A = \alpha$ for endpoint B

Table 1.2 Error inflation due to different numbers of endpoints

Level α_A	Level α_B	Number of analyses	FWER
		1	0.050
		2	0.098
0.05	0.05	3	0.143
		5	0.226
		10	0.401

The strong FWER α control requires that

$$FWER = \sup_{H_o} P\left(\text{rejecting } H_o\right) \leq \alpha. \tag{1.7}$$

On the other hand, the weak FWER control requires only α control under the global null hypothesis. We will focus on the strong FWER control for the rest of this chapter.

Local alpha: A local alpha is the type-I error rate allowed (often called the size of a local test) for individual H_{oi} testing. In most hypothesis test procedures, the local α is numerically different from (smaller than) the global (familywise) α to avoid FWER inflation. Without the adjusted local α, FWER inflation usually increases as the number of tests in the family increases.

Suppose we have two primary endpoints in a two-arm, active-control, random-ized trial. The efficacy of the drug will be claimed as long as one of the endpoints is statistically significant at level α. In such a scenario, the FWER will be inflated. The level of inflation is dependent on the correlation between the two test statistics (Table 1.1). The maximum error rate inflation occurs when the endpoints are independent. If the two endpoints are perfectly correlated, there is no alpha inflation. For a correlation as high as 0.75, the inflation is still larger than 0.08 for a level 0.05 test. Hence, to control the overall α, an alpha adjustment is required for each test. Similarly, to study how alpha inflation is related to the number of analyses, simulations are conducted for the two independent endpoints, A and B. The results are presented in Table 1.2. We can see that alpha is inflated from 0.05 to 0.226 with five analyses and to 0.401 with ten analyses.

Closed family: A closed family is one for which any subset intersection hypothesis involving members of the testing family is also a member of the family. For example, a closed family of three hypotheses H_1, H_2, H_3 has a total of seven members, listed as follows: H_1, H_2, H_3, $H_1 \cap H_2$, $H_2 \cap H_3$, $H_1 \cap H_3$, $H_1 \cap H_2 \cap H_3$.

Closure principle: This was developed by Marcus et al. (1976). This principle asserts that one can ensure strong control of FWER and coherence (see below) at the same time by conducting the following procedure. Test every member of the closed family using a local α-level test (here, α refers to the comparison-wise error rate, not the FWER). A hypothesis can be rejected provided (1) its corresponding test was significant at the α-level, and (2) every other hypothesis in the family that implies it has also been rejected by its corresponding α-level test.

Closed testing procedure: A test procedure is said to be closed if and only if the rejection of a particular univariate null hypothesis at an α-level of significance implies the rejection of all higher-level (multivariate) null hypotheses containing the univariate null hypothesis at the same α-level. The procedure can be described as follows (Bretz et al. 2006):

1. Define a set of elementary hypotheses, $H_1; \ldots ; H_K$, of interest.
2. Construct all possible $m > K$ intersection hypotheses, $H_I = \cap \; H_i, I \subseteq \{1, \ldots, K\}$.
3. For each of the m hypotheses find a suitable local α-level test.
4. Reject H_i at FWER α if all hypotheses H_I with $i \in I$ are rejected, each at the (local) α-level.

This procedure is not often used directly in practice. However, the closure principle has been used to derive many useful test procedures, such as those of Holm (1979), Hochberg (1988), Hommel (1988), and gatekeeping procedures.

α-exhaustive procedure: If P (Reject H_I) $= \alpha$ for every intersection hypothesis $H_I, I \subseteq \{1, \ldots, K\}$, the test procedure is α-exhaustive.

Partition principle: This is similar to the closed testing procedure with strong control over the familywise α-level for the null hypotheses. The partition principle allows for test procedures that are formed by partitioning the parameter space into disjointed partitions with some logical ordering. Tests of the hypotheses are carried out sequentially at different partition steps. The process of testing stops upon failure to reject a given null hypothesis for predetermined partition steps (Hsu 1996; Dmitrienko et al. 2010, pp. 45–46). We will discuss this more later in this chapter.

Coherence and *consonance* are two interesting concepts in closed testing procedures. *Coherence* means that if hypothesis H implies H^*, then whenever H is retained, so must be H^*. *Consonance* mean that whenever H is rejected, at least one of its components is rejected, too. Coherence is a necessary property of closed test procedures; consonance is desirable but not necessary. A procedure can be coherent but not consonant because of asymmetry in the hypothesis testing paradigm. When H is rejected we conclude that it is false. However, when H is retained, we do not conclude that it is true; rather, we say that there is not sufficient evidence to reject it. Multiple comparison procedures that satisfy the closure principle are always coherent but not necessarily consonant (Westfall et al. 1999).

Adjusted p-value

The adjusted p-value for a hypothesis test is defined as the smallest significance level at which one would reject the hypothesis using the multiple-testing procedure (Westfall and Young 1993). If p_I denotes the p-value for testing intersection hypothesis H_I, the adjusted p-value for H_{oi} is given by

$$p_i^{adj} = \max_{I:i \in I} p_I. \tag{1.8}$$

If $p_i^{adj} \leq \alpha$, H_{oi} is rejected.

Simultaneous confidence interval

It is well known that a two-sided $(1 - \alpha)\%$ confidence interval for parameter θ consists of all parameter values for which the hypothesis $H_o : \theta = 0$ is retained at level α. This concept can be applied to multiple-parameter problems to form a confidence set or a simultaneous confidence interval.

1.2 Multiple-Testing Approaches

1.2.1 Single-Step Procedures

The commonly used single-stage procedures include the Sidak method (Sidak 1967), the simple Bonferroni method, the Simes-Bonferroni method (Global test: Simes 1986), and Dunnett's test for all active arms against the control arm (Dunnett 1955). In the single-step procedure, to control the FWER, the unadjusted p-values are compared against the adjusted alpha to make the decision to reject or not reject the corresponding null hypothesis. Alternatively, we can use the adjusted p-values to compare against the original α for decision-making.

1.2.1.1 Sidak Method

The Sidak method is derived from the simple fact that the probability of rejecting at least one null hypothesis is equal to $1-$ Pr (all null hypotheses are correct). To control the FWER, the adjusted alpha α_k for the null hypothesis H_{ok} $(k = 1, \ldots, K)$ can be found by solving the following equation:

$$\alpha = 1 - (1 - \alpha_k)^K. \tag{1.9}$$

Therefore, the adjusted alpha is given by

$$\alpha_k = 1 - (1 - \alpha)^{1/K} . \tag{1.10}$$

If the p-value is less than or equal to α_k, reject H_{ok}. Alternatively we can calculate the adjusted p-value:

$$\tilde{p}_k = 1 - (1 - p_k)^K . \tag{1.11}$$

If the adjusted p-value $\tilde{p}_k$ is less than or equal to α, then reject H_{ok}.

1.2.1.2 Bonferroni Method

The simple Bonferroni method is a simplification of the Sidak method that uses the Bonferroni inequality:

$$P(\cup_{k=1}^K H_k) \le \sum_{k=1}^K P(H_k). \tag{1.12}$$

Based on (1.12), we can conservatively use the adjusted alpha,

$$\alpha_k = \frac{\alpha}{K}, \tag{1.13}$$

and the adjusted p-value,

$$\tilde{p}_k = K p_k.$$

This is a very conservative approach without consideration of any correlations among p-values.

The alpha doesn't have to be split equally among all tests. We can use the so-called weighted Bonferroni tests, for which the adjusted alpha and p-value are given by

$$\alpha_k = w_k \alpha \text{ and } \tilde{p}_k = \frac{p_k}{w_k}, \tag{1.14}$$

where the weight $w_k \ge 0$ and $\sum_{k=1}^K w_k = 1$. The weight w_k can be determined based on the clinical importance of the kth hypothesis or the power of the kth hypothesis test.

1.2.1.3 Simes Global Testing Method

The Simes-Bonferroni method is a global test in which the type-I error rate is controlled for the global null hypothesis (1.3). We reject the null hypothesis H_o if

$$p_{(k)} \le \frac{k\alpha}{K} \text{ for at least one } i = 1, \dots, K, \tag{1.15}$$

where $p_{(1)} < \dots < p_{(K)}$ are the ordered p-values.

The adjusted p-value is given by

$$\tilde{p} = \max_{k \in \{1,\ldots,K\}} \left\{ \frac{K}{k} p_{(k)} \right\}. \tag{1.16}$$

If $\tilde{p} \leq \alpha$, the global null hypothesis (1.3) is rejected.

1.2.1.4 Dunnett's Method

Dunnett's method can be used for multiple comparisons of active groups against a common control group, which is often done in clinical trials with multiple parallel groups. Let n_0 and n_i $(i = 1, \ldots, K)$ be the sample sizes for the control and the ith dose group; the test statistic (one-sided) is given by Westfall et al. (1999, p. 77)

$$T = \max_i \frac{\bar{y}_i - \bar{y}_0}{\sigma \sqrt{1/n_i + 1/n_0}}, \tag{1.17}$$

The multivariate t-distribution of T in (1.17) is called one-sided Dunnett distribution with $v = \sum_{i=1}^{K+1} (n_i - 1)$ degrees of freedom. The cdf is defined by

$$F(x|K, v) = P(T \leq x). \tag{1.18}$$

The calculation of (1.18) requires numerical integrations (Hochberg and Tamhane 1987, p. 141). Tabulation of the critical values is available from the book by Kanji (2006), and in software such as SAS.

The adjusted p-value corresponding to t_i is given by

$$\tilde{p}_i = 1 - F(t_i|K, v). \tag{1.19}$$

If $\tilde{p}_i < \alpha$, H_i is rejected, $i = 1, \ldots, K$.

1.2.1.5 Fisher-Combination Test

To test the global null hypothesis $H_o = \cap_{i=1}^{K} H_{oi}$, we can use the so-called Fisher combination statistic,

$$\chi^2 = -2 \sum_{i=1}^{K} \ln(p_i), \tag{1.20}$$

where p_i is the p-value for testing H_{oi}. When H_{oi} is true, p_i is uniformly distributed over [0,1]. Furthermore, if the p_i $(i = 1, \ldots, K)$ are independent, the test statistic χ^2 is distributed as a chi-square statistic with $2K$ degrees of freedom. Thus H_o is rejected if $\chi^2 \geq \chi^2_{2K,1-\alpha}$. Note that if the p_i are not independent or H_o is not true (e.g., one of the H_{oi} is not true), then χ^2 is not necessarily a chi-square distribution.

1.2.2 Stepwise Procedures

Stepwise procedures are different from single-step procedures in the sense that a stepwise procedure must follow a specific order to test each hypothesis. In general, stepwise procedures are more powerful than single-step procedures. There are three categories of stepwise procedures which are dependent on how the stepwise tests proceed: stepup, stepdown, and fixed-sequence procedures. The commonly used stepwise procedures include the Bonferroni-Holm stepdown method (Holm 1979), the Sidak-Holm stepdown method (Westfall et al. 1999, p. 31), Hommel's procedure (Hommel 1988), Hochberg's stepup method (Hochberg and Benjamini 1990), Rom's method (Rom 1990), and the sequential test with fixed sequences (Westfall et al. 1999).

1.2.2.1 Stepdown Procedure

A stepdown procedure starts with the most significant p-value and ends with the least significant. In this procedure, the p-values are arranged in ascending order,

$$p_{(1)} \leq p_{(2)} \leq \cdots \leq p_{(K)}, \tag{1.21}$$

with the corresponding hypotheses

$$H_{(1)}, H_{(2)}, \ldots, H_{(K)}.$$

The test proceeds from $H_{(1)}$ to $H_{(K)}$. If $p_{(k)} > C_k \alpha$ $(k = 1, \ldots, K)$, retain all $H_{(i)}$ $(i \geq k)$; otherwise, reject $H_{(k)}$ and continue to test $H_{(k+1)}$. The critical values C_k are different for different procedures.

The adjusted p-values are

$$\begin{cases} \tilde{p}_1 = C_1 p_{(1)}, \\ \tilde{p}_k = \max\left(\tilde{p}_{k-1}, C_k p_{(k)}\right), k = 2, \ldots, n. \end{cases} \tag{1.22}$$

Therefore an alternative test procedure is to compare the adjusted p-values against the unadjusted α. After adjusting p-values, one can test the hypotheses in any order.

1.2.2.2 Stepup Procedure

A stepup procedure starts with the least significant p-value and ends with the most significant p-value. The procedure proceeds from $H_{(K)}$ to $H_{(1)}$. If, $P_{(k)} \leq C_k \alpha$ $(k = 1, \ldots, K)$, reject all $H_{(i)}$ $(i \leq k)$; otherwise, retain $H_{(k)}$ and continue to test $H_{(k-1)}$. The critical values C_k for the Hochberg stepup procedure are $C_k = K - k + 1$ $(k = 1, .., K)$.

The adjusted p-values are

$$\begin{cases} \tilde{p}_K = C_K p_{(K)}, \\ \tilde{p}_k = \min\left(\tilde{p}_{k+1}, C_k p_{(k)}\right), \ k = K-1,\ldots,1. \end{cases} \tag{1.23}$$

Therefore, an alternative test procedure is to compare the adjusted p-values against the unadjusted α.

The Hochberg stepup method does not control the FWER for all correlations, but it is a little conservative when p-values are independent (Westfall et al. 1999, p. 33). The Rom method (Rom 1990) controls α exactly for independent p-values. However, the calculation of C_k is complicated.

1.2.2.3 Fixed-Sequence Test

This procedure is a stepdown procedure with the order of hypotheses predetermined:

$$H_1, H_2, \ldots, H_K.$$

The test proceeds from H_1 to H_K. If $p_k > \alpha$ $(k = 1,\ldots,K)$, retain all H_i $(i \geq k)$. Otherwise, reject H_k and continue to test H_{k+1}.

The adjusted p-values are given by

$$\tilde{p}_k = \max\left(p_1,\ldots,p_k\right), \ k = 1,..,K. \tag{1.24}$$

The sequence of the tests can be based on the importance of hypotheses or the power of the tests. Note that if the previous test is not significant, the next test will not proceed even if its p-value is extremely small.

1.2.2.4 Dunnett Stepdown Procedure

A commonly used stepdown procedure is the Dunnett stepdown procedure. The adjusted p-values are formulated as follows. First, p-values are arranged in a descending order,

$$t_{(1)} \geq t_{(2)} \geq \cdots \geq t_{(K)},$$

with the corresponding hypotheses

$$H_{(1)}, H_{(2)}, \ldots, H_{(K)}.$$

Based on (1.18), we calculate $p_k^* = 1 - F\left(t_{(k)} | K - k + 1, v\right)$, where the second argument in $F(\cdot)$ is $K - k + 1$ instead of K as in the single-step Dunnett test. The adjusted p-values are then calculated as follows:

$$\tilde{p}_k = \begin{cases} p_1^* \\ \max\left(\tilde{p}_{k-1}, p_k^*\right) \text{ if } k = 2,\ldots,K. \end{cases} \tag{1.25}$$

The decision rule can be specified as: if $\tilde{p}_k < \alpha$, reject $H_{(k)}$.

1.2.2.5 Holm Stepdown Procedure

Suppose there are K hypothesis tests H_i ($i = 1, \ldots, K$). The Holm stepdown procedure (Holm 1979; Dmitrienko et al. 2010) can be outlined as follows:

Step 1. If $p_{(1)} \leq \alpha/K$, reject $H_{(1)}$ and go to the next step; otherwise retain all hypotheses and stop.

Step i ($i = 2, \ldots, K - 1$). If $p_{(i)} \leq \alpha/(K - i + 1)$, reject $H_{(i)}$ and go to the next step; otherwise retain $H_{(i)}, \ldots, H_{(K)}$ and stop.

Step K. If $p_{(K)} \leq \alpha$, reject $H_{(K)}$; otherwise retain $H_{(K)}$.

The adjusted p-values are given by

$$\tilde{p}_k = \begin{cases} p_{(K)} & \text{if } k = K \\ \min\left(\tilde{p}_{k+1}, (K - k + 1)\, p_{k+1}\right) & \text{if } k = K - 1, \ldots, 1. \end{cases} \tag{1.26}$$

1.2.2.6 Shaffer Procedure

Shaffer (1986) and Dmitrienko et al. (2010) uses logical dependencies between the hypotheses to improve the Holm procedure. The dependency means that the truth of certain hypotheses implies the truth of other hypotheses. To illustrate, suppose a trial with four dose levels and a placebo group has a treatment mean μ_i for the ith group ($i = 0$ for the placebo). If the null hypotheses under consideration are $H_{ij}: \mu_i = \mu_j$, then H_{12} and H_{13} imply H_{23}. The steps of the Shaffer procedure are similar to those for the Holm procedure, but replace the divisors $(K - i + 1)$ by k_i. Here k_i is the maximum number of hypotheses $H_{(i)}, \ldots, H_{(K)}$ that can be simultaneously true, given that $H_{(1)}, \ldots, H_{(i-1)}$ are false. Thus, at the ith step, reject $H_{(i)}$ if

$$p_{(j)} \leq \frac{\alpha}{k_j}, \ j = 1, \ldots, i. \tag{1.27}$$

As an example, for the five-group dose-response study, there can be $k_1 = \binom{5}{2} = 10$ pairwise comparisons (the same as for the Holm procedure). After $H_{(1)}$ is rejected, there are $k_2 = \binom{4}{2} = 6$ possible pairwise comparisons (compared to $K - i + 1 = 9$ in the Holm procedure).

1.2.2.7 Fallback Procedure

The Holm procedure is based on a data-driven order of testing, while the fixed-sequence procedure is based on a prefixed order of testing. A compromise between them is the so-called fallback procedure. The fallback procedure was introduced by Wiens (2003) and was further studied by Wiens and Dmitrienko (2005) and Hommel and Bretz (2008). The test procedure can be outlined as follows:

Suppose hypotheses H_i ($i = 1, \ldots, K$) are ordered according to (1.22). We allocate the overall error rate α among the hypotheses according to their weights

w_i, where $w_i \geq 0$ and $\sum_i w_i = 1$. For Fixed-Sequence test, $w_1 = 1$ and $w_2 = \ldots = w_K = 0$.

1. Test H_1 at $\alpha_1 = \alpha w_1$. If $p_1 \leq \alpha_1$, reject this hypothesis; otherwise retain it. Go to the next step.
2. Test H_i at $\alpha_i = \alpha_{i-1} + \alpha w_i$ ($i = 2, \ldots, K-1$) if H_{i-1} is rejected and at $\alpha_i = \alpha w_i$ if H_{i-1} is retained. If $p_i \leq \alpha_i$, reject H_i; otherwise retain it. Go to the next step.
3. Test H_K at $\alpha_K = \alpha_{K-1} + \alpha w_K$ if H_{K-1} is rejected and at $\alpha_K = \alpha w_K$ if H_{K-1} is retained. If $p_K \leq \alpha_K$, reject H_K; otherwise retain it.

Example 1.4. Suppose that a dose-finding trial has been conducted to compare low (L), medium (M), and high (H) doses of a new antihypertension drug. The primary efficacy variable is diastolic blood pressure (DBP). The mean reduction in DBP is denoted by μ_P, μ_L, μ_M, and μ_H for the placebo, and low, medium, and high doses, respectively. The global null hypothesis of equality, $\mu_P = \mu_L = \mu_M = \mu_H$, can be tested using an F-test from a model such as analysis of covariance (ANCOVA). However, for strong FWER control, this F-test is not sufficient. We illustrate how to apply various multiple-testing procedures to this problem. One is interested in three pairwise comparisons (one for each dose) against a placebo (P) with null hypotheses: $H_1 : \mu_P = \mu_L$, $H_2 : \mu_P = \mu_M$, and $H_3 : \mu_P = \mu_H$. Denote the p-values for these tests by p_1, p_2, and p_3, respectively. A one-sided significance level α of 2.5% is used for the trial.

In the following methods or procedures (1)–(8), we assume $p_1 = 0.009$, $p_2 = 0.0085$, and $p_3 = 0.008$.

Weighted Bonferroni Procedure

Suppose we suspect the high dose may be more toxic than the low dose. Unless the high dose is more efficacious than the low dose, we will choose the low dose as the target dose. For this reason, we want to spend more alpha in the low-dose comparison than in the high-dose comparison. Specifically, we choose one-sided significance levels $\alpha_1 = 0.01$, $\alpha_2 = 0.008$, and $\alpha_3 = 0.007$ ($\alpha_1 + \alpha_2 + \alpha_3 = \alpha$), which will be used to compare p_1, p_2, p_3, respectively, for rejecting or accepting the corresponding hypotheses. Since $p_1 = 0.009 < \alpha_1$, $p_2 = 0.0085 > \alpha_2$, and $p_3 = 0.008 > \alpha_3$, we will reject H_1 but accept H_2 and H_3.

Simes-Bonferroni Method

We first order the p-values: $p_{(1)} = p_3 < p_{(2)} = p_2 < p_{(3)} = p_1$; the adjusted p-values calculated from (1.16) are $\tilde{p} = \max\{\frac{3}{1}p_{(1)} = 0.024, \frac{3}{2}p_{(2)} = 0.01275, \frac{3}{3}p_{(3)} = 0.009\} = 0.024 < \alpha$. Therefore the global hypotheses ($\mu_P = \mu_L = \mu_M = \mu_H$) are rejected and we conclude that one or more dose levels are effective, but the testing procedure has not indicated which one.

Fisher Combination Method

This method usually requires independent p-values; otherwise, the test may be on the conservative or liberal side. However, for illustrating the calculation procedure, let's pretend the p-values are independent. From (1.20), we can calculate the Chi-square value: $\chi^2 = -2\ln((0.009)(0.0085)(0.008)) = 28.62$ with six degrees of freedom. The corresponding p-value is $0.0001 < \alpha$. Thus the global null hypothesis is rejected.

Fixed-Sequence Procedure

Suppose we have fixed the test sequence as H_3, H_2, H_1 before we see the data. Since $p_3 < \alpha$, we reject H_3 and continue to test H_2. Because $p_2 < \alpha$, we reject H_2 and continue to test H_1. Since $p_1 < \alpha$, we reject H_1.

Holm Procedure

Since $p_{(1)} = p_3 = 0.008 < \alpha/K = 0.025/3$, reject H_3 and continue to test H_2. Because $p_{(2)} = p_2 = 0.0085 < \alpha/(K-2+1) = 0.025/2 = 0.0125$, reject H_2 and continue to test H_1. Since $p_1 = 0.009 < \alpha/(K-3+1) = 0.025$, H_1 is rejected.

Shaffer Procedure

Since $p_{(1)} = p_3 = 0.008 < \alpha/k_1 = 0.025/3$, reject H_3. After H_3 is rejected, H_1 and H_2 can be simultaneously true, but $k_2 = 2$ and $p_{(2)} = p_2 = 0.0085 < \alpha/k_2 = 0.025/2 = 0.0125$, so reject H_2. We have only H_1 left, and thus $k_3 = 1$ and $p_1 = 0.009 < \alpha/(K-3+1) = 0.025$; H_1 is rejected. We can see that in this case the Holm and Shaffer procedures are equivalent. This is because we are not interested in the other possible comparisons: μ_1 versus μ_2, μ_2 versus μ_3, and μ_3 versus μ_1.

Fallback Procedure

Choose equal weights $w_i = 1/K = 1/3$. $\alpha_1 = \alpha/3 = 0.00833$, $\alpha_2 = \alpha_1 + \alpha/3 = 0.0167$, and $\alpha_3 = \alpha_2 + \alpha/3 = \alpha = 0.025$. Since $p_1 = 0.009 > \alpha_1$, $p_2 = 0.0085 < \alpha_2$, and $p_3 = 0.008 < \alpha_3$, H_1 is retained but H_2 and H_3 are rejected.

Hochberg Stepup Procedure

Since $p_{(3)} = 0.009 < \alpha = 0.025$, we reject all three hypotheses, H_1, H_2, and H_3. The adjusted p-values $\tilde{p}_1$, $\tilde{p}_2$, and $\tilde{p}_3$ can be calculated using (1.23).

Dunnett's Procedure

Suppose the adjusted p-values calculated from (1.19) (requiring a software package) are $\tilde{p}_1 = 0.027 > \alpha$, $\tilde{p}_2 = 0.021 < \alpha$, and $\tilde{p}_3 = 0.019 < \alpha$. Then, we reject H_2 and H_3 but retain H_1.

Dunnett's Stepdown Procedure

Suppose the test statistics $t_{(1)} = t_3 > t_{(2)} = t_2 > t_{(3)} = t_1$ for the three hypotheses H_3, H_2, and H_1. Assume that the p-values are $p_1^* = 0.019$, $p_2^* = 0.018$, and $p_3^* = 0.0245$ for the hypotheses $H_{(1)} = H_3$, $H_{(2)} = H_2$, and $H_{(3)} = H_1$, respectively. The adjusted p-values can be calculated from (1.25): $\tilde{p}_1 = p_1^* = 0.019 < \alpha$, $\tilde{p}_2 = \max\left(\tilde{p}_1, p_2^*\right) = 0.019 < \alpha$, $\tilde{p}_3 = \max\left(\tilde{p}_2, p_1^*\right) = 0.0245 < \alpha$. Then, we reject H_3, H_2, and H_1.

1.2.3 Common Gatekeeper Procedure

The gatekeeper procedure (Dmitrienko et al. 2005, pp. 106–127) is an extension of the fixed-sequence method. The method is motivated by the following hypothesis-testing problems in clinical trials. (1) Benefit of secondary endpoints can be claimed in the drug label only if the primary endpoint is statistically significant. (2) If there are coprimary endpoints (multiple primary endpoints), secondary endpoints can be claimed only if one of the primary endpoints is statistically significant. (3) In multiple-endpoint problems, the endpoints can be grouped based on their clinical importance.

Suppose there are K null hypotheses to test. We group them into m families. Each family is a composite of hypotheses. The null hypotheses in the ith$(i = 1, \ldots, m_i)$ family are denoted by either a serial gatekeeper

$$F_i = H_{i1} \cup H_{i2} \cup \ldots \cup H_{im_i} \tag{1.28}$$

or a parallel gatekeeper

$$F_i = H_{i1} \cap H_{i2} \cap \ldots \cap H_{im_i}. \tag{1.29}$$

The hypothesis test proceeds from the first family, F_1, to the last family, F_m. To test F_i $(i = 2, \ldots, m)$, the test procedure has to pass $i - 1$ previous gatekeepers, i.e., reject all F_k $(k = 1, \ldots, i - 1)$ at the predetermined level of significance α.

For a parallel gatekeeper we can either weakly or strongly control the familywise type-I error. For a serial gatekeeper, we always strongly control the familywise error. The serial gatekeeping procedure is straightforward: test each family of null hypotheses sequentially at a level α with any strong α-control method.

The stepwise procedure of parallel gatekeeping proposed by Dmitrienko and Tamhane (2007) can be described as follows. The procedure is built around the concept of a rejection gain factor. At the kth stage, the significance test is performed at the $\rho_k \alpha$ level, $k = 1, 2, \ldots, m$, where α is the FWER, and the rejection gain factor, $0 \leq \rho_k \leq 1$ (with $\rho_1 = 1$), depends on the number and importance of the hypotheses rejected at the earlier stages.

The stepwise parallel gatekeeping procedure for testing the null hypotheses in $F_1, \ldots, F_m$ can be performed as follows:

1. Family F_k, $k = 1, \ldots, m - 1$: Test the null hypotheses using the Bonferroni test at the $\rho_k \alpha$ level.
2. Family F_m: Test the null hypotheses using the weighted Holm test at the $\rho_m \alpha$ level.

The rejection gain factors ρ_i are given by

$$\rho_1 = 1, \rho_k = \prod_{i=1}^{k-1} \left(\sum_{j=1}^{m_i} r_{ij} w_{ij} \right), k = 2, \ldots, m, \qquad (1.30)$$

where the weights $w_{ij} \geq 0$ with $\sum_{j=1}^{n_i} w_{ij} = 1$ represent the importance of the null hypotheses in F_i, and $r_{ij} = 1$ if H_{ij} is rejected and 0 otherwise. For equally weighted hypotheses ($w_{ij} = 1/m_i$), the formula for ρ_k reduces to

$$\rho_k = \prod_{i=1}^{k-1} \left(\frac{r_i}{m_i} \right), k = 2, \ldots, m, \qquad (1.31)$$

where $r_i = \sum_j r_{ij}$ is the number of rejected hypotheses in F_i. Thus, ρ_k is the product of the proportions of previously rejected hypotheses in F_1 through F_{k-1}.

The modified adjusted p-value for H_{ij}, $i = 2, \ldots, m$, is given by $p_{ij}^* = \tilde{p}_{ij}/\rho_i$, where $\tilde{p}_{ij}$ is the usual adjusted p-value produced by the multiple tests within F_i. Inferences in $F_2, \ldots, F_m$ can be performed by p_{ij}^* to the prespecified FWER, α.

Example 1.5. This example was given by Dmitrienko and Tamhane (2007). The trial was designed to compare a single dose of an experimental drug with a placebo. Two families of endpoints were considered in this trial. F_1 consisted of two hypotheses related to the primary endpoints, P1 (lung function) and P2 (mortality), and F_2 consisted of two hypotheses related to the secondary endpoints, S1 (ICU-free days) and S2 (quality of life). The raw p-values p_{ij} for the endpoints P1, P2, S1, and S2 are 0.048, 0.003, 0.026, and 0.002, respectively. F_1 was chosen as a parallel gatekeeper. P1 was deemed more important than P2 in F_1 with weights $w_{11} = 0.9$ and $w_{12} = 0.1$, respectively; S1 and S2 were considered equally important with weight $w_{21} = w_{22} = 0.5$. The FWER is to be controlled at $\alpha = 0.05$.

To apply the stepwise parallel gatekeeping procedure, one first considers the adjusted p-values produced by the weighted Bonferroni test and the Holm test for the null hypotheses in F_1 and F_2, respectively. The adjusted p-values $\tilde{p}_{ij}$ for the endpoints P1, P2, S1, and S2 are $0.048/0.9 = 0.053$ (the weighted Bonferroni test), $0.003/0.1 = 0.03$ (the weighted Bonferroni test), 0.026 (the Holm test), and $0.002 \times 2 = 0.004$, respectively. Next, since $\rho_1 = 1$, the primary hypotheses are tested at the full $\alpha = 0.05$ level. The P2 comparison is significant at this level, whereas the P1 comparison is not. Therefore, the rejection gain factor for the secondary family based on (1.31) is $\rho_2 = w_{12} = 0.1$, and the adjusted p-values for S1 and S2 are $0.026/\rho_2 = 0.260$ and $0.004/\rho_2 = 0.040$, respectively. It is clear that only the hypothesis concerning S2 is rejected.

1.2.4 Tree Gatekeeping Procedure

The tree gatekeeping procedure (TGP) is a stepwise procedure that combines the characteristics of both the parallel and series gatekeeping methods. For each individual hypothesis H_{ij} in family F_i, where $i = 2, \ldots, m$, $j = 1, \ldots, n_i$, we define two associated hypothesis sets: the serial rejection set, R_{ij}^S, and the parallel rejection set, R_{ij}^P. These sets consist of some hypotheses from $F_1, \ldots, F_{i-1}$; at least one of them is non-empty. Without loss of generality, we assume R_{ij}^S and R_{ij}^P do not overlap.

Dmitrienko et al. (2007) developed Bonferroni-based and resampling-based tree gatekeeping procedures. The Bonferroni-based tree-gatekeeping procedure is described as follows.

Let H be any non-empty intersection of the hypotheses H_{ij} and let $w_{ij}(H)$ be the weight assigned to the hypothesis $H_{ij} \in H$. From (1.14), we know that the Bonferroni (adjusted) p-value for testing H is given by $p(H) = \min_{i,j}\{\frac{p_{ij}}{w_{ij}(H)}\}$. Because there can be more than one H that includes each H_{ij}, we need to further adjust the p-value $p(H)$. The multiplicity-adjusted p-value for the null hypothesis H_{ij} is defined as $\tilde{p}_{ij} = \max_H \{p(H)\}$, where the maximum is taken over all intersection hypotheses H such that $H_{ij} \subseteq H$. The rejection rules are: reject H_{ij} if $\tilde{p}_{ij} \leq \alpha$; and retain H_{ij} otherwise.

The testing procedure above for the adjusted p-value is based on the closure principle, which requires us to construct the weight $w_{ij}(H)$ appropriately. For convenience, we define two indicator variables: let $\delta_{ij}(H) = 0$ if $H_{ij} \in H$ and 1 otherwise, and let $\xi_{ij}(H) = 0$ if H contains any hypothesis from R_{ij}^S or all hypotheses from R_{ij}^P and 1 otherwise. The following three conditions together for the weights will constitute a sufficient condition for using the closure principle, and thus for the TGP, also.

Condition 1: For any intersection hypothesis H, $w_{ij}(H) \geq 0$, $\sum_{j=1}^{m_i} w_{ij}(H) \leq 1$ and $w_{ij}(H) = 0$ if $\delta_{ij}(H) = 0$ or $\xi_{ij}(H) = 0$.

Condition 2: $w_i(H) = (w_{i1}(H), \ldots, w_{im_i}(H))$ is a vector function of the weights $w_1(H), \ldots, w_{i-1}(H)$ $(i = 2, \ldots, m)$ and does not depend on $w_{i+1}(H), \ldots, w_m(H)$ $(i = 1, \ldots, m-1)$.

Condition 3: The weights for $F_1, \ldots, F_{m-1}$ meet the monotonicity condition, i.e.
$w_{ij}(H) \leq w_{ij}(H^*)$, $i = 1, \ldots, m-1$, if $H_{ij} \in H$, $H_{ij} \in H^*$, and $H^* \subseteq H$.

1.2.4.1 Implementation of a Tree Gatekeeping Procedure

The authors developed the following algorithm for the weight assignments that meets conditions 1–3. Here we define $0/0 = 0$.

Step 0: Choose Bonferroni weights $\tilde{w}_{ij} > 0$ satisfying $\sum_{j=1}^{m_i} \tilde{w}_{ij} = 1$ and the serial rejection set R_{ij}^S and the parallel rejection set R_{ij}^P for $i = 2, \ldots, m$, $j = 1, \ldots, m_i$.

Step 1: Family F_1. Let $w_{1j}(H) = w_1^*(H)\tilde{w}_{1j}\delta_{1j}(H)$, $j = 1, \ldots, m_1$, where $w_1^*(H) = 1$ and $w_2^*(H) = w_1^*(H) - \sum_{j=1}^{m_1} w_{1j}(H)$.

Step $i = 2, \ldots, m-1$: Family F_i. Let $w_{ij}(H) = w_i^*(H)\tilde{w}_{ij}\delta_{ij}(H)\xi_{ij}(H)$, $j = 1, \ldots, m_i$, and $w_{i+1}^*(H) = w_i^*(H) - \sum_{j=1}^{m_i} w_{ij}(H)$.

Step m: Family F_m. Let

$$w_{mj}(H) = \frac{w_m^*(H)\tilde{w}_{mj}\delta_{mj}(H)\xi_{mj}(H)}{\sum_{k=1}^{m_m} \tilde{w}_{mk}\delta_{mk}(H)\xi_{mk}(H)}, \quad j = 1, \ldots, m_m. \qquad (1.32)$$

After each w_{ij} is determined, we can calculate the adjusted p-value

$$\tilde{p}_{ij} = \max_H \min_{i,j} \left\{ \frac{p_{ij}}{w_{ij}(H)} \right\}. \qquad (1.33)$$

If $\tilde{p}_{ij} \leq \alpha$, reject H_{ij}; otherwise, accept H_{ij}.

1.2.5 Generalized FWER and Partitioning Testing

Let $H_{oi} : \theta \in \Theta_{oi}, i = 1, \ldots, K$, be a family of null hypotheses, where the parameter subspace Θ_{oi} constitutes the null parameter subspace $\Theta_o = \cup\Theta_{oi}$. The complementary set of Θ_{oi}, denoted by Θ_{ai}, constitutes of the alternative parameter subspace $\Theta_a = \cup\Theta_{ai}$. The parameter space is therefore $\Theta = \Theta_o \cup \Theta_a$. The generalized FWER (gFWER) is defined as the probability of making strictly more than $\eta \geq 0$ false rejections in multiple-hypothesis testing. We define gFWER by

$$\vartheta(\eta) = \sup_{\theta \in \Theta_0} P(v > \eta | \theta), \qquad (1.34)$$

where v is the number of different null hypotheses rejected. FWER is the special case of gFWER when $\eta = 0$.

1.2.5.1 Single-Step Test

Let p_i be the raw p-value associated with the null hypothesis $H_{oi}, i = 1, \ldots, K$. Define the adjusted p-value as

$$\tilde{p}_i = \sum_{j=\eta+1}^{k} \binom{k}{j} p_i^j (1 - p_i)^{k-j} . \qquad (1.35)$$

The procedure, which rejects H_{oi} if $\tilde{p}_i \leq \alpha$ and retains it otherwise, will control gFWER(η) at level α in the strong sense for the single hypothesis $H_{oi}, i = 1, \ldots, K$, if the p_i are independently distributed. See the Ph.D. dissertation by Xu (2005).

Lehmann and Romano (2005) proposed the following generalized Bonferroni procedure.

Reject H_{oi} if the adjusted p-value $\tilde{p}_i \leq \alpha$, where

$$\tilde{p}_i = \min \left\{ \frac{K}{\eta + 1} p_i, 1 \right\} , i = 1, \ldots, K.$$

When $\eta = 0$, the Lehmann-Romano procedure degenerates to the common Bonferroni test.

1.2.5.2 Partitioning Testing Principle

1. Let $I = \{1, \ldots, K\}$. Partition Θ into disjoint $\Theta_J^*, J \subseteq I$, based on different combinations of the null parameter subspace Θ_{oi} and the alternative parameter subspace Θ_{ai}, i.e., for each $J \subseteq I$, let $\Theta_J^* = \bigcap_{i \in J} \Theta_{oi} \cap \left(\bigcap_{j \notin J} \Theta_{aj} \right)$. Then $\{\Theta_J^*, J \subseteq I\}$ and $\Theta_\emptyset = \bigcap_{j \in I} \Theta_{aj}$ partition the parameter space Θ.
2. Test each null hypothesis $H_{oJ}^P : \theta \in \Theta_J^*$ at level α. There are no multiplicity adjustments needed because the $H_{oJ}^P, J_* \subseteq I$ are disjoint.
3. For all $J \subseteq I$, infer $\theta \notin \Theta_J^*$ if all $H_{oJ'}^P$ such that $J \subseteq J'$ are rejected. That is, reject the intersection null hypothesis H_{oJ} if all null hypotheses $H_{oJ'}^P$ implying it are rejected, particularly rejecting $H_{oi}, i \in I$, if all H_{oJ}^P such that $i \in J$ are rejected.

As discussed earlier, the closed testing principle can be stated as:

1. Let $I = \{1, \ldots, K\}$. For every $J \subseteq I, J \neq \emptyset$, define $\Theta_J = \bigcap_{i \in J} \Theta_i$ and the intersection null hypothesis $H_{oJ} : \theta \in \Theta_J$.
2. Test each $H_{oJ} : \theta \in \Theta_J$ at level α.
3. For all $J \subseteq I$, infer $\theta \notin \Theta_J$ if all $H_{oJ'}^P$ such that $J \subseteq J'$, are rejected, i.e., reject the intersection null hypothesis H_{oJ} if all hypotheses implying it are rejected.

Comparing the partitioning testing principle with the closed testing principle, we can see that in the partitioning testing principle Θ_J^* consists of all null parameter subspaces Θ_{oi} for which $i \in J$ and all alternative parameter subspaces Θ_{aj} for which $j \notin J$ (There are $\sum_{j=\eta+1}^{K} \binom{K}{j} = 2^K - 2^\eta$ such Θ_J^*s.) In the closed testing procedure, Θ_J is the parameter subspace, for which $H_{oi}, i \in J$, are true. This is the essential difference between the two principles.

1.2.5.3 Generalized Partitioning Testing Principle for Controlling gFWER

Xu (2005) proposed the following procedure for the gFWER:

1. Partition Θ into disjoint Θ_J^*, $J \subseteq I = \{1, \dots, K\}$, such that, for each $J \subseteq I$,

$$\Theta_J^* = \bigcap_{i \in J} \Theta_{oi} \cap \left(\bigcap_{j \notin J} \Theta_{aj} \right).$$

2. In each Θ_J^*, reject all $H_{oi}, i \notin J$, and test $H_{oJ}^P = \{H_{oi} : \theta_i \in \Theta_i, i \in J\}$ at level gFWER α, controlling $\sup_{\theta \in \Theta_J^*} P(v > \eta | \theta) \le \alpha$.

3. For $i \in J \subseteq I$, define H_{oi} to be J-rejected to mean H_{oi} is rejected in Θ_J^*. Reject H_{oi} if H_{oi} is J-rejected for any $J \subseteq I$.

1.2.5.4 Stepdown Partitioning Testing

As we stated earlier there are $2^K - 2^\eta$ tests with the partitioning principle. Xu (2005) proposed a stepdown procedure that reduces the maximum number of tests required to no more than $K - \eta$. This reduction is significant for larger K, such as in microarray analysis. A set of sufficient conditions for such a reduction to be valid is specified as:

S1 All tests are based on a set of statistics $\{T_i, i = 1, \dots, K\}$ whose values do not depend on which Θ_J^* is being tested.

S2 The tests are performed in each of the disjoint Θ_J^*s, defined previously.

S3 For $|J| > \eta$, where $|J|$ denotes the cardinality of J, the critical values C_J have the property that if $J \subset J'$, then $C_J \le C_{J'}$, and $C_J = C_{J'}$ if $|J| = |J'|$.

As an example, consider the test statistics $T_i = 1 - p_i, i = 1, \dots, k$, where p_i is a suitably defined p-value for testing H_{oi}. Define the critical values as

$$C_J = 1 - \frac{(\eta + 1)\alpha}{|J|}. \tag{1.36}$$

Since C_J is dependent on $|J|$, it can be denoted by $C_{|J|}$. Let $T_{(1)} \le \dots \le T_{(K)}$ be the test statistics that associate the hypotheses $H_{(1)}, \dots, H_{(K)}$. The stepdown procedure is specified as follows:

1. Reject $H_{(K)}, \dots, H_{(K-\eta+1)}$.

2. For $i = \eta, \ldots, K - 1$, if $T_{(K-i)} \geq C_{K-i}$, reject $H_{(K-i)}$ and continue; otherwise retain $H_{(K-i)}$ and stop.

Xu's stepdown procedure includes Lehmann and Romano's (2005) procedure as a special case.

1.2.5.5 General Stopping Boundary

Suppose the stepdown testing condition **S1** holds and the distribution of T_i when the null hypothesis H_{0i} is true is the same for all i. Denote by F the common marginal null distribution and by P_0 the probability computed based on the assumption of the null hypotheses involved. Let $\alpha_c = F\left(C_{|J|-\eta}\right)$. If the test statistics are independent, then

$$P_0\left(\nu > \eta\right) = 1 - \sum_{j=0}^{\eta} \binom{|J|}{j} \alpha_c^j \left(1 - \alpha_c\right)^{|J|-j}. \tag{1.37}$$

In general, Markov's inequality holds

$$P_0\left(\nu > \eta\right) \leq \frac{|J|\alpha_c}{\eta + 1}. \tag{1.38}$$

Keep in mind that neither (1.37) nor (1.38) is necessarily the upper bound of the gFWER or FWER when the dependence of T_i is not specified. The rejection boundary C_i can be determined using either simulation or numerical methods.

1.2.6 Procedures Controlling False Discovery Rate

1.2.6.1 Type-I Error Rate Versus False Discovery Rate

The false discovery rate (FDR) is the expected proportion of false rejections among all rejections. The FDR is defined to be zero when the total number of rejections equals zero (Benjamini and Hochberg 1995; Westfall et al. 1999, p. 21)

$$FDR = E\left(\frac{\nu}{\max\left(R, 1\right)}\right), \tag{1.39}$$

where R denotes the number of rejected hypotheses and ν is the number of falsely rejected hypotheses.

FDR-controlling procedures may lead to more type-I errors and fewer type-II errors than FWER-controlling procedures. However, increasing the number of true positive drugs in the market is as important as reducing the number of false drugs, because a reduction in FDR will increase the probability of treating patients with the right drugs. FDR is more relevant than the type-I error rate for increasing the probability of patients getting the right drugs. Therefore, controlling the proportion of false drugs in the market may be more meaningful than type-I error rates. However, be cautious. In the FDR procedure, one can purposely include some hypotheses that are known to be rejected in the set of hypotheses to be tested, and this will increase the test level for the hypothesis of main interest (Finner and Roter 2001).

It is informative to investigate the relationship between FDR and the type-I rate α. If we denote by P_e the proportion of effective test compounds and by P_w the power for the pivotal trials, then the expected proportion of ineffective drugs in the market is (neglecting other factors such as drug disapproval due to safety issues)

$$FDR = \frac{(1 - P_e)\alpha}{(1 - P_e)\alpha + P_e P_w}. \tag{1.40}$$

The FDR is a monotonic function of α.

From (1.40) we know that when $P_e = 0$ the FDR is 100% and so is the type-I error rate. In other words, if all test drugs in the pivotal trials are ineffective, then regardless of the α value, 100% of the approved drugs are no more effective than the control. On the other hand, if all drugs in the pivotal trials are effective ($P_e = 1$), then regardless of α, 100% of the approved drugs are effective ($FDR = 0$).

1.2.6.2 Benjamini-Hochberg Procedure

Let $p_{(i)}$ be the p-value associated with the hypothesis $H_{(i)}$, where $p_{(1)} \leq \ldots \leq p_{(K)}$. The Benjamini and Hochberg (1995) linear stepup (LSU) procedure can be described as: reject all $H_{(i)}$, $i = 1, \ldots, K^*$, where K^* is the largest i for which $P_{(i)} \leq \frac{i}{K}\alpha$. This procedure will control the FDR strongly at level α when the p-values are independent or positively dependent (Benjamini and Yekutieli 2001). In fact, the FDR of the LSU is bounded by $\pi_0\alpha$, where π_0 is the proportion of true null hypotheses. Moreover, if the p-values associated with the true null hypotheses are exactly distributed as a uniform distribution, the linear stepup procedure has an FDR exactly equal to $\pi_0\alpha$ (Blanchard and Roquain 2009).

1.2.6.3 Blanchard-Roquain Procedure

Under an unspecified dependence of the family of p-values p_i for H_i ($i = 1, \ldots K$), and β being a shape function of the form

$$\beta(r) = \int_0^r u\,dv(u), \tag{1.41}$$

where v is some fixed prior probability distribution on $(0, \infty)$ and $r > 0$, Blanchard and Roquain (2009) proved that the procedure that rejects H_i if $p_i < C_i = \alpha\beta(i)/K$ has an FDR bounded above by $\alpha\pi_0$.

This general result can be used to develop different testing procedures depending on different estimations of $\hat{\pi}_0$. Such a procedure that includes an estimating π_0 is called an adaptive procedure. As an example, if the p-values are independent and $\lambda \in (0, 1)$ is fixed, then the following procedure will control the FDR at level α: reject H_i if the p-value $p_i \leq C_i$, where $C_i = \min\left((1-\lambda)\frac{\alpha i}{K-i+1}, \lambda\right)$.

Theorem 1.1. *(Blanchard and Roquain 2009) Let β be a fixed shape function given by (1.41), and $0 < \alpha_0 < \alpha_1 < 1$. Denote by R_0 the stepup procedure with critical values $C_{0i} = \frac{\alpha_0\beta(i)}{K}$. Then the adaptive stepup procedure R with data-dependent critical values $C_{1i} = \frac{\alpha_1\beta(i)}{K}F_\zeta\left(\frac{|R_0|}{K}\right)$ has an FDR bounded above by $\alpha_1 + \zeta\alpha_0$, where $\zeta \geq 2$ and*

$$F_\zeta(x) = \begin{cases} 1 & \text{if } x \leq 1/\zeta, \\ \frac{2/\zeta}{1-\sqrt{1-4(1-x)/\zeta}} & \text{otherwise.} \end{cases} \tag{1.42}$$

1.2.6.4 Storey-Taylor-Siegmund Procedure

If the rejection rule for H_i is $p_i \leq \gamma$, then a conservative FDR is given by

$$FDR = \frac{K\hat{\pi}_0\gamma}{\max(R(\gamma), 1)}, \tag{1.43}$$

where $\hat{\pi}_0 = (\#\{p_i \geq \lambda\} + 1)/[(1-\lambda)K]$ is an estimator of π_0 and $R(\gamma)$ is the number of rejected hypotheses. Here $\#\{p_i \geq \lambda\}$ denotes the number of p-values exceeding $\lambda \in [0, 1)$. The larger λ is, the smaller the bias of $\hat{\pi}_0$ will be (at the cost of a larger variance). The critical value is chosen as the maximal $\gamma \leq \lambda$ such that the estimated $FDR(\gamma) \leq \alpha$. This procedure controls the FDR at the nominal level α if the p-values corresponding to the true null hypotheses are independent and are obtained from conservative tests (Storey et al. 2004).

1.2.6.5 Sequential Testing Method

Suppose an experiment has K hypotheses and up to N stages. Denote the p-value of hypothesis i at stage t by p_{it}, which is computed from the data accumulated for hypothesis i up to stage t. Let τ denote the random variable determining the stage where the trial is stopped. The stopping time τ may be a function of the collected data (e.g., p_{it}) but may also depend on external information. Posch et al. (2009) proved that the following procedure asymptotically ($K \to \infty$) controlled the FDR at level α.

For the stopping stage τ, define the critical value γ_τ to be the maximal $\gamma_\tau \leq \lambda$ such that $F\hat{D}R_\tau(\gamma_\tau) \leq \alpha$, where $F\hat{D}R_\tau$ is defined as in (1.43) with p_i replaced by p_{it}. Here λ is assumed to be a fixed prior. All null hypotheses with $p_{i\tau}$ $\leq \gamma_\tau$ are rejected. Furthermore, sampling is stopped for all hypotheses at the same interim analysis, and the test in the final analysis solely determines which hypotheses are rejected; we restrict early stopping to interim analyses where at least a certain fraction of null hypotheses can be rejected. No stopping rule needs to be prespecified, but one can flexibly decide at every interim analysis to stop the trial or change the sample size.

1.3   Controversies and Challenges

1.3.1   Family of Errors

We want to control the familywise type-I error rate in a multiple-testing problem. However, how should we determine the "family" of errors? Should the family chosen be an experiment (e.g., a clinical trial) even when two completely different hypotheses (a single drug treating two different diseases, two drugs treating the same disease, or two drugs treating two different diseases) are included in the same experiment? Why should we adjust multiplicity when hypotheses are addressed in the same experiment but not when they are addressed in two different experiments? Does this discourage people who use a more efficient way (one experiment) to do scientific research? Keep in mind that the concept of "an experiment" is subjective. We can define two experiments as a super-experiment. We can even consider the whole life of an individual an experiment and all the errors one has made in his life the family of errors. The difference in the definition of the family of errors could lead to completely different adjustments of p-values and conclusions. On the other hand, controlling alpha beyond the scope of the (commonly defined) experiment is difficult because we don't know what types of studies and how many of them we are going to conduct.

We should be aware that the same term, type-I error, does not necessarily mean the same thing at different times. As a result, $\alpha = 2.5\%$ may not imply the same criterion at different times. The first drug for an indication may be tested against a placebo. Newer compounds are being tested each year against better and better drugs in the market. It appears that $\alpha = 2.5\%$ doesn't change, but in fact the bar is set higher and higher because different competitors are used.

As we mentioned earlier, a reduction in FDR will increase the chance of treating patients with the right drugs. Thus, it seems reasonable to consider FDR control in place of the type-I error control α. However, one can purposely include some hypotheses known to be rejected in the set of hypotheses to be tested and therefore increase the test level for the hypothesis of main interest.

Furthermore, not all type-I errors have the same impact. Why do we control the error rate, and not the impact of the errors (Chap. 2)?

1.3.2 Interpretation of Multiple-Testing Results

Remember that all stepwise testing procedures can be expressed in a single-step fashion using adjusted p-values (Chang 2009). In general, for any given data and any stepwise test procedure, the rejection criterion associated with the null hypothesis H_{ok} at the kth step can be written as

$$p_k \le \alpha_k(\alpha, p_1, p_2, \dots, p_{k-1}), k = 1, 2, \dots K, \qquad (1.44)$$

where the critical point $\alpha_k(\alpha, p_1, p_2, \dots, p_{k-1})$ is a function of the overall alpha and the previous p-values in the procedure. By solving for α, (1.44) is equivalent (leads to the same decision) to

$$Q_k(p_1, p_2, \dots, p_k) \le \alpha, k = 1, 2, \dots K, \qquad (1.45)$$

where the function $Q_k(p_1, p_2, \dots, p_k)$ usually is not continuous in the p_i. Note that the right-hand side of (1.45) is the constant α for all ks and can be used in any order of k, just as in a single-step test procedure.

Formulation (1.45) suggests that all stepwise procedures in fact implicitly use some form of "composite endpoint" – rejection of H_{ok} is dependent on a certain combination of $p_1, p_2, \dots, p_k$ for the k "endpoints." This type of "composite endpoint," unlike a common endpoint (e.g., ACR50 for rheumatoid arthritis), often makes little sense scientifically or clinically, so interpretations of "composite endpoints" are difficult. In light of this, why shouldn't we use direct p-value combinations with clear clinical meanings for the test statistics (e.g., $T_k = \sum_i^K w_{ki} p_i$, where $w_{ki} \ge 0$ and $\sum_{i=1}^K w_{ki} = 1$)?

1.3.3 The Spring Water Paradox

If controlling the type-I error rate is a critical goal for an experiment, the following is a paradox. An experiment is to be conducted to test the hypothesis that spring water is effective compared with a placebo in a certain disease population. To carry out the trial at a minimal cost, we will need a coin and two patients with the disease. To control type-I error, the coin is used; i.e., zero patients are needed. To have an unbiased point estimate, a sample size of two patients is required (for a higher precision, more patients are needed). The trial is carried out as follows:

1. Randomize two patients: one takes the placebo and the other drinks spring water. The unbiased estimate of the treatment difference is given by $y - x$, where x and y are the clinical responses from the placebo and the spring water, respectively.

2. If $y - x > 0$, we will proceed with the hypothesis test $H_o : \mu_y - \mu_x \leq 0$ at a level of one-sided $\alpha = 0.05$. To perform the hypothesis test, we flip the coin 100 times. If the number of heads (n) appears at least 95 times, the efficacy of spring water will be claimed.

Suppose the spring water is presumably very safe. This is a cost-effective approach (two patients $+$ a coin), even though there is only approximately a 5% power and approximately a 2.5% probability of making the efficacy claim.

What if all pharmaceutical companies test such water-like compounds, over and over again, in their drug development? There will be many ineffective drugs on the market. In fact, this scenario could happen for two reasons: (1) A small α makes it difficult to show statistical significance for compounds that have small to moderate effects, so testing water-like compounds is more cost-effective. (2) Many companies screen the same compound libraries without multiple-testing adjustments. Therefore, a smaller α (more stringent type-I error control) could lead to more ineffective compounds flowing into the drug development pipeline and to the market.

1.3.4 A Patient's Dilemma with Multiple-Testing

Andy is a biochemists and Mike is a statistician working for a pharmaceutical company. They both had cancer and were hospitalized in the same room on the same day. Their doctor was discussing their treatment options: drug A or drug B. Both have been tested on 500 patients, drug A prolongs survival by 6 months and drug B prolongs survival by 2 years. Andy preferred drug B without a second thought. Mike proceeded cautiously, asking: "Was there any interim analysis and multiplicity adjustment?" The doctor told him that the raw p-value was 0.04 for A and 0.01 for B. However after the multiplicity adjustment, the p-value for B was close to significance ($p = 0.055$); no adjustment was needed for drug A. After listening to the details, Mike chose drug A. He thought B was not even statistically significant. Andy asked Mike: "Why did you pick A? Do you believe the statistical testing procedure will damage the chemical structure of the compound?" Mike replied: "The false positive rate will be very high if you choose drugs this way!" Andy was wondering: "Everyone only has one life; we don't have many chances to repeat this! Also, the selection of the type-I error rate 5% is a somewhat arbitrary value; why did Mike take this literally?" Later, however, Mike learned that there was an interim analysis showing that B was better than the control in the trial. Mike informed Andy about this, and asked him if he wanted to switch the treatment to drug A. What would be your answer if you were Andy (Fig. 1.1)?

Fig. 1.1 A personal dilemma

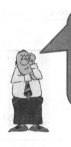

I don't think the p-value should be adjusted for multiplicity since the hypothesis test procedure will not damage the drug. However, if the p-value is not adjusted, the false positive rate could be very high. Adjust or not adjust?

1.4 Exercises

1.1. Suppose there are six hypotheses in an experiment with the associated p-values (one-sided): 0.0001, 0.0018, 0.009, 0.021, 0.034, and 0.052. Use the single-step testing procedures in Sect. 1.2.1 to test the six hypotheses with a familywise type-I error rate of $\alpha = 0.05$ (one-sided).

1.2. Given the same p-values as in Exercise 1.1, perform the hypothesis test using the Holm, Shaffer, and fallback procedures (one-sided $\alpha = 0.05$).

1.3. (Dmitrienko and Tamhane 2007) Suppose a parallel-group trial is conducted to compare a new formulation of an insulin therapy (formulation A) with a standard formulation (formulation B) in patients with Type 2 diabetes. Patients are allocated to three treatment groups (A, B, and $A + B$), and the efficacy analysis is based on the mean change in hemoglobin $A1c$ from baseline to a 6-month endpoint. The three pairwise comparisons among the treatment groups are ordered according to their clinical relevance. The primary objective of the study is to compare the new formulation with the standard one (A versus B). After that, the combination is compared with the standard formulation ($A + B$ versus B) and the new formulation ($A + B$ versus A). Each comparison begins with a noninferiority test, followed by a superiority test if noninferiority is established. According to this strategy, the six null hypotheses are grouped into four families:

Family $F1 = \{H_1\}$, where H_1 states that A is inferior to B.

Family $F2 = \{H_2, H_3\}$, where H_2 states that A is not superior to B and H_3 states that $A + B$ is inferior to B.

Family $F3 = \{H_4, H_5\}$, where H_4 states that $A + B$ is not superior to B and H_5 states that $A + B$ is inferior to A.

Family $F4 = \{H_6\}$, where H_6 states that $A + B$ is not superior to A.

The raw p-values are presented in Table 1.3. Please draw the decision tree (diagram) for the testing procedure and complete the table by filling in the adjusted p-values. The adjusted p-values are then compared with $\alpha = 0.05$ for rejecting or accepting the corresponding hypothesis.

1.4. Do you believe the FDR, the type-I error rate, or another efficacy criterion should be used in the regulatory approval of a drug? Why?

Table 1.3 Tree gatekeeping procedure based on the Bonferroni test

Family	Hypothesis	Serial rejection set	Raw p-value	Adjusted p-value
F_1	H_1	NA	0.011	
F_2	H_2	H_1	0.023	
F_2	H_3	H_1	0.006	
F_3	H_4	H_3	0.018	
F_3	H_5	H_3	0.042	
F_4	H_6	H_5	0.088	

Note: The parallel rejection sets are empty

1.5. In Sect. 1.3.2, we stated that any stagewise testing procedure implies an adoption of a "composite endpoint." Do you agree? Why? How do you interpret the results from a stepwise testing procedure?

1.6. If you faced the dilemma presented in Sect. 1.3.4, which drug would you take? Why?

Further Readings and References

Bauer, P., Rohmel, J., Maurer, W., Hothorn, L.: Testing strategies in multi-dose experiments including active control. Stat. Med. **17**, 2133–2146 (1998)

Benjamini, Y., Hochberg, Y.: Controlling the false discovery rate: A practical and powerful approach to multiple testing. J. R. Stat. Soc. B **57**(2), 289–300 (1995)

Benjamini, Y., Liu, W.: A step-down multiple hypotheses testing procedure that controls the false discovery rate under independence. J. Stat. Plan. Inference **82**, 163–170 (1999)

Benjamini, Y., Yekutieli, D.: The control of the false discovery rate in multiple testing under dependency. Ann. Stat. **29**(4), 1165–1188 (2001)

Berger, R.L.: Multiparameter hypothesis testing and acceptance sampling. Technometrics **24**, 295–300 (1982)

Birnbaum, A.: On the foundations of statistical inference (with discussion). J. Am. Stat. Assoc. **57**, 269–326 (1962)

Blanchard, G., Roquain, E.: Adaptive false discovery rate control under independence and dependence. J. Mach. Learn. Res. **10**, 2837–2871 (2009)

Bretz, F., Schmidli1, H., König, F., Racine1, A., Maurer, W.: Confirmatory seamless phase II/III clinical trials with hypotheses selection at interim: General concepts. Biom. J. **48**:4.48, 623–634 (2006)

Bretz, F., Hothorn, T., Westfall, P.: Multiple Comparison Using R. CRC Press, Boca Raton (2010)

Chang, M.: Adaptive Design Theory and Implementation Using SAS and R. Chapman and Hall/CRC, Boca Raton (2007)

Chang, M.: Limitations of hypothesis testing in clinical trials: Discussion of "Some Controversial Multiple Testing Problems in Regulatory Applications." J. Biopharm. Stat. **19**, 35–41 (2009)

Chang, M., Chow, S.C.: Analysis strategy of multiple-endpoint adaptive design. J. Biopharm. Stat. **17**, 1189–1200 (2007)

Chen, X., Luo, X., Capizzi, T.: The application of enhanced parallel gatekeeping strategies. Stat. Med. **24**, 1385–1397 (2005)

Dmitrienko, A., Offen, W.W., Westfall, P.H.: Gatekeeping strategies for clinical trials that do not require all primary effects to be significant. Stat. Med. **22**, 2387–2400 (2003)

Dmitrienko, A., Molenberghs, G., Chuang-Stein, C., Offen, W.: Analysis of Clinical Trials Using SAS: A Practical Guide. SAS, Cary (2005)

Dmitrienko, A., Offen, W., Wang, O., Xiao, D.: Gatekeeping procedures in dose–response clinical trials based on the Dunnett test. Pharm. Stat. **5**, 19–28 (2006a)

Dmitrienko, A., Tamhane, A.C., Wang, X., Chen, X.: Stepwise gatekeeping procedures in clinical trial applications. Biom. J. **48**, 984–991 (2006b)

Dmitrienko, A., Wiens, B.L., Westfall, P.H.: Fallback tests in dose–response clinical trials. J. Biopharm. Stat. **16**, 745–755 (2006c)

Dmitrienko, A., Tamhane, A.C.: Gatekeeping procedures with clinical trial applications. Pharma. Stat. **6**, 171–180 (2007)

Dmitrienko, A., Wiens, B.L., Tamhane, A.C., Wang, X.: Tree-structured gatekeeping tests in clinical trials with hierarchically ordered multiple objectives. Stat. Med. **26**, 2465–2478 (2007)

Dmitrienko, A., Tamhane, A.C., Bretz, F.: Multiple Testing Problems in Pharmaceutical Statistics. Chapman and Hall/CRC, Boca Raton (2010)

Dunnett, C.W.: A multiple comparison procedure for comparing several treatments with a control. J. Am. Stat. Assoc. **50**, 1096–1121 (1955)

European Medicines Agency: ICH Topic E 9 Statistical Principles for Clinical Trials. Step 5. http://www.ema.europa.eu (1998). Accessed 8 Jan 2011

Finner, H., Roter, M.: On the false discovery rate and expected type I errors. Biom. J. **43**, 985–1005 (2001)

Ghosh, J.K., Delampady, M., Samanta, T.: An Introduction to Bayesian Analysis. Springer, New York (2006)

Grechanovsky, E., Hochberg, Y.: Closed procedures are better and often admit a shortcut. J. Stat. Plan. Inference **76**, 79–91 (1999)

Hochberg, Y.: A sharper Bonferroni procedure for multiple tests of significance. Biometrika **75**, 800–802 (1988)

Hochberg, Y., Benjamini, Y.: More powerful procedures for multiple significance testing. Stat. Med. **9**, 811–818 (1990)

Hochberg, Y., Tamhane, A.C.: Multiple Comparison Procedures. Wiley, New York (1987)

Holm, S.: A simple sequentially rejective multiple test procedure. Scand. J. Stat. **6**, 65–70 (1979)

Hommel, G.: A stagewise rejective multiple test procedure based on a modified Bonferroni test. Biometrika **75**, 383–386 (1988)

Hommel, G., Bretz, F.: Aesthetics and power considerations in multiple testing – a contradiction? Biom. J. **50**, 657–666 (2008)

Hommel, G., Bretz, F., Maurer, W.: Powerful shortcuts for multiple testing procedures with special reference to gatekeeping strategies. Stat. Med. **99**, 25–41 (2007)

Hsu, J.C.: Multiple Comparisons: Theory and Methods. Chapman and Hall, London (1996)

Hung, H.M.J.: Some controversial multiple testing problems in regulatory applications. J. Biopharm. Stat. **4**, 1–25 (2008)

Huque, M., Röhmel, J.: Multiplicity problems in clinical trials: A regulatory perspective. In: Dmitrienko, A., Tamhane, A.C., Bretz, F. (eds.) Multiple Testing Problems in Pharmaceutical Statistics. Chapman and Hall/CRC, Boca Raton (2010)

Kanji, G.K.: 100 Statistical Tests, 3rd edn. Sage Publications, London (2006)

Lehmacher, W., Wassmer, G., Reimeir, P.: Procedure for two-sample comparisons with multiple endpoints controlling the experimentwise error rate. Biometrics **47**, 511–521 (1991)

Lehmann, E.L., Romano, J.P.: Generalizations of the familywise error rate. Ann. Stat. **33**, 1138–1154 (2005)

Marcus, R., Peritz, E., Gabriel, K.R.: On closed testing procedures with special reference to ordered analysis of variance. Biometrika **63**, 655–660 (1976)

Lemuel, A.M.: Multiple analysis in clinical trials. Springer-Verlag, New York (2003)

Pocock, S., Geller, N., Tsiatis, A.: Analysis of multiple endpoints in clinical trials. Biometrics **43**, 487–498 (1987)

Posch, M., Zehetmayer, S., Bauer, P.: Hunting for significance with the false discovery rate. J. Am. Stat. Assoc. **104**(486), 832–840 (2009)

Quan, H., Luo, X., Capizzi, T.: Multiplicity adjustment for multiple endpoints in clinical trials with multiple doses of an active control. Stat. Med. **24**, 2151–2170 (2005)

Rom, D.M.: A sequentially rejective test procedure based on a modified Bonferroni inequality. Biometrika **77**, 663–665 (1990)

Roy, S.N.: On a heuristic method for test construction and its use in multivariate analysis. Ann. Stat. **24**, 220–238 (1953)

Sarkar, S.K., Chang, C.K.: Simes' method for multiple hypothesis testing with positively dependent test statistics. J. Am. Stat. Assoc. **92**, 1601–1608 (1997)

Shaffer, J.P.: Modified sequentially rejective multiple test procedures. J. Am. Stat. Assoc. **81**, 826–831 (1986)

Sidak, Z.: Rectangular confidence regions for the means of multivariate normal distributions. J. Am. Stat. Assoc. **62**, 626–633 (1967)

Simes, R.J.: An improved Bonferroni procedure for multiple tests of significance. Biometrika **63**, 655–660 (1986)

Storey, J., Taylor, J., Siegmund, D.: Strong control, conservative point estimation and simultaneous conservative consistency of false discovery rates: A unified approach. J. R. Stat. Soc. Ser. B, **66**(1), 187–205 (2004)

Tsong, Y., Wang, S.J., Hung, H.M.J., Cui, L.: Statistical issues on objective, design, and analysis of noninferiority active-controlled clinical trial. J. Biopharm. Stat. **13**, 29–41 (2003)

Wang, X.: Gatekeeping procedures for multiple endpoints. Ph.D. Dissertation, Department of Statistics, Northwestern University, Evanston (2006)

Westfall, P.H., Krishen, A.: Optimally weighted, fixed-sequence and gatekeeper multiple testing procedures. J. Stat. Plan. Inference **99**, 25–41 (2001)

Westfall, P.H., Tobias, R.D., Rom, D., Wolfinger, R.D., Hochberg, Y.: Multiple Comparisons and Multiple Tests Using the SAS System. SAS Institute, Cary (1999)

Westfall, P.H., Young, S.S.: Resampling-Based Multiple Testing: Examples and Methods for p-value Adjustment. Wiley, New York (1993)

Wiens, B.L.: A fixed-sequence Bonferroni procedure for testing multiple endpoints. Pharm. Stat. **2**, 211–215 (2003)

Wiens, B., Dmitrienko, A.: The fallback procedure for evaluating a single family of hypotheses. J. Biopharm. Stat. **15**, 929–942 (2005)

Xu, H.: Using the partitioning principle to control generalized familywise error rate. Ph.D. Dissertation, The Ohio State University, Columbus (2005)

Chapter 2
Pharmaceutical Decision and Game Theory

2.1 Pharmaceutical Decisions

A pharmaceutical or biopharmaceutical company is a commercial business licensed to research, develop, market, and/or distribute drugs, most commonly in the context of healthcare. It is subject to a variety of laws and regulations regarding the patenting, testing, and marketing of drugs, particularly prescription drugs.

Drug development involves large, lengthy collaborations among people from dozens of disciplines. The entire development process includes multiple stages or phases from discovery, preclinical, and clinical trials, to phase IV commitment or marketing. It is estimated that, on average, a drug takes 10–12 years from initial research to the commercialization stage. The cost of this process is estimated to be more than US$500 million. At each stage of research and development, decisions have to be made. A correct decision will lead to successful of drug development, the mitigation of risks, or a cost reduction. A wrong decision can have a significant negative impact. Thus, drug development can be viewed as a sequence of decision processes, which can be modeled statistically by Markov decision processes. We will give many examples later, after we introduce the concept of a Markov decision process.

2.1.1 Markov Decision Process

A Markov decision process (MPP) is similar to a Markov chain, but there are also actions and utilities (rewards or gains, see Fig. 2.1). MDPs provide a powerful mathematical framework for modeling the decision-making process in situations where outcomes are partly random and partly under the control of the decision-maker. They are useful in studying a wide range of optimization problems solved via dynamic programming and reinforced learning. Since the 1950s, when MDP first became known (Bellman, 1957a), it has been widely used in robotics, automated

Fig. 2.1 Markov sequential
decision-making

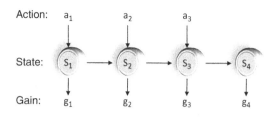

control, economics, business management, nursing system, and manufacturing
(Gosavi 2003; Bertsekas 1995).

There are two types of MDPs: finite and infinite horizon problems. In a finite
horizon problem, the transition probabilities (from state s at time t to state s' at time
$t + 1$) vary over time,

$$T\left(s, a, s'\right) = \Pr\left(s_{t+1} = s' | s_t = s, a_t = a\right), \tag{2.1}$$

whereas in the infinite horizon MDP problem, the system reaches a steady state and
the transition probability is only dependent on the two states (s and s') and the
action taken, a, but is independent of the time when the transition occurs. Thus, the
transition probability can be simplified as

$$T\left(s, a, s'\right) = \Pr\left(s' | s, a\right). \tag{2.2}$$

We will focus our discussions on infinite horizon MDPs.

Suppose a dynamic system (Fig. 2.1) moves over states $s_i \in S, i = 1, 2, \ldots, N$
and the motion is controlled by choosing a sequence of actions $a_i \in A, i =$,
$1, 2, \ldots N$. There is a net numerical gain (immediate reward or cost) $g_i\left(\alpha_i\right)$
associated with each action a_i. The goal is to find a policy (strategy) that maximizes
the total expected gain. This problem can be formalized as a Markov decision
process.

An infinite horizon Markov decision process is a 4-tuple of four elements
$\{S, A, \Pr\left(S, A\right), g\left(S, A\right)\}$ with the following properties:

1. Finite (N) set of states, S.
2. Set of actions, A (can be conditioned on the state s).
3. Policy/strategy/action rule – action mapping to state s.
4. Discount rate for future rewards $0 < \gamma < 1$.
5. Immediate reward (utility or gain function) $g : S \times A \to \Re, g\left(s, a\right) =$ immediate
   reward by reaching the state s and taking action a.
6. Transition model (dynamics) $T : S \times A \times S \to [0, 1]\ T(s, a, s') =$ probability
   of going from s to s' under action a.

$$T\left(s, a, s'\right) = \Pr\left(s' | s, a_i = a\right). \tag{2.3}$$

7. The goal is to find a policy $\pi^* = \{a_i^*, i = 1, \ldots, N\}$ that maximizes the total
   expected reward over the course of motion, which is subject to some initial
   conditions and possible constraints. Note that action a often associates with
   state s. We may write a_s for action at state s.

Here are examples of Markov decision processes in drug development (Fig. 2.1):

1. s_1 = drug discovery phase, s_2 = preclinical phase, s_3 = clinical development phase, and s_4 = regulatory approval and marketing. The a_i represents the general decision rules or action rules for moving from the ith phase to the next phase in the drug development process.
2. s_1 = Preclinical phase, s_i = the ith phase clinical trial ($i = 1, 2, 3$), and a_i has a similar meaning as in (1).
3. s_1 = initiation of a clinical trial, s_i = interim and final analyses for the $(i - 1)$th phase trial ($i = 2, 3, 4$); the actions, a_i, are the stopping and adaptive rules (see the details in Chap. 4).

2.1.2 Dynamic Programming

2.1.2.1 Bellman's Optimality Principle

An optimal policy has the property that, whatever the initial state and initial decision, the remaining decisions must constitute an optimal policy with regard to the state resulting from the first decision (Bellman 1957a).

This principle can be applied to the stochastic decision problems here, but the optimal policy is regarded as the expected gain (loss) as opposed to loss in a deterministic sense.

Computationally, stochastic decision problems are usually solved using the so-called Bellman equations in terms of value $V(s)$:

$$V(s) = \max_{a_s \in A} \left(g(s, a) + \gamma \sum_{s' \in S} \Pr(s'|s, a_s) \cdot V(s') \right). \qquad (2.4)$$

The optimal policy, $\pi^* = \{a_1^*, a_2^*, \ldots, a_N^*\}$, for the MDP is a vector whose components are defined by

$$a_s^* = \arg\max_{a_s} \left\{ g(s, a_s) + \gamma \sum_{s' \in S} \Pr(s'|s, a_s) \cdot V(s') \right\}. \qquad (2.5)$$

Equation 2.4 can be written in matrix form:

$$V_\pi = g_\pi + \gamma P_\pi V_\pi. \qquad (2.6)$$

The solution to (2.6) can be written in matrix form:

$$V_\pi = (I - \gamma P_\pi)^{-1} g_\pi. \qquad (2.7)$$

Fig. 2.2 Markov decision
process for CDP

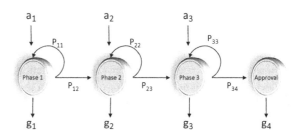

We can optimize policy π among all possible policy options to maximize V_π in (2.7). However, a more efficient way is to use the Bellman equations (2.4) as the dynamic programming algorithm (a backward induction algorithm) to obtain the optimal policy. The iterations will go from the last state to the first state (Chang 2010).

2.1.3 Clinical Development Program

The success of a pharmaceutical company depends on integrating scientific, clinical, regulatory, and marketing approaches into the development and commercialization of therapies. The MDP-based clinical development program design can eliminate unnecessary or redundant clinical trials that are used for internal decision-making, identify and address critical path issues that could delay development timelines, and ensure that clinical programs focus quickly and unambiguously on key attributes of the compound.

A stochastic decision process can provide a rational basis for decision-making and help optimize the compound's regulatory strategy and determine its commercial position and value. Simulation of the clinical development program (CDP) can increase confidence in decision-making and help to define and track critical success factors and their uncertainties.

Let's study how to model a clinical development program using a Markov decision process.

A typical drug development program includes phases I–IV clinical trials that are conducted in a sequence. At the end of each phase the decision is made regarding whether to stop the program (the "No-Go" decision) or to carry on to the next phase (the "Go" decision). Each action is associated with an estimated net gain (Fig. 2.2). Formally, it can be modeled by the following MDP:

1. A finite set of states, S. For the case in Fig. 2.2, the state space is given by $S = \{$phase I, phase II, phase III, NDA approval$\}$.
2. A set of actions, A_s (state-dependent action space). The choice of the action set can be $A_s = \{$Go, No-Go$\}$ and/or sample size n_i for the ith phase.
3. Action rules. The action rule or decision rule is typically a set of values, $A_i = \{a_{ij}, j = 1, 2, \ldots m, i = 1, 2, 3\}$, where a_{ij} can be a set of sample size options

($j = 1, \ldots, m$) for the ith phase trial or $A_i = [a_{\min}, a_{\max}]$ as the range of the cutpoint for "Go or No-Go" decision-making. The action space can also be a vector, e.g., corresponding to efficacy and safety requirements or to the point estimate and confidence interval of a parameter (or a p-value). The goal is to find the optimal policy $A_i^* = \{a_{1*}, a_{2*}, a_{3*}\}$ that maximizes the expected gain.

4. A discount factor for future rewards, $0 < \gamma \leq 1$.
5. Immediate reward. In the simplest case, the immediate reward g_i ($a_i = a$), or g_i (a) for simplicity, at the ith state (phase) can be a cost c_{i+1} and a reward from NDA approval or the value of out-licensing of the new molecular entity (NME).
6. Transition dynamics $T : S \times A \times S \rightarrow [0, 1]$.

The transition probability of going from the ith phase to the $(i + 1)$th phase is a function of the action rule A_i, written as

$$T(s_i, a, s_{i+1}) = \Pr(s_{i+1}|s_i, A_i). \tag{2.8}$$

We now use a numerical example to illustrate the process.

Example 2.1. Optimal Sample Size for Trials in a Clinical Development Plan: Suppose the CDP team wants to develop a clinical development program for a disease indication that includes phases I–III trials (Fig. 2.2). Phase I is a single-arm toxicity study; the phases II and III trials are two-group efficacy studies with two parallel groups. A common and important question is how to determine the optimal sample size for each trial so that the success or the expected overall gain for the CDP is maximized. Let's build, step by step, a Markov decision process for this problem.

1. State space

$$S = \{\text{phase I, phase II, phase III, NDA approval}\}$$

2. Action space

In practice, there are limits for the sample size. For simplicity, assume the limits (i.e., the action space) are independent of state (the phase):

$$A = \{10, \ldots, 1,000\}.$$

3. Discount rate

Based on typical trial durations, assume that the discount rate is

$$\gamma = 0.95.$$

4. Immediate reward and cost

In calculating immediate gains in phases I–III trials, the costs are approximately proportional to the corresponding sample size. After approval for marketing, there is a commercial/advertising cost. The net gains (cost) for phases I–III can be written as functions of sample size or simply the sample sizes themselves:

$$g_i(n_i) = n_i, i = 1, 2, 3, \tag{2.9}$$

and the net gain for marketing the drug (less commercial cost) is assumed to be $g_4 = 10,000$.

5. Decision rules and transition probabilities

Assume the decision rule for the phase I trial is that if the toxicity rate $r_1 \leq \eta_1 = 0.2$, the study will continue to phase II; otherwise stop. The decision rules for phase II are based on a hypothesis test for treatment differences in efficacy. Specifically, if the one-sided p-value for the test is $p_2 \leq \eta_2 = 0.1$, the study will continue and a phase III trial will be launched; otherwise, the clinical program will stop after phase II. Similar to phase II, phase III is a parallel two-group active-controlled trial. The decision rule is that if the one-sided p-value for the efficacy test is $p_3 < \eta_3 = 0.025$, the drug will be approved for marketing, otherwise, the NDA will fail.

From these decision rules, we can determine the transition probabilities. The transition probability from phases I to II can be calculated using the binomial distribution

$$p_{12}(n_1) = \sum_{i=0}^{\lfloor \eta_1 n_1 \rfloor} B(i; p_0, n_1) = \sum_{i=0}^{\lfloor \eta_1 n_1 \rfloor} \binom{n_1}{i} p_0^i (1 - p_0)^{n_1 - i}, \qquad (2.10)$$

where p_0 is the toxicity rate of the NME, $B(i; p_0, n_1)$ is the binomial probability mass function (p.m.f.). and the floor function $\lfloor x \rfloor$ gives the integer part of x.

The transition probability p_{23} from phases II to III is the power of the hypothesis test in the phase II trial at the one-sided alpha level of $\eta_2 = 0.1$,

$$p_{23}(n_2) = \Phi \left(\frac{\sqrt{n_2}}{2} \delta - z_{1-\eta_2} \right), \qquad (2.11)$$

where δ is the standardized treatment difference and Φ is the standard normal c.d.f.

Similarly, the transition probability from phase III to NDA approval is given by

$$p_{34}(n_3) = \Phi \left(\frac{\sqrt{n_3}}{2} \delta - z_{1-\eta_3} \right). \qquad (2.12)$$

Note that there is no repeated trial, even though p_{ii} in Fig. 2.2 seems to represent a transition loop. Keep in mind that in this simple case each state has only one immediately proceeding state. The rest of the transition probabilities can be easily calculated as follows:

$$\begin{cases} p_{11} = 1 - p_{12}, \\ p_{22} = 1 - p_{23}, \\ p_{33} = 1 - p_{34}. \end{cases} \qquad (2.13)$$

6. Dynamic programming

We are now ready to use dynamic programming to solve this problem. Start with Bellman's equation:

$$\begin{cases} V_4 = g_4, \\ V_i = \max\limits_{n_i \in A} \{g_i(n_i) + \gamma p_{i,i+1}(n_i) V_{i+1}\}, i = 3, 2, 1. \end{cases} \quad (2.14)$$

Example 2.2. In Example 2.1, we are only concerned with the optimization of sample size, but in practice it is also important to optimize the cutpoints $\{\eta_1, \eta_2, \eta_3\}$ simultaneously. Let's build the MDP for the decision problem:

1. State space

$$S = \{\text{phase I, phase II, phase III, NDA approval}\}.$$

2. Action space

$$A_i = u_i \times v_i, \quad (2.15)$$

where the sample size space and cutpoint space are given, respectively, by

$$u_i = \{n_{i,\min}, \dots, n_{i,\max}\} \text{ and } v_i = [\eta_{i,\min}, \eta_{i,\max}], i = 1, 2, 3.$$

3. Discount rate

Let $\gamma = 1$ for simplicity.

4. Immediate reward and cost

Assume the rewards have the form

$$g_i(a_i) = c_{0i} + n_i, i = 1, 2, 3, \quad (2.16)$$

where c_{0i} is a constant.

The net gain for marketing the drug (less commercial cost) is assumed to be a linear function of the estimated treatment effect $\hat{\delta}$,

$$g_4 = g_0 + b\hat{\delta}, \quad (2.17)$$

where g_0 and b are constants.

5. Decision rules and transition probabilities

Assume the decision rules are similar to those in Example 2.1, specified as follows:

phase I: If the observed toxicity rate is $r_1 \leq \eta_1$, the study will continue to phase II; otherwise stop.

phase II: If the one-sided p-value for the efficacy test is $p_2 \leq \eta_2$, launch a phase III trial; otherwise, stop.

phase III: If the one-sided p-value for the efficacy test is $p_3 < 0.025$ (0.025 is a regulatory requirement for approval and therefore is not considered a variable), the drug will be approved for marketing; otherwise, the NDA will fail.

The expressions for the transition probabilities are the same as in Example 2.1. For clarity, we rewrite p_{ij} as a function of both the sample size n_i and the cutpoint η_i,

$$p_{12}(n_1, \eta_1) = \sum_{i=0}^{\lfloor \eta_1 n_1 \rfloor} B(i; p_0, n_1), \tag{2.18}$$

where p_0 is the toxicity rate of the NME.

The transition probability p_{23} from phases II to III is the power of the hypothesis test in the phase II trial (Chang 2008; Chang and Chow 2006),

$$p_{23}(n_2, \eta_2) = \Phi\left(\frac{\sqrt{n_2}}{2}\delta - z_{1-\eta_2}\right). \tag{2.19}$$

Similarly, the transition probability from phase III to approval is given by

$$p_{34}(n_3) = \Phi\left(\frac{\sqrt{n_3}}{2}\delta - z_{1-0.025}\right). \tag{2.20}$$

The rest of the transition probabilities can be calculated using (2.13).

6. Dynamic programming

We are now ready to use dynamic programming to solve this problem. Start with Bellman's equation:

$$\begin{cases} V_4 = g_4, \\ V_i = \max_{n_i \in u_i, \eta_i \in v_i} \{g_i(n_i) + p_{i,i+1}(n_i) V_{i+1}\}, i = 3, 2, 1. \end{cases} \tag{2.21}$$

So far, we have not considered the action rules (policy) that concern efficacy and safety jointly. In most realistic settings, they have to be considered simultaneously at some point (e.g., in phases II and III trials). The key is to construct the transition probabilities using the policy with efficacy and safety components. We may consider another common situation, multiple optional paths in clinical development plans. This will be illustrated in the next section.

2.1.4 R & D Portfolio Optimization

Most pharmaceutical research efforts have focused on four major disease areas: central nervous system, cancer, cardiovascular, and infectious disease. Increasingly, researchers will have to search for products in poorly understood and more complex therapeutic areas such as autoimmune diseases and genitourinary conditions (Bernard 2002; Hu et al. 2007). The increasing failure rate and cost in pharma R & D (5,000 patients per NDA based on data from 1999 to 2003) alert pharmaceutical companies to be extremely cautious in their decision-making. They have to carefully

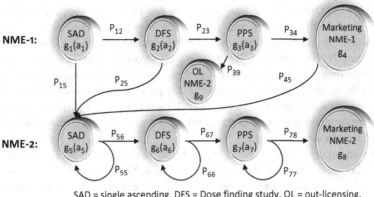

SAD = single ascending, DFS = Dose finding study, OL = out-licensing,
JV = Joint venture, PPS = Pivotal phase 3 study

Fig. 2.3 Decision modeling for two new molecular entities

evaluate their core competencies, technological advantages, competitive barriers, and financial resources before committing to develop a drug to fulfill the unmet need. They have to weigh their options carefully from the perspectives of market potential, patent, intellectual property portfolio, competitive forces and regulatory status, and core competencies, and build their R & D portfolio accordingly.

In this regard, many new technologies can be used in conjunction with traditional methods to accelerate the R & D process and reduce the cost. The following example illustrates how to use MDPs in the product development program.

Example 2.3. Suppose a biotech company has identified two leading compounds (NME-1 and NME-2) from drug discovery and preclinical studies. Due to financial constraints, the management team proposed the following strategy for evaluations: If the NME-1 phases I or II trial fails, we will consider launching the NME-2 trials. If the phases I and II trials are successful but the NME-1 phase III fails, the sponsor doesn't have enough cash to invest in the NME-1 clinical trials and NME-2 will be considered for out-licensing. However, if phase III is successful for drug marketing, the company will consider investigating NME-2 in clinical trials. Other options such as joint ventures are, for simplicity, not considered. This strategy is plotted as an MDP in Fig. 2.3.

What the working team needs to do is to develop an MDP with specific action rules that optimize the MDP and evaluate the maximum expected net gain.

Example 2.4. Risk Aversion and Pick-Winner Strategy: Risk aversion is a concept in economics, finance, and psychology related to the behavior of consumers and investors in the face of uncertainty. Risk aversion is the reluctance of a person to accept a bargain with an uncertain payoff rather than another bargain with more certainty but possibly a lower expected payoff. This concept is also applicable to the pharmaceutical industry. Risk aversion is measured as the additional marginal reward required for an investor to accept additional risk, which is measured as the standard deviation of the return on investment.

Risk aversion is reflected in the diversity of the pharmaceutical portfolio. With multiple leading NMEs in the drug discovery and preclinical pipeline, an optimal strategy to pick the winners and carry them forward to clinical development becomes critically important. We can do this by means of an MDP. Suppose there are n leading NMEs identified. If n is relatively small, we can launch all n NMEs at the same time. In the development process (preclinical to phase III trials), an MDP can be used to tune the decision rule for picking the winner so that the gain is optimized. If n is large, a subset of the NMEs can be tested first and losers (bad NMEs) are dropped over time in the development process. Then, more NMEs can be tested later in development.

There are many criteria (i.e., decision rules) that can be used for picking the winners. For example, pick the safest m_0 out of n NMEs, based on the observed toxicity rate (aggregated toxicity rate from multiple components) in the preclinical phase, for further testing in the phase I; pick m_1 best responses out of m_0 NMEs in the phase I trial and carry on to the phase II trial. The criteria for the best response can be measured by some utility index that consists of safety and efficacy biomarkers. After a set of decision rules is formed, the corresponding transition probabilities can be constructed as well as gain/reward functions. Finally, the optimal policy can be found using the dynamic programming algorithm to maximize the gain or success.

2.1.5 Prescription Drug Marketing

A pharmaceutical company usually starts its marketing strategy research before the drug gets approval for marketing. There are several key factors to consider in making the strategy: (1) company marketing positioning; (2) characteristics of the prescription drug and its competitors, including efficacy, safety, convenience, and cost; (3) target patient segmentation and mapping to the drug characteristics in (2); (4) physician prescription behavior of the drug class; (5) behavior characteristics of the competitors; (6) financial condition of the company and its competitors; and (7) availability of the marketing force.

Example 2.5. Suppose we do marketing consulting for the company and need to decide marketing strategies, and there are three patient segments (inferior, mixed, and prime) that are determined for the overall patient population. For each of the patient segments, we have to decide on x dollars for advertising. If $x = 0$, it means no direct advertising at all for that segment; if $x = D_{\max}$, it reaches the financial constraint.

It is important to fully realize that the outcomes of the advertisement are not only dependent on the company's advertising strategy but are also influenced by the behavior of other game players (competitors).

Let's build the Markov decision process. For the current problem (Fig. 2.4), there are three states, $S = \{s_1, s_2, s_3\}$, for each patient segment: (1) the inferior, patients

Fig. 2.4 Markov decision
process for marketing

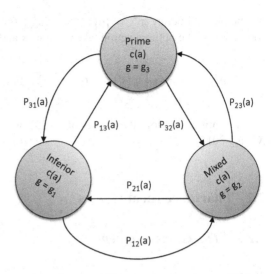

Table 2.1 Probabilities
of strategy matching

		Competitor		
		SC	LA	DN
Sponsor	SC	$\tilde{p}_{ss}$	$\tilde{p}_{sl}$	$\tilde{p}_{sd}$
	LA	$\tilde{p}_{ls}$	$\tilde{p}_{ll}$	$\tilde{p}_{ld}$
	DN	$\tilde{p}_{ds}$	$\tilde{p}_{dl}$	$\tilde{p}_{dd}$

who will mostly use the competitor's drug (the gain at this state is $g = g_1 = 0$); (2) the mixed, patients who will use both our client's and the competitor's drugs (the gain at this state is $g = g_2(\xi)$, which is dependent on the patient segment ξ); and (3) the prime, patients who will virtually use only our client's drug.

At each stage, we have to make a decision on whether to launch a strong campaign (SC), do limited advertising (LA), or do nothing (DN); i.e., the action space is $A = \{SC, LA, DN\}$. A cost is associated with each action taken, specifically $C = \{c_1, c_2, c_3\}$ corresponding to $A = \{SC, LA, DN\}$. No discount γ will be considered.

The transition probabilities $p_{ij}(a)$ can be estimated using the information about the competitor's possible strategies. We can use Table 2.1 to illustrate this conceptually. The probability that both the sponsor and the competitor have a strong marketing campaign is $\tilde{p}_{ss}$, and the conditional transition probability from state i to state j under this campaign condition is $\hat{p}_{ij}(ss)$. Therefore, the transition probability is given by

$$p_{ij} = \sum_{a \in A \times A} \tilde{p}_a \hat{p}_{ij}(a). \tag{2.22}$$

Bellman's equation can be written as

$$V(s) = \max_{a \in A} \left(g(s') - c(a) + \gamma \sum_{s' \in S} \Pr(s'|s, a) \cdot V(s') \right). \tag{2.23}$$

The optimal policy $\pi^* = \{a_1^*, a_2^*, \ldots, a_N^*\}$ for the MDP is a vector whose ith component is the optimal action taken at state s and is defined by

$$a_s^* = \arg\max_{a_s} \left\{ g\left(s'\right) - c\left(a\right) + \gamma \sum_{s' \in S} \Pr\left(s'|s, a_s\right) \cdot V\left(s'\right) \right\}. \tag{2.24}$$

The implementation algorithms of (2.23) and (2.24) can be found elsewhere (Chang 2010).

2.2 Pharmaceutical Games

2.2.1 The Game Concept

A game is a formal description of a strategic situation. *Game theory* is the formal study of decision-making wherein several players must make choices that potentially affect the interests of the other players. A player is an agent who makes decisions in a game.

Tucker's Prisoners' Dilemma is one of the most influential examples in economics and the social sciences. It is stated like this: Two criminals, Bob and John, are captured at the scene of their crime. Each has to choose whether or not to confess and implicate the other. If neither man confesses, then both will serve 2 years. If both confess, they will go to prison for 10 years each. However, if one of them confesses and implicates the other, and the other does not confess, the one who has collaborated with the police will go free while the other will go to prison for 20 years on the maximum charge.

The strategies offered in this case are confess or don't confess. The payoffs or penalties are the sentences served. We can express all this in a standard *payoff table* in game theory (Table 2.2).

Let's discuss how to solve this game. Assume both prisoners are rational and try to minimize the time they spend in jail. Bob might reason as follows: If John confesses, I will get 20 years if I don't confess and 10 years if I do, so in that case it's best to confess. On the other hand, if John doesn't confess, I will go free if I confess and get 2 years if I don't confess. Therefore, either way, it's better (best) if I confess. John reasons in the same way. Therefore, they both confess and get 10 years. This is the solution or equilibrium for the game. This solution

Table 2.2 The Prisoners' Dilemma		John (Player B)	
		Confess	Don't
Bob	Confess	(10, 10)	(0, 20)
(Player A)	Don't	(20, 0)	(2, 2)

Fig. 2.5 Braess's Paradox

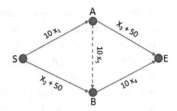

is a noncooperative solution; it is a solution to a noncooperative game in which no communication is allowed and thus no collaboration exists between the players. However, we can see in this example that it is better for both players if they both don't confess, which is a solution of a cooperative game and will be discussed later.

We now introduce an important concept in game theory: Nash equilibrium. Nash equilibrium, named after John Forbes Nash, is a solution concept of a game involving two or more players in which no player can benefit by changing his strategy unilaterally. If each player has chosen a strategy and no player can benefit by changing his or her strategy while the other players keep theirs unchanged, then the current set of strategy choices and the corresponding payoffs constitute a Nash equilibrium (see Nash 1951). The Nash equilibrium is a pretty simple idea: we have a Nash equilibrium if each participant chooses the best strategy, given the strategies chosen by other participants. In the Prisoners' Dilemma, the pair of strategies {confess, confess} constitutes the equilibrium of the game.

Another well-known example is the so-called Braess's Paradox: eliminating a road, rather than building a road, will sometimes improve traffic conditions.

When 42nd Street in New York City was temporarily closed to traffic, rather than the expected gridlock resulting, traffic flowed more easily. In fact, it was reported in the September 2, 2002, edition of The New Yorker that in the 23 American cities that added the most new roads per person during the 1990s, traffic congestion rose by more than 70% (Havil 2008). Braess's Paradox was named after the German mathematician Dietrich Braess, who published a paper (Braess 1969) in which he showed that, under the appropriate conditions, building new roads to ease congestion actually makes the problem worse.

Suppose there are initially two alternative roads to E from S: $S \rightarrow A \rightarrow E$ and $S \rightarrow B \rightarrow E$. The one-way relief road $A \rightarrow B$ was added with the intention of easing congestion. The time taken on each route is shown in Fig. 2.5, where x_i is the number of vehicles on that road. Assume that each driver is completely aware of the traffic situation at all times and selfishly chooses the route that minimizes his time of driving.

Suppose there are six cars. Let's look into the process consisting of six cars with and without the relief road.

1. Without the relief road $A \rightarrow B$, there will be three cars on route $S \rightarrow A \rightarrow E$ and three cars on route $S \rightarrow B \rightarrow E$. The average driving time is $10(3) + 3 + 50 = 83$.

2. With road $A \rightarrow B$, we assume all six cars line up at the starting point (S) one by
one. Because each driver takes the shortest route available at the moment, the first
two cars will be on $S \rightarrow A \rightarrow B \rightarrow E$ with the drivers' perceived driving time
60 min, shorter than the alternative routes. The third and fourth cars will be on
$S \rightarrow A \rightarrow E$ and $S \rightarrow B \rightarrow E$, with the drivers' perceived driving time 81 min,
one on each route; the fifth and sixth cars will also be on $S \rightarrow A \rightarrow E$ and
$S \rightarrow B \rightarrow E$, with the drivers' perceived driving time 92 (minutes). However,
the drivers' perceived time is not the actual time because they didn't consider the
drivers behind them. The actual drive time should be based on the actual number
of cars on the routes: $x_1 = 4$ cars on $S \rightarrow A$, $x_2 = 2$ cars on $S \rightarrow B$, $x_3 = 2$
cars on $A \rightarrow E$, $x_4 = 4$ cars on $B \rightarrow E$, and $x_1 = 2$ cars on $A \rightarrow B$. The
driving time on route $S \rightarrow A \rightarrow E$ or $S \rightarrow B \rightarrow E$ is $10(4) + 2 + 50 = 92$.
The driving time on route $S \rightarrow A \rightarrow B \rightarrow E$ is $10(4) + 10(2) + 10(4) = 100$.
It is interesting that the first two drivers, who think they are getting the best deal
for being the first two making the choice, are actually getting the worst result, or
the longest driving time.

Braess's Paradox can be found in any network, such as water flow, computer data
transfer, electrical and electronic networks, and telephone exchanges. In 1990, the
British Telecom network suffered in such a way when its "intelligent" exchanges
reacted to blocked routes by rerouting calls along "better" paths. This in turn caused
later calls to be rerouted with a cascade effect, leading to a catastrophic change in the
network's behavior (Havil 2008). Can you identify examples of Braess's Paradox in
the pharmaceutical and health industries?

Game theory is a distinct and interdisciplinary approach to the study of human
behavior. Game theory addresses interactions using the metaphor of a game: in
these serious interactions, the individual's choice is essentially a choice of strategy,
and the outcome of the interaction depends on the strategies chosen by each of the
participants. The significance of game theory is dignified by the three Nobel Prizes
to researchers whose work is largely game theory: in 1994 to Nash, Selten, and
Harsanyi, in 2005 to Aumann and Schelling, and in 2007 to Maskin and Myerson.

Most game theories assume three conditions: common knowledge, perfect
information, and rationality. A fact is common knowledge if all players know it, and
know that they all know it, and so on. The structure of the game is often assumed to
be common knowledge among the players. A game has perfect information when at
any point in time only one player makes a move and knows all the actions that have
been made until then. A player is said to be rational if he seeks to play in a manner
that maximizes his own payoff. It is often assumed that the rationality of all players
is common knowledge. A payoff is a number, also called the utility, that reflects the
desirability of an outcome to a player, for whatever reason. When the outcome is
random, payoffs are usually weighted with their associated probabilities. Note that
the expected payoff incorporates the player's attitude toward risk.

There are games that have more than one Nash equilibrium point. The following
example contains multiple equilibria.

Table 2.3 Payoffs with
multiple equilibria

| | | Diagnosis (Player B) | |
		Go	No-Go
Biotech	Go	$(10, 5)$	$(-5, 0)$
(Player A)	No-Go	$(0, -3)$	$(0, 0)$

Example 2.6. Suppose a biotech company has identified a drug compound that is expected to effectively treat cancer patients with certain genetic markers or biomarkers. However, there is no commercial screening tool currently available to test the biomarker. Luckily, a diagnostic company has the capability to develop the screen tool. The two companies now face a Go or No-Go decision.

If the biotech company (player A) decides to develop the drug (the Go decision) and the diagnostic company (player B) also decides to develop the screen tool (the Go decision), then if both are approved by the regulatory agency, the drug can be marketed and made available to cancer patients. As a result, the gains for player A and Player B are 10 and 5, respectively. If player A chooses "Go" and player B chooses "No-Go," then the drug may be available but the biotech company doesn't have the screening tool to identify the right patients to treat. Therefore, the drug can't be marketed. In such a case, the payoffs for players A and B are -5 and 0, respectively. Player A has a negative payoff due to the development cost. If player B chooses "Go" and player A chooses "No-Go," then the biomarker patient population can be identified but no drug is available. Therefore, no one wants to buy the screening tool. The payoffs for A and B are 0 and -3, respectively. If both companies choose "No-Go," then there is a zero payoff for both of them. The payoffs are summarized in Table 2.3.

There are two Nash equilibria, at the upper left {Go,Go} and the lower right {No-Go, No-Go}. Starting from the upper left, either the column player (B) or the row player (A) will be worse off if she changes strategies unilaterally. Similarly, starting from the lower right, either of the players will be worse off if he changes strategies unilaterally. In either case, they don't want to change unilaterally. In other words, there are two Nash equilibria. However, if communication is allowed so that either of the players can learn immediately when the other player makes a move, then {Go,Go} is the only equilibrium. This is because under open communication player A or B is willing to make the first move or Go decision by knowing that the other will immediately follow her and make the same Go decision.

A Nash equilibrium is reached if neither player can be better off changing strategy unilaterally. However, even though the outcome {No-Go, No-Go} is a Nash equilibrium, it is clearly inferior to {Go, Go}.

A game in *strategic form*, also called normal form, is a compact representation of a game in which players simultaneously choose their strategies. The resulting payoffs are presented in a table with a cell for each strategy combination.

Definition 2.1. A *strategy* is a complete contingent plan for a player in the game.

A typical strategy profile is a vector of strategies $s = (s_1, \ldots s_n)$, where s_i is the strategy of player i $(i = 1, \ldots, n)$.

A two-person win-lose game can be played on a so-called graph, $G = (X, F)$, by stipulating a starting position $x_0 \in X$ and using the following rules:

1. Player 1 moves first, starting at x_0.
2. Players alternate moves.
3. At position x, the player whose turn it is to move chooses a position $y \in F(x)$.
4. The player who is confronted with a terminal position at his turn, and thus cannot move, loses.

A game is often solved efficiently using so-called backward induction. Backward induction is a technique to solve a game of perfect information. It first considers the moves that are the last in the game and determines the best move for the player in each case. Then, taking these as given future actions, it proceeds backward in time, again determining the best move for the respective player, until the beginning of the game is reached.

Among various types of games, a simple and well-studied type of game is the zero-sum game. A zero-sum game is a game in which one player's winnings are equal to the other player's losses.

We have discussed the *pure game*, where there is no probability involved regarding strategy selection. However, in reality we more often encounter mixed strategy games, where each player's strategy selection involves a probability distribution.

Definition 2.2. If a player in a game chooses among two or more strategies randomly according to specific probabilities, this choice is called a *mixed strategy*.

The game of matching pennies has a solution in mixed strategies. The game rules are: The two players involved show their pennies at the same time; if both are heads or tails, player A wins, and if one is a head and one is a tail, player B wins. In such a game, neither player wants his opponent to know what to show. In other words, they both should randomly choose heads or tails with a probability of 0.5.

We may be curious about the existence of an equilibrium in a game. The following well-known theorem by John Nash answers the question.

Theorem 2.1. *(Nash 1951). Every finite pure or mixed game with a finite number of players and a finite strategy space has at least one Nash equilibrium.*

2.2.2   Multiple-Player Game

In the prisoner's game, there are two players and each has only two options. The solution of the game can be found intuitively. However, in practice there are usually more than two options for each player. To solve such games, the following theorem is a very powerful tool.

Theorem 2.2. *(Dresher 1961, p. 43). Suppose all pure strategies for each player in a two-person zero-sum matrix game are active (i.e., no dominance or saddle point*

Fig. 2.6 Mechanism
of competition

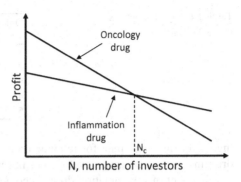

exists in the game) and the matrix of the game is square and nonsingular. Then a unique optimal mixed strategy for each player can be computed using

$$q^* = \frac{\left(A'\right)^{-1}1}{1'A^{-1}1} \ and \ p^* = \frac{A^{-1}1}{1'A^{-1}1}, \tag{2.25}$$

where $A = \{a_{ij}\}_{n\times n}$ is a nonsingular payoff matrix of the game, $1 = (1, 1, \ldots, 1)'$ is an $n \times 1$ column vector, and the column vectors q^* and p^* are the optimal mixed strategies for the players with row and column strategies in the matrix game, respectively. The value of the game to the row player using q^* is $u = 1'A^{-1}1$.

One way of phrasing this theorem is that player A searches for a strategy that makes player B indifferent as to which of the (good) pure strategies to use. Similarly, player B should play in such a way as to make player A indifferent among his (good) strategies. This is called the *Principle of Indifference*.

2.2.3 Queuing Game

Queuing theory deals with providing a service on a waiting line (queue). In a queuing game, the order of a player benefiting more is based on his order in the queue. Economic competition and highway congestion are two common examples. When the number of players, N, is larger, we traditionally simplify with some assumptions such as the *representative agent model*, in which we assume that all players are identical, have the same strategy options, and get symmetrical payoffs. We also assume that the payoff to each player depends only on the number of other players who choose each strategy and not on which agent chooses which strategy.

Example 2.7. An example of the representative agent model is shown in Fig. 2.6, where each investor has to decide whether to invest in inflammation or oncology drug development but the return on investment (ROI) is dependent on the number of investors in the product. In this hypothetical example, at the beginning the ROI is

Table 2.4 Payoff structures in a queuing game

Order served	Gross payoff	Cost of standing	Expected net payoff .
1	20	3	17
2	17	3	14
3	14	3	11
4	11	3	8
5	8	3	5

higher for oncology than for inflammation drugs. When the number of oncology drug investors increases, development becomes expensive and at the same time development of inflammation drugs becomes less expensive in comparison. Note that when more drugs become available for treating one disease, the chance of having or dying from other diseases increases.

Suppose the objective is to maximum the ROI. The equilibrium is reached at the intersection of the two profit lines in Fig. 2.6. From the figure, it is obvious that the first N_c investors will be interested in investing in oncology drugs but investors who come after will be interested in investing in inflammation drugs. This is a queuing game in which multiple players are involved and payoffs are dependent on the order of the player's engagement.

The following is another example of a queuing game.

Example 2.8. Suppose there are five customers trying to receive a service. They all want to get the service as early as possible, but at the same time they don't like to stand in line. To quantify, we make the following assumptions that apply to all five players: The gross payoffs and cost of standing depend on the order served as listed in Table 2.4. Net payoffs are the difference between the gross payoff and the cost of standing (Table 2.4).

Those who do not stand in line are chosen randomly for service, after those standing in line have been served. Therefore, the expected payoff for anyone not standing in the line is their average gross payoff. The player's decision on whether to stand in line or not is driven by the maximization of his net payoff. The game can be analyzed as follows:

1. If no one stands in line, then each person will have an equal probability of being served first, second, ..., and fifth. The expected payoff is $(20 + 17 + 14 + 11 + 8)/5 = 14$. However, such a case can be improved since an individual can improve his payoff by standing first in line. The net payoff to the person first in line is $(20 - 3) = 17 > 14$, so someone will get up and stand in line.
2. If no more persons stand in line, the expected payoff is $(17 + 14 + 11 + 8)/4 = 12.5$ for the four remaining. Since the second person in line gets a net payoff of $14 > 12.5$, someone will get up and stand in the second place in line.
3. This leaves the average payoff at 11 for the three remaining. Since the third person in line gets a net payoff of 11, there may or may not be someone standing in the third place in line. When either two or three persons stand in the line, the Nash equilibrium is reached, i.e., there are two equilibria.

4. If no one stands in the third place, the game is over; if there is a third person in line, then the remaining two have the expected payoff of 9.5 for not standing in line and 8 for standing in line. Therefore, no one wants to stand in the fourth place. The game is definitely over.

With two or three people standing in the line, a Nash equilibrium is reached. The total net payoff for queuing is $17 + 14 + 11 + 9.5 + 9.5 = 61$, which is less than 70 for not queuing at all. We call such a case inefficient queuing. To prevent this from happening, the authority (e.g., an airline) can simply ignore the queue and, let's say, pass out lots for order of service at the time of each customer's arrival, and no standing in line will be necessary.

2.2.4 Cooperative Games

Games in which the participants cannot make commitments to coordinate their strategies are *noncooperative games*. In a noncooperative game, the rational person's problem is to answer the question "What is the rational choice of strategy when other players will try to choose their best responses to my strategy?" In contrast, games in which the participants can make commitments to coordinate their strategies are *cooperative games*.

In noncooperative games, the solution from an individual perspective often leads to inferior outcomes, as in the Prisoners' Dilemma. It is preferable, in many cases, to define a criterion to rank outcomes for the group of players as a whole. The Pareto criterion is one of this kind: an outcome is better than another if at least one person is better off and no one is worse off. If an outcome cannot be improved upon (i.e., if no one can be made better off without making somebody else worse off), then we say that the outcome is *Pareto optimal*. A Pareto optimization for the drug price, if it exists, would be the price value such that any change to this price will either make the pharmaceutical company less profitable or provide less benefit to patients.

Example 2.9. Suppose two companies are in a position to decide whether to develop competitive drugs for anemia – a decrease in the normal number of red blood cells (RBCs) or less than the normal quantity of hemoglobin in the blood. Since hemoglobin (found inside RBCs) normally carries oxygen from the lungs to the tissues, anemia's leading symptoms are nonspecific symptoms: a feeling of weakness or fatigue, general malaise and sometimes poor concentration.

The cost (including opportunity loss) for developing such a drug is presumably C_a for company A and C_b for company B. The probability of success of such an indication for marketing is denoted by p; if the drug gets regulatory approval, gross profit for the successful company is dependent on the success of the other company for the same indication. Assume that the total profit for the two companies is fixed and equals G billion dollars if at least one is successful in developing the drug; if both companies are successful in developing drugs for anemia, they get $G/2$

Table 2.5 Expected net profits

		Company B	
		Go	No-Go
Company A	Go	$(0, 0)$	$(0.5, 0)$
	No-Go	$(0, 0.5)$	$(0, 0)$

Note: $G = \$10B$, $C_a = C_b = 0.5$, $p = 0.1$

billion dollars each. If both companies make the Go decision (develop the drug), the expected net profits will be $pG/2 - C_a$ and $pG/2 - C_b$ for companies A and B, respectively. If only one company, say company A, made the Go decision and company B made the No-Go decision, the net profit for company A is $pG - C_a$ and that for company B is zero. Similarly, we can calculate the net profits for the two other scenarios as summarized in Table 2.5.

{Go, Go} is a Nash equilibrium (can you explain why?) with an expected net profit of $0 for each company. Remember that the values for the parameters in this example more or less reflect the realities in the pharmaceutical industry.

Other than by internal development, a firm can acquire necessary resources through partnerships with other stakeholders in the pharmaceutical industry such as pharmas, biotechs, CROs, academicians, policy-makers, and government. Common forms of partnerships include (1) spot market exchanges, (2) contractual agreements and alliances, and (3) mergers and acquisitions.

In Example 2.9, companies A and B can make a joint venture to develop the two drug candidates sequentially; i.e., if one fails, then the second will be invested in the clinical trials. This will reduce the risk and increase the success of development.

2.2.5 Sequential Game

2.2.5.1 Compulsory Licensing and Parallel Importation

Compulsory licenses are licenses that are granted by a government to regulate the use of patents, copyrighted works, and other types of intellectual property. Compulsory licenses are an essential government instrument to intervene in the market and limit patent and other intellectual property rights, in order to correct market failures. As concerns public health and compulsory licensing, the restrictions imposed by the intellectual property rights (IPRs) system on access to (patented) drugs must be reasonable, not creating situations where entire populations are denied access to known therapies. Therefore, the 1994 WTO TRIPs agreement contains provisions on safeguards, exceptions, and mechanisms to protect essential public health interests. The TRIP provides for compulsory licenses of patents but also provides a number of restrictions on the use of compulsory licenses.

The propriety of parallel trade is a matter of intense policy debate in a number of countries and in the World Trade Organization (WTO). Presently, WTO provisions allow member countries to establish their own rules for the "exhaustion" of intellectual property rights (IPRs). If a country opts for national exhaustion of IPRs, a rights holder there may exclude parallel imports because intellectual property rights continue until such time as a protected product is first sold in that market. If a country instead chooses international exhaustion of IPR, parallel imports cannot be blocked because the rights of the patent, copyright, or trademark holder expire when a protected product is sold anywhere in the world. The United States practices national exhaustion for patents and copyrights, but permits parallel imports of trademarked goods except when the trademark owner can show that the imports are of different quality from goods sold locally or otherwise might cause confusion for consumers. The European Union provides for regional exhaustion of IPR, whereby goods circulate freely within the trading bloc but parallel imports from nonmember countries are banned. Japanese commercial law permits parallel imports except when such trade is explicitly excluded by contract provisions or when the original sale is made subject to foreign price controls (Grossman and Lai 2008).

When parallel trade comes into play, the regulated price cap becomes a strategic variable in an international setting. Parallel trade is an arbitrage mechanism through which the drugs produced in a low-price market flow into a high-price market, reestablishing nearly uniform prices in the presence of a large number of parallel traders. The price difference mainly results from the transportation and transaction costs for the reimportation.

Opponents of parallel trade are concerned that such trade undermines manufacturers' intellectual property rights. The prevailing wisdom, expressed for example by Barfield and Groombridge (1998), Chard and Mellor (1989), and Danzon and Towse (2003), is that parallel trade impedes the ability of research-intensive firms such as those in the pharmaceutical industry to reap an adequate return on their investments in new technologies. Grossman and Lai (2008) challenge the prevailing wisdom that parallel trade is induced by different national price controls. They argue that the existing policy discussions and formal modeling overlook an important effect of national policy regarding the exhaustion of IPRs. First, the admissibility of parallel trade introduces the possibility that a manufacturer will eschew low-price sales in the foreign market in order to mitigate or avoid reimportation. When arbitrage is impossible, the manufacturer is willing to export at any price above the marginal production cost. But when the potential for arbitrage exists, the manufacturer may earn higher profits by selling only in the unregulated (or high-price) market than by serving both markets at the lower, foreign-controlled price. Accordingly, a switch from a regime of national exhaustion to one of international exhaustion can induce an increase in the controlled price as the foreign government seeks to ensure that its consumers are adequately served. Second, the admissibility of parallel trade mitigates the opportunity for one government to free-ride on the protection of IPRs granted by another.

Example 2.10. In this example, we will discuss how to model drug marketing using a sequential game. Suppose a sequential game consists of three stages specified as follows, where we use North and South to represent two countries with and without an intellectual property, respectively.

Fig. 2.7 Extensive form
of drug marketing game

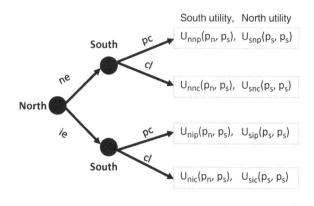

Stage 1: North decides to go for national exhaustion (ne) or international exhaustion (ie).

Stage 2: South decides to exercise a price control (pc), i.e., set up a price cap p_c or a compulsory license (cl).

Stage 3: North decides the price for North and South, p_n and p_s.

The extensive form of the sequential game is shown in Fig. 2.7.

A *non-cooperative solution* is the solution to the game when the players take actions to maximize each individual gain. Let $U_{nij}(\cdot, \cdot)$ be North's utility when North takes strategy i and South takes strategy j; let $U_{sij}(\cdot, \cdot)$ be South's utility when North takes strategy i and South takes strategy j, as illustrated in Fig. 2.7.

Using backward induction, South will take the action A_{sk} (price control or compulsory license) to maximize its utility U_{sk} such that $U_{sk} = \max(U_{skp}(p_n, p_s), U_{skc}(p_s, p_s))$, where $k = n$ for national exhaustion or $k = i$ for international exhaustion. After knowing South will take action A_{sk}, North will take action A_{nk} to maximize its utility.

If $\max U_{nnp}(p_n, p_s) > \max U_{nnc}(p_n, p_s) > \max U_{nip}(p_n, p_s) > \max U_{nic}(p_n, p_s)$, $\max U_{snp}(p_n, p_s) < \max U_{snc}(p_n, p_s)$, and $\max U_{sip}(p_n, p_s) > \max U_{sic}(p_n, p_s)$, then South will decide to exercise the compulsory license if North opts for national exhaustion of IPRs. On the other hand, South will exercise price control if North opts for international exhaustion, which implies North either has utility $\max U_{nnc}(p_n, p_s)$ under national exhaustion or $\max U_{nip}(p_n, p_s)$ under international exhaustion. Knowing this fact and that $\max U_{nnc}(p_n, p_s) > \max U_{nip}(p_n, p_s)$, North will exercise national exhaustion.

The noncooperative solution can often be improved. We use an example to illustrate how to find a Pareto optimum for the cooperative game in Fig. 2.5. Suppose $\max U_{nip}(p_n, p_s) = 10 > \max U_{nnp}(p_n, p_s) = 8 > \max U_{nnc}(p_n, p_s) = 5 > \max U_{nic}(p_n, p_s) = 1$ and $\max U_{snp}(p_n, p_s) = 2 < \max U_{snc}(p_n, p_s) = 3 < \max U_{sip}(p_n, p_s) = 7 < \max U_{sic}(p_n, p_s) = 10$. In such a case, South will exercise the compulsory license regardless of North's action (national or international exhaustion), which implies North either has utility $\max U_{nnc}(p_n, p_s) = 4$ under national exhaustion or $\max U_{nic}(p_n, p_s) = 1$ under international exhaustion. It is obvious that North will exercise national exhaustion with a utility of 5 and South will have a utility of 3. However, the result can be improved through an agreement that North will use international exhaustion and South will use the price control. This is the only Pareto optimum for the game, which gives North 10 and South 7 for the utility.

2.3 Implementation Challenges

The most fundamental step in pharmaceutical decision-making and game modeling is to quantify a utility function based on the objective and to understand the process of the problem to be modeled. For different objectives, the assumptions made about the process are different because an assumption may be quite suitable for one purpose but not suitable at all for another. Model building is an abstract thinking process in which the model builder tries to capture the most important factors and simplify or convert the problem into a decision or game model. The selection of factors to be included in the model is a dimension-reduction process using knowledge beyond statistics, which is different from and not replaceable by statistical modeling approaches such as stepwise elimination in a linear regression. Pharmaceutical decision modeling here is beyond traditional modeling. It is large-scale, cross-discipline modeling directed by decision and game theory.

Decision modeling requires strong collaborations among people from different disciplines, in which the statistician plays the critical role of the "project coordinator." He or she has to know what information is needed, and where and how to acquire it. Furthermore, the statistician should have a good sense about the precision or variability of the information. For example, to determine the utility of developing a drug, we have to determine the value proposition and project the short-term and long-term market values, which can usually be obtained by working with the commercial/marketing group of the company. The statistician may be asked to design clinical development programs, which involve multiple phases in clinical trials.

The success of decision-process modeling will also include the campaign of the proposed model, which requires diverse skills, including presentation and interpersonal skills. Such soft skills are critical but unfortunately often neglected by statisticians. Statistics alone can, in this case, only make things look good on paper. Note that the campaign for the project is itself a game.

The utility in the Markov decision process will direct the choice of the optimal design. Years ago, a colleague of mine told me that he had tried different pharmaceutical decision models in a certain clinical trial but the maximization of utility always led to an infinitely large sample size or a Go decision. I suspect that the reason behind this is an overly optimistic model. This overly optimistic attitude is a general trend in the pharmaceutical industry. I am going to elaborate upon this and discuss how pharmaceutical decision modeling can be made realistic and successful.

A study (Pearlman, 2007) shows that big pharma has consistently been the single most profitable industry of all 47 represented in the Fortune 500. However, this kind of comparison may not be very informative, as we know that investment in pharmaceutical R & D has a high risk. The success rate in the pharmaceutical industry is very low: there are many failures and bankruptcies; only a small proportion of the NMEs can make it all the way to market. The profitability for successful big pharma is naturally higher. Just like playing lotteries, if the profitability is calculated based only on the winners, it will be much higher than that for the real-life pharmaceutical industry. However, the expected profit of playing any lottery game is negative. Because "the winner talks all," we often overestimate the value of a new drug. This optimism may sometimes be used as a strategy of a team to get the financial support they need. Not only is the drug's value over-projected, but also the probability of success (I will provide an example soon). Optimism adversely inflates the probability of moving the project forward but eventually fails with high costs.

The most obvious example, but surprisingly not well recognized, concerns the power calculation in clinical trial designs. We know that the phase III trial approval rate has been about 40% in the past 10 years, including the reason of failing to demonstrate efficacy. However, phase III trials are commonly designed at approximately a 90% power, which means that about 90% (81% if two independent trials are required) will demonstrate statistical significance. Why is there such a big difference, 90 versus 40%? There are several reasons: (1) overestimating the treatment effect or using the minimal clinical difference inappropriately to calculate the power, (2) underestimating the variance, and (3) the commonly used methods for power calculation do not consider variability of the treatment effect (see Chap. 10).

The Markov decision processes we have discussed so far have known transition probabilities, so that calculation can be carried out. What if the probability is unknown, or is too complicated and becomes intractable? In our previous examples of clinical development, both the transition probabilities and the expected overall gain are heavily dependent on the toxicity rate p_0 and the treatment effect δ, two unknown parameters. If the assumptions about the two parameters change, the overall expected gain will change. In other words, the optimal action rules will depend on the assumptions around the parameters. To solve this dilemma, several methods are proposed, including Q-learning and the one-step-forward approach.

Q-Learning (Gosavi 2003) is a form of model-free reinforcement learning. It is a forward induction and an asynchronous dynamic programming. The power of reinforcement learning lies in its ability to solve the Markov decision process without computing the transition probabilities that are needed in value and policy iteration.

One of the popular approaches in robotics is to let the agent randomly choose an action with the selection probability proportional to the potential gain from each action. The idea behind this approach is to modify the randomization probability gradually in such a way that when our initial judgment about expected gains is wrong, the action will be corrected over time. This has motivated the one-step-forward approach, which has the transition probability

$$ p_{ij} = \frac{g_j}{\sum_k g_k}, $$

where the summation is performed over all nodes that can be reached by one step forward from node i. We will use this concept in designing adaptive trials, i.e., the response-randomization trials in Chap. 4.

However, both the Q-learning and one-step-forward approaches are effective only when the same experiments can be repeated many times, which does not happen for any single drug candidate.

Most game theories are developed under the assumption of common knowledge. However, such an assumption generally does not hold because each pharmaceutical company is very protective of its intellectual properties. In such a scenario, the complexity of the game increases, and we have to distinguish between what our opponent actually knows and what we think they know.

In collaborative games, many details about partnerships between the two or multiple players cannot be specified in the contract; the actions and associated consequences have great uncertainties. Therefore, probability theory, including Bayesian approaches (Chap. 10), plays an important role here. Pharmaceutical decision and game modeling often require simulation for support (see Chap. 9).

2.4 Exercises

2.1. Braess illustrated his paradox using an example in Fig. 2.5, but the time taken on the relief road $A \rightarrow B$ was $10 + x_5$ instead of $10x_5$. Solve this game (Braess Paradox). If there are generally a total of n cars, solve the game. Hint: At Nash equilibrium, the times taken on each road of the three routes ($S \rightarrow A \rightarrow E$, $S \rightarrow A \rightarrow B \rightarrow E$, and $S \rightarrow B \rightarrow E$) will be the same; furthermore, $x_1 = x_3 + x_5$ and $x_2 + x_5 = x_4$.

2.2. Table 2.6 represents the actual success rates of different phases of clinical trials. Success is defined as the launch of the next phase, with the exception of phase III. Success for a phase III trial means NDA approval. Please discuss how to use this prior to your clinical development program (CDP) modeling using the stochastic decision process.

2.3. Explain the terms: game, strategy, player, zero-sum game, mixed strategy game, matrix game, queuing game, cooperative and non-cooperative games, equilibrium in a game, Nash equilibrium, Pareto optimum, and strategic and extensive forms.

Table 2.6 Success rates of various phases of trials

	Year					
	1990	1992	1994	1996	1998	2000
Preclinical	0.24	0.24	0.19	0.21	0.18	0.21
Phase I	0.55	0.60	0.52	0.55	0.55	0.50
Phase II	0.47	0.44	0.42	0.47	0.39	0.28
Phase III	0.78	0.79	0.73	0.60	0.65	0.43

Source: Chang (2010)

2.4. Find the Pareto optimal solution set for the following cooperative game (McCain, 2009).

Suppose that Joey has a bicycle. Joey would rather have a game machine than a bicycle, and he could buy a game machine for $80 but doesn't have any money. We express this by saying that Joey values his bicycle at $80. Mikey has $100 and no bicycle, and would rather have a bicycle than anything else he can buy for $100. We express this by saying that Mikey values a bicycle at $100. Analyze the game, construct a 2 × 2 payoff table, and solve the game. You can make assumptions as necessary.

2.5. Elaborate how Bellman's backward induction algorithm can improve the efficiency of simulations in the CDP.

2.6. Discuss different forms of alliances, their advantages, and their disadvantages.

2.7. Elaborate on the three common assumptions in game theory, and discuss the fitness of those assumptions in situations of interest.

2.8. For the two-player pharmaceutical game (Table 2.3), discuss the following cooperative game: The two companies make strategic alliances in which they agree to jointly develop a drug for an indication using one of the NMEs. If it is successful, the second NME will not be studied; if it fails, they will bring the second one to the development pipeline.

Further Readings and References

Barfield, C.E., Groombridge, M.A.: The economic case for copyright and owner control over parallel imports. J. World Intellect. Prop. **1**, 903–939 (1998)

Bellman, R.: A Markovian decision process. J. Math. Mech. **6**, 23–35 (1957a)

Bellman, R.: Dynamic Programming. Princeton University Press, Princeton (1957b)

Berger, J.: Statistical Decision Theory and Bayesian Analysis. Springer, New York (1985)

Bernard, S.: The drug drought, Pharmaceutical Executive, November 1 (2002). www.design-and-determination.com. Accessed 15 June 2010

Bertsekas, D.: Dynamic Programming and Optimal Control, vol. 2. Athena, Belmont (1995)

Braess, D.: Über ein Paradoxon aus der Verkehrsplanung. Unternehmensforschung **12**, 258–268 (1969)

Cambridge Pharma Consultancy: Pricing and Reimbursement Review 2003. IMS Health-Management Consulting, Cambridge (2004)

Chang, M.: Biomarker development. In: Statistics for Translational Medicine. Taylor and Francis, New York (2008)

Chang, M., Chow, S.C.: Power and sample size for dose response studies. In: Ting, N. (ed.) Dose Finding in Drug Development. Springer, New York (2006)

Chang, M.: Monte Carlo Simulation for the Pharmaceutical Industry. Chapman and Hall/CRC, Boca Raton (2010)

Chard, J.S., Mellor, C.J.: Intellectual property rights and parallel imports. World Econ. **12**, 69–83 (1989)

Danzon, P., Towse, A.: Differential pricing for pharmaceuticals: Reconciling access, R&D and patents. Int. J. Health Care Finance Econ. **3**, 183–205 (2003)

Gosavi, A.: Simulation-based Optimization: Parametric Optimization Techniques and Reinforcement Learning. Springer, Boston (2003)

Dresher, M.: Games of Strategy. Prentice-Hall, Englewood Cliffs (1961)

Grossman, G., Lai, E.: Parallel imports and price controls. RAND J Econ. **39**(2), 378–402 (2008)

Havil, J.: Impossible? Surprising Solutions to Counterintuitive Conundrums. Princeton University Press, Priceton (2008)

Hu, M., Schultz, K., Sheu, J., Tschopp, D.: The Innovation Gap in Pharmaceutical Drug Discovery & New Models for R&D Success. www.kellogg.northwestern.edu/academic/biotech/faculty/articles/NewRDModel.pdf (2007). Accessed 2 Mar 2009

McCain, R.: Strategy and Conflict: An Introductory Sketch of Game Theory. http://william-king.www.drexel.edu (2009). Accessed 20 June 2009

Nash, J.: Non-coorperative games. Ann. Math. **5**, 286–295 (1951)

Parmigiani, G., Inoue, L.: Decision Theory: Principles and Approaches. Wiley, Hokoken (2009)

Pearlman, J.B.: The commercialization of medicine. http://www.google.com (2007). Accessed 10 Sep 2009

Powell, W.B.: Approximate Dynamic Programming: Solving the Curses of Dimensionality. Wiley-Interscience, New York (2007)

Watson, J.: Strategy. W.W. Norton and Company, New York (2008)

Chapter 3
Noninferiority Trial Design

3.1 Concept of Noninferiority Trial

3.1.1 Needs for Noninferiority Design

Superiority and noninferiority (NI) trials are two common types of clinical trials. Superiority means, in layman's language, that the test drug is better than the comparative drug (active comparator or active-control), whereas noninferiority suggests that the test drug may not be as good as the comparative drug, but the difference is not clinically significant. If a test drug is noninferior to an active-control, it must be at least superior to a placebo (Fig. 3.1).

Statistically, the hypothesis tests for superiority and noninferiority are expressed, respectively, as

$$H_o : \theta_T - \theta_C \leq 0 \text{ versus } H_a : \bar{H}_o$$

and

$$H_o : \theta_T - \theta_C \leq -\delta_{NI} \text{ versus } H_a : \bar{H}_o,$$

where θ_T and θ_C are treatment effects for the test and control groups, respectively. Here the so-called noninferiority margin δ_{NI} is usually defined based on clinical and statistical considerations (see details later in this chapter).

As the European regulatory agency, Committee for Medicinal Products for Human Use (CHMP 2005) stated, "Many clinical trials comparing a test product with an active comparator are designed as noninferiority trials. The term 'noninferiority' is now well established, but if taken literally could be misleading. The objective of a noninferiority trial is sometimes stated as being to demonstrate that the test product is not inferior to the comparator. However, only a superiority trial can demonstrate this. In fact a noninferiority trial aims to demonstrate that the test product is not worse than the comparator by more than a pre-specified, small amount. This amount is known as the noninferiority margin, or delta."

Until recent years, the majority of clinical trials were designed for superiority to a comparative drug (the control group). A statistic shows that only 23% of all NDAs

M. Chang, *Modern Issues and Methods in Biostatistics*, Statistics for Biology and Health, DOI 10.1007/978-1-4419-9842-2_3, © Springer Science+Business Media, LLC 2011

Fig. 3.1 Superiority versus noninferiority

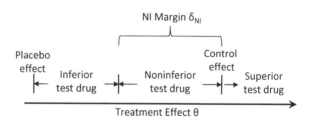

from 1998 to 2002 were innovative drugs, and the rest were accounted for as "me-too" drugs (Chang, 2010). Those me-too drugs are based on noninferiority criteria. The increasing popularity of noninferiority trials is a reflection of the regulatory and industry adjustments in response to the increasing challenges in drug development.

The emerging trend of more noninferiority trials than superiority trials can be attributed to the following causes:

1. When many efficacious treatments are available, the use of placebo-control trials for the evaluation of new medical treatments in clinical trials is ethically problematic.
2. Test and control drugs are expected to have a similar magnitude of efficacy, but they may have different mechanics of action and hence will work for different (at least partially) populations.
3. A new test drug may be safer, cheaper, more convenient or easy to administrate, or have a better taste, different interactions with other drugs, or other kinds of benefits to patients.
4. There is growing interest among third-party payers and some regulatory authorities, on both cost-effectiveness and medical grounds, in the comparative effectiveness of treatments.
5. The "low-hanging fruits" in drug development are much less available than in prior years. When we continue to make more effective and/or safer drugs, the chance of finding a compound better than the "best" in the market is smaller and the efforts required to find such a compound are bigger.
6. There are great attractions to develop generic drugs after patent expiration of innovative drugs.

CHMP (2005) pointed out the situations in which NI trials may be used, which include:

1. Applications based upon essential similarity in areas where bioequivalence studies are not possible, e.g., modified release products or topical preparations;
2. Products with a potential safety advantage over the standard might require an efficacy comparison to the standard to allow a risk-benefit assessment to be made;
3. Cases where a direct comparison against the active comparator is needed to help assess risk/benefit;
4. Cases where no important loss of efficacy compared to the active comparator would be acceptable;
5. Disease areas where the use of a placebo arm is not possible and an active-control trial is used to demonstrate the efficacy of the test product.

However, there are concerns and challenges in design, conduct, and analysis and interpretation of a noninferiority trial, such as active-control selection, the noninferiority margin determination, and inclusion of a placebo arm. We will discuss these issues in later sections.

3.1.2 Noninferiority Lingo

1. *Noninferiority margin:* The noninferiority active-control trial should demonstrate that the new treatment T is within the noninferiority margin δ_{NI} of the active-control C. This margin should have clinical relevance. The determination of the NI margin is a major challenge in designing an NI trial.
2. *Assay sensitivity:* Assay sensitivity, a property of a clinical trial, refers to the ability of the trial to distinguish effective drugs from ineffective ones. Assay sensitivity depends on the effect size one needs to detect. A trial may have assay sensitivity for an effect of ten but not an effect of five. One therefore needs to know the effect of the control drug (Temple 2002). Assay sensitivity is the assurance that the active-control would have been superior to a placebo if a placebo had been employed in the noninferiority trial. Establishing assay sensitivity is a basic requirement in an NI trial, which is usually accomplished using an adequate NI margin that is based on past placebo-control trials.
3. *Constancy:* The constancy assumption means that the historical difference between the active-control and placebo is assumed to hold in the setting of the new trial if a placebo control was used. The populations in the historical trial and the current NI trial are similar (D'Agostino et al. 2003).
4. *Putative placebo:* The term "putative placebo" is often used in a situation where no placebo has actually been used. Since an NI trial often does not include a placebo group, to establish the assay sensitivity it is then necessary to use C versus T data in conjunction with C versus P, the historical placebo-controlled trial data, to demonstrate that T is superior to P. This process is called the putative placebo comparison.
5. *Biocreep:* Biocreep refers to the phenomenon that can occur when a slightly inferior treatment becomes the active-control for the next generation of noninferiority trials, and so on. Eventually the active controls become no better than a placebo.
6. Noninferiority design methods include the fixed-effect method, λ-method, synthesis method, NI95-H95 method, and others.

3.1.3 Noninferiority Design Methods

There are three major sources of uncertainty about the conclusions from an NI study: (1) the uncertainty of the active-control effect over a placebo, which is estimated from historical data, (2) the control effect may change over time, violating the "constancy assumption," and (3) that the risk of making a wrong decision from the test of the noninferiority hypothesis in the NI study, i.e., the type-I error. These three uncertainties have to be considered in developing a noninferiority design method.

Most commonly used noninferiority trials are based on parallel, two-group designs. Three-group designs with a placebo may sometimes be used, but they are not very cost-effective and often face ethical challenges by including a placebo group, especially in the United States.

We now discuss five commonly used hypothesis-testing methods for noninferiority trials: the fixed-margin method, the λ-portion method, and three synthesis methods (one in original scale and two in log scale). In the rest of the chapter, we will denote the test and the active-control groups by subscripts T and C, respectively. Where there is no confusion, T will also be used for test statistics. We will use the hat "^" to represent an estimate of the corresponding parameter, e.g., $\hat{\theta}$ is an estimate of θ.

3.1.3.1 Fixed-Margin Method

The null hypothesis for the fixed-margin method is given by

$$H_o : \theta_T - \theta_C + \delta_{NI} \leq 0, \tag{3.1}$$

where θ can be the mean, hazard rate, adverse event rate, recurrent events rate, or the mean number of events. The constant noninferiority margin $\delta_{NI} \geq 0$ is usually determined based on a historical placebo-control study (see more discussions later). When $\lambda_{NI} = 0$, (3.1) becomes a null hypothesis test for superiority.

The rejection of (3.1) can be interpreted in layman's terms: The test drug T is not inferior to C by δ_{NI} or more.

3.1.3.2 λ-Portion Method

The null hypothesis for the λ-portion method is given by

$$H_o : \theta_T - \lambda_{NI}\theta_C \leq 0, \tag{3.2}$$

where $0 < \lambda_{NI} < 1$. For the superiority test, $\lambda_{NI} = 1$.

The rejection of (3.2) can be interpreted in layman's terms: Drug T is at least $100\lambda_{NI}\%$ as effective as drug C.

3.1.3.3 Synthesis Method

The null hypothesis for the synthesis method is given by

$$H_o : \frac{\theta_T - \theta_P}{\theta_C - \theta_P} - \lambda_{NI} \leq 0. \tag{3.3}$$

Assuming we have proved $\theta_C - \theta_P > 0$, (3.3) is then equivalent to

$$H_o : \theta_T - \theta_C + (1 - \lambda_{NI})(\theta_C - \theta_P) \leq 0, \tag{3.4}$$

where $0 < \lambda_{NI} < 1$. For the superiority test, $\lambda_{NI} = 1$.

The rejection of (3.3) can be interpreted in layman's terms: The test drug T is at least $100\lambda_{NI}\%$ as effective as C after subtracting the placebo effect. When $\lambda_{NI} = 0$, (3.3) represents a null hypothesis for a putative placebo-control trial.

3.1.3.4 Synthesis Method in Log Form

Drug effect is often measured by the hazard ratio (relative risk) or odds ratio, i.e., $\frac{\theta_T}{\theta_C}$ and $\frac{\theta_C}{\theta_P}$. These ratios are often expressed in log scale, so that their distributions are close to normal distributions. In such cases, we can use the NI null hypothesis

$$H_o : \frac{\theta_T/\theta_C}{\theta_C/\theta_P} - \lambda_{NI} \leq 0, \tag{3.5}$$

where $0 < \lambda_{NI} < 1$ if a larger value of θ_i indicates a better result and $\lambda_{NI} > 1$ if a smaller θ_i indicates a better result.

Taking the logarithm, (3.5) becomes

$$H_o : \ln\left(\frac{\theta_T}{\theta_C}\right) - \ln\left(\frac{\theta_C}{\theta_P}\right) - \lambda_{NI}^* \leq 0, \tag{3.6}$$

where $\lambda_{NI}^* = \ln \lambda_{NI}$. Thus $\lambda_{NI}^* < 0$ if a larger value of θ_i indicates a better result and $\lambda_{NI}^* > 0$ if a smaller θ_i indicates a better result.

The rejection of (3.5) can be interpreted in layman's terms: The incremental effect of test drug T over the active-control is at least $100\lambda_{NI}\%$ of the effect $\left(\frac{\theta_C}{\theta_P}\right)$ of the active versus placebo. Note that θ_T/θ_C is addressed in the current NI trial, whereas θ_C/θ_P is addressed in the historical trial.

3.1.3.5 Synthesis Method for Time-to-Event Endpoint

Rothmann et al. (2003) proposed the noninferiority test method for the time-to-event analysis with the null hypothesis being

$$H_o : \ln\frac{\theta_T}{\theta_C} + \lambda_{NI}^* \ln\frac{\theta_C}{\theta_P} \leq 0, \tag{3.7}$$

where $0 < \lambda_{NI}^* \ll 1$ if a smaller θ_i indicates a better result and $\lambda_{NI}^* < 0$ if a larger θ_i indicates a better result. Hypothesis (3.7) can also be used for a hazard ratio test for a binary (not time-to-event) endpoint. The advantage of (3.7) is small variance and higher power in comparison with (3.6), but interpretation is not intuitive.

We can rewrite the hypothesis tests (3.1)–(3.7) above in a general form,

$$H_o : L\left(\hbar\left(\boldsymbol{\theta}\right)\right) \leq 0 \text{ versus } H_a : \bar{H}_o, \tag{3.8}$$

where $\bar{H}_o$ is the negation of H_o, $L(\cdot)$ is a linear function, function $\hbar(\cdot)$ can be, for example, the natural logarithm function, and vector $\boldsymbol{\theta}$ can be, for example, means, proportions, or hazard rates.

For hypothesis (3.8), we can define the test statistic as

$$T = \frac{L\left(\hbar\left(\hat{\boldsymbol{\theta}}\right)\right)}{v}, \tag{3.9}$$

where $\hat{\boldsymbol{\theta}}$ can be an estimate of $\boldsymbol{\theta}$ with variance

$$v^2 = \text{var}\left(L\left(\hbar(\hat{\boldsymbol{\theta}})\right)\right). \tag{3.10}$$

The asymptotic distribution of the test statistic T given by (3.9) usually has a normal distribution,

$$T \sim N\left(\frac{\varepsilon}{v}, 1\right), \tag{3.11}$$

where $\varepsilon = L\left(\hbar(\boldsymbol{\theta})\right) = E\left(L\left(\hbar(\hat{\boldsymbol{\theta}})\right)\right)$.

Under the null hypothesis boundary $\varepsilon = 0$, the test statistic has the standard normal distribution $T \sim N(0, 1)$. Therefore, the power can be expressed as

$$1 - \beta = \Phi\left(\frac{\varepsilon}{v} - z_{1-\alpha}\right), \tag{3.12}$$

where β is the type-II error rate, $\Phi(\cdot)$ is the standard normal c.d.f., and $z_{1-\alpha} = \Phi^{-1}(1-\alpha)$.

Solving (3.12) for $1/v$, we have

$$\frac{1}{v} = \frac{(z_{1-a} + z_{1-\beta})}{\varepsilon}. \tag{3.13}$$

Where, under a large-sample assumption, v can usually be expressed as $v = \frac{\sigma}{\sqrt{n}}$, where σ is independent of the total sample size n. Therefore, the sample size can be obtained from (3.13),

$$n = \frac{(z_{1-a} + z_{1-\beta})^2 \sigma^2}{\varepsilon^2}, \tag{3.14}$$

where the "equivalent variance," σ^2, will be discussed later for each particular case.

Remark. The rejection of the null hypothesis $H_o : \theta \leq 0$ implies concluding the general condition $\theta > 0$ (the negation of H_o) but not concluding any particular value of $\theta = \varepsilon$ even if we have written the alternative hypothesis as $H_a : \theta = \varepsilon$. Therefore, in this chapter, we always use the negation of H_o as the alternative hypothesis in hypothesis-testing. However we have to assume a particular value for $\theta = \varepsilon$ for the purpose of power or sample size calculation.

3.1.4 Analysis of Noninferiority Trials

In superiority trials, the intent-to-treat (ITT) population is the primary analysis population because of the ITT principle and is also a conservative approach. However, for the NI trial, both ITT and per protocol analyses are equally important, according to CPMP (2000), partially because ITT analysis does not necessarily provide conservative results.

P-values for the NI hypothesis-test and confidence interval are usually presented. The two methods are equivalent in terms of making the positive or negative claim about the test drug. The confidence interval consists of all the possible values of the parameter (e.g., $\theta_T - \theta_C$, θ_T/θ_C, etc.) that will not lead to the rejection of the null hypothesis. Theorem 3.1 and its converse, Proposition 3.1, assert the equivalence. In practice, the confidence interval (CI) method is used more often because it is a common view that it is more informative than the p-value. In fact, CHMP (2005) suggests applicants provide CIs both for each treatment group separately, and for the difference between the groups.

Theorem 3.1. *(Shao, 2003, p. 477) For each $\theta_0 \in \Theta$ (parameter space), let T_{θ_0} be a test for $H_o : \theta - \theta_0 = 0$ versus $H_a : \bar{H}$ with significance level α and acceptance region $A(\theta_0)$. For each x in the range of X, define*

$$C(x) = \{\theta : x \in A(\theta)\}.$$

Then $C(x)$ is a level $1 - \alpha$ confidence set for θ.

Proof. Under the given condition,

$$\sup_{\theta=\theta_0} P(X \notin A(\theta_0)) = \sup_{\theta=\theta_0} P(T_{\theta_0} = 1) \leq \alpha$$

is the same as

$$1 - \alpha \leq \inf_{\theta=\theta_0} P(X \in A(\theta_0)) = \inf_{\theta=\theta_0} P(\theta_0 \in C(X)).$$

Since this holds for all θ_0, the result follows from

$$\inf_{P \in \wp} P(X \in C(X)) = \inf_{\theta_0 \in \Theta} \inf_{\theta=\theta_0} P(\theta_0 \in C(X)) \geq 1 - \alpha.$$

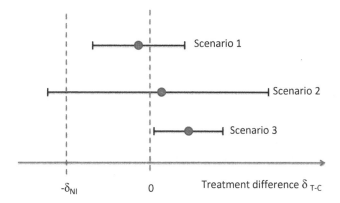

Fig. 3.2 Determination of superiority and noninferiority with CI

The converse of Theorem 3.1 is the following proposition.

Proposition 3.1. *Let $C(X)$ be a confidence set for θ with significance level $1 - \alpha$. For any $\theta_0 \in \Theta$, define a region $A(\theta_0) = \{x : \theta_0 \in C(x)\}$. Then the test $T(X) = 1 - I_{A(\theta_0)}(X)$ has a significance level α for testing $H_o : \theta = \theta_0$ versus $\bar{H}_a$.*

However, the equivalence between the CI method and hypothesis-testing may not hold for sequential or multiple-testing; e.g., in a multiple-endpoint NI trial. In such a case, we may use the methods discussed in Chap. 1.

We have illustrated the concepts of noninferiority and superiority in terms of the true treatment effect (parameter). However, because the true effect can't be known exactly, the confidence method is illustrated in Fig. 3.2. In scenario 1, the lower 95% confidence bound is larger than the NI margin $(-\delta_{NI})$, indicating the test drug is effective (NI demonstrated). In scenario 2, the point estimate favors the test drug but the lower 95% confidence bound is smaller than the NI margin $(-\delta_{NI})$, indicating unacceptable loss of the control effect (assume a larger treatment difference is better). In scenario 3, the test drug is superior to the active-control because the lower 95% confidence bound is larger than 0.

3.2   Two-Arm Design

3.2.1   Fixed-Margin Method

Based on the fixed-margin method, a hypothesis test for a noninferiority test for two independent parallel-group designs can be specified as

$$H_o : \theta_T - \theta_C + \delta_{NI} \leq 0 \text{ versus } H_a : \bar{H}_o. \tag{3.15}$$

The test statistic is defined as

$$T = \frac{\hat{\varepsilon}\sqrt{n}}{\hat{\sigma}}, \tag{3.16}$$

where

$$\begin{cases} \hat{\varepsilon} = \hat{\theta}_T - \hat{\theta}_C + \delta_{NI}, \\ \hat{\sigma} = \sqrt{\dfrac{\hat{\sigma}_T^2}{f_T} + \dfrac{\hat{\sigma}_C^2}{f_C}}, \end{cases} \tag{3.17}$$

with $\hat{\sigma}_i^2$ being the sample variance ($i = T, C$), n being the total sample size, and sample size fractions $f_i = n_i/n$ ($i = T, C$).

For a large sample size, T has the standard normal distribution of $N(0, 1)$ on the boundary of the null hypothesis domain ($\theta_T - \theta_C + \delta_{NI} = 0$) and has the normal distribution $N(\frac{\varepsilon\sqrt{n}}{\sigma}, 1)$ under the condition $\theta_T - \theta_C + \delta_{NI} = \varepsilon$.

For the mean endpoint μ_i, $\hat{\sigma}_T$ and $\hat{\sigma}_C$ are the sample standard deviations. For the proportion endpoint p_i, the standard deviations are

$$\hat{\sigma}_i^2 = \hat{p}_i(1 - \hat{p}_i), i = T, C. \tag{3.18}$$

For the survival endpoint, $\hat{\theta}_i = \hat{\lambda}_i, i = T, C$, where λ_i is the population hazard rate for group i. The standard deviation for $\hat{\lambda}_i$, under exponential distribution, is given by (e.g., Chang 2007b):

$$\sigma_i^2 = \lambda_i^2 \left[1 + \frac{e^{-\lambda_i T_s}(1 - e^{\lambda_i T_0})}{T_0 \lambda_i} \right]^{-1}, \tag{3.19}$$

where T_0 and T_s are the accrual time period and the total trial duration, respectively.

Under an exponential survival model, the relationship between hazard (λ), median (T_{median}), and mean (T_{mean}) survival time is very simple:

$$T_{Median} = \frac{\ln 2}{\lambda} = (\ln 2)T_{mean}.$$

The rejection rule is specified as follows (assume larger θ is preferred):

$$\begin{cases} \text{Reject } H_o \text{ if } T \geq z_{1-\alpha}, \\ \text{Accept } H_o \text{ otherwise.} \end{cases} \tag{3.20}$$

Equivalently, we can use the confidence interval of ε:

$$\begin{cases} \text{Reject } H_o \text{ if } \hat{\varepsilon} - z_{1-\alpha}\frac{\hat{\sigma}}{\sqrt{n}} \geq 0, \\ \text{Accept } H_o \text{ otherwise.} \end{cases} \tag{3.21}$$

The power of the test statistic T under a particular H_a can be expressed as

$$1 - \beta = \Phi\left(\frac{\varepsilon\sqrt{n}}{\sigma} - z_{1-\alpha}\right), \tag{3.22}$$

where ε and σ are estimated by (3.17).

Solving (3.22) for the sample size, we obtain

$$n = \frac{\left(z_{1-\alpha} + z_{1-\beta}\right)^2 \sigma^2}{\varepsilon^2}. \tag{3.23}$$

Equation 3.23 is a general sample size formulation for the two-group designs with a normal, binary, or survival endpoint (Chang 2007a).

For the test statistic given by (3.16), the p-value is given by

$$p = 1 - \Phi\left(\frac{\hat{\varepsilon}\sqrt{n}}{\hat{\sigma}}\right). \tag{3.24}$$

Remark. A common misconception is that for an NI trial the sample size calculation must assume $\theta_T - \theta_C = 0$, which is not true at all. One could choose an NI design because the difference $\theta_T - \theta_C > 0$ is too small for superiority testing with reasonable power. The treatment difference can be positive or negative depending on the particular situation. The power and sample size calculation should be based on the best knowledge about the value of $\theta_T - \theta_C$, and this knowledge should not change because of the different choice of hypothesis test. Therefore, for a given value of $\theta_T - \theta_C$ and power, superiority testing always requires a smaller sample size than noninferiority testing.

Example 3.1. Arteriosclerotic Vascular Disease Trial: Cholesterol is the main lipid associated with arteriosclerotic vascular disease. The purpose of cholesterol testing is to identify patients at risk for arteriosclerotic heart disease. The liver metabolizes cholesterol to its free form and transports it to the bloodstream via lipoproteins. Nearly 75% of the cholesterol is bound to low-density lipoproteins (LDLs) – "bad cholesterol" and 25% is bound to high-density lipoproteins (HDLs) ("good cholesterol"). Therefore, cholesterol is the main component of LDLs and only a minimal component of HDLs and very-low-density lipoproteins. LDL is the substance most directly associated with increased risk of coronary heart disease (CHD).

Suppose we are interested in a phase III trial for evaluating the effect of a test drug on cholesterol in patients with CHD. A two-group (test versus control) parallel design is chosen for the trial, with LDL as the primary endpoint. The treatment difference in LDL is estimated from the previous phase II trial to be $\theta_T - \theta_C = 5\%$ (LDL reduction $\hat{\theta}_T = 25\%$ and $\hat{\theta}_C = 20\%$) with a standard deviation of $\hat{\sigma} = 2\hat{\sigma}_T = 2\hat{\sigma}_C = 0.3$ (sample size fraction $f_T = f_C = 0.5$ for the balance design, $\hat{\sigma}_C = 0.15$). For power = 90% and one-sided $\alpha = 0.025$, the total sample required for superiority can be calculated:

$$n = \frac{4(1.96 + 1.28)^2 \left(0.3^2\right)}{0.05^2} = 1{,}512.$$

For a noninferiority test with a margin $\delta_{NI} = -0.01$, the total sample size is given by (2.23):

$$n = \frac{4(1.96 + 1.28)^2 \left(0.3^2\right)}{(0.05 + 0.01)^2} = 1{,}050.$$

We can see that the required sample size is smaller for the noninferiority test than for a superiority test under the same assumption of treatment effect $\theta_T - \theta_C$. However, if we assume the treatment difference is $\theta_T - \theta_C = 0$ instead of 5%, the sample size for the noninferiority trial will be

$$n = \frac{4(1.96 + 1.28)^2 \left(0.3^2\right)}{0.01^2} = 27{,}791,$$

which means that if the test drug has the same effect as the control, $\theta_T = \theta_C$, it is not feasible for a superiority trial ($n = \infty$) or noninferiority trial ($n = 27{,}791$). In practice, if the estimate $\theta_T - \theta_C = 5\%$ is reliable, we may design the noninferiority trial with 90% power ($n = 1{,}050$). The trial will be tested both for noninferiority and superiority claims at one-sided $\alpha = 0.025$. With the same size of $n = 1{,}050$, the power for the superiority test is 77%.

3.2.2 λ-Portion Method

For the λ-portion method, the hypothesis is given by

$$H_o : \theta_T - \lambda_{NI} \theta_C \leq 0 , \tag{3.25}$$

where $0 < \lambda_{NI} < 1$ (assume that a larger θ is better).

The test statistic is defined in the same way as in (3.16), where

$$\begin{cases} \hat{\varepsilon} = \hat{\theta}_T - \lambda_{NI} \hat{\theta}_C, \\ \hat{\sigma}^2 = \dfrac{\hat{\sigma}_T^2}{f_T} + \lambda_{NI}^2 \dfrac{\hat{\sigma}_C^2}{f_C}. \end{cases} \tag{3.26}$$

With $\hat{\varepsilon}$ and $\hat{\sigma}$ given by (3.25), the calculations for the p-value (3.24), the rejection rule (3.21), power formulation (3.22), and the sample size formulation (3.23) are still valid.

The λ-portion method is usually more powerful than the fixed-margin method because the variance given by (3.26) is usually smaller than the corresponding variance (3.17) for the fixed-margin method.

Example 3.2. For the LDL trial in Example 3.1, the estimated $\hat{\varepsilon} = \hat{\theta}_T - \hat{\theta}_C + \delta_{NI} = 0.06$. For the purpose of comparison with the fixed-margin method, assume $\lambda_{NI} = 0.95$ such that the estimated

$$\hat{\varepsilon} = \hat{\theta}_T - \lambda_{NI}\hat{\theta}_C = 25\% - 0.95(20\%) = 0.06.$$

From (3.26), we can obtain

$$\hat{\sigma}^2 = \sqrt{0.15^2/0.5 + 0.95^2(0.15^2/0.5)} = 0.293.$$

Therefore, the total sample size required can be obtained from (3.14),

$$n = \frac{4(1.96 + 1.28)^2\,(0.293^2)}{0.06^2} \approx 1{,}000,$$

which is smaller than the sample size ($n = 1{,}050$) required for the fixed-margin method.

For the survival endpoint, the logarithm of the hazard ratio ($\ln\theta$) is often used in the hypothesis test. The standard error of $\ln\theta$ is conveniently expressed as a function of events (deaths),

$$\mathrm{SE}_{\ln\hat{\theta}} = \int_0^1 \left(\frac{n_T \cdot n_C}{n_C + n_T \theta \eta^{(\theta-1)/\theta}} \right)^{1/2} d\eta \approx \left(\frac{1}{d_T} + \frac{1}{d_C} \right)^{1/2},$$

where d_T and d_C are the number of deaths for the test and control groups, respectively. The approximate upper limit of the confidence interval of θ is given by

$$UL = \exp\left(\ln\hat{\theta} + z_{1-\alpha}\mathrm{SE}_{\ln\hat{\theta}} \right).$$

If the $UL \leq \theta_{\lambda_{NI}}$ (the cut point for NI, e.g., $\theta_{\lambda_{NI}} = 1.25$), noninferiority will be claimed.

3.2.3 Synthesis Method

1. With the synthesis method, the hypothesis test for noninferiority with two-group designs can be specified as

$$H_o : \theta_T - \theta_C + (1 - \lambda_{NI})\,(\theta_C - \theta_P) \ \leq 0 \text{ versus } H_a : \bar{H}_o. \tag{3.27}$$

The test statistic is again defined as in (3.16), where

$$\begin{cases} \hat{\varepsilon} = \hat{\theta}_T - \hat{\theta}_C + (1 - \lambda_{NI})\,\hat{\delta}_{C-P}, \\ \hat{\sigma}^2 = \left(\dfrac{\hat{\sigma}_T^2}{f_T} + \dfrac{\hat{\sigma}_C^2}{f_C} + (1 - \lambda_{NI})\,s_e^2 n \right), \end{cases} \tag{3.28}$$

and σ_i ($i = T, C$) is the same as given earlier for the fixed-margin approach for different endpoints, mean proportion, and hazard rate. Both $\hat{\delta}_{C-P} = \hat{\theta}_C - \hat{\theta}_P$ and the standard error s_e of $\hat{\delta}_{C-P}$ are obtained from the historical placebo-control trial(s). The standard error s_e can be estimated by

$$se = \sqrt{\hat{\theta}_C \left(1 - \hat{\theta}_C\right)/n_C + \hat{\theta}_P \left(1 - \hat{\theta}_P\right)/n_P},$$

where n_i ($i = C, P$) are the sample sizes in the treatment groups C and P of the historical trial, respectively.

For a large sample size, $T \sim N(\frac{\varepsilon\sqrt{n}}{\sigma}, 1)$, where

$$\varepsilon = \theta_T - \theta_C + (1 - \lambda_{NI})\delta_{C-P}. \qquad (3.29)$$

Therefore, using (3.28) and (3.29), the calculations for the p-value (3.24) and rejection rules (3.21) are still valid; so are the power (3.22) and sample size (3.23). However, because σ involves n, the sample size needs to be reformulated for easy calculation.

The sample size can be obtained through iterations based on the following formulation:

$$n = \frac{\left(z_{1-\alpha} + z_{1-\beta}\right)^2 \left(\frac{\sigma_T^2}{f_T} + \frac{\sigma_C^2}{f_C} + (1 - \lambda_{NI})\,s_e^2\,n\right)}{\varepsilon^2}. \qquad (3.30)$$

Alternatively, we can solve (3.30) for n. We can obtain

$$n = \frac{\eta_0 \left(\frac{\sigma_T^2}{f_T} + \frac{\sigma_C^2}{f_C}\right)}{1 - (1 - \lambda_{NI})\,s_e^2\,\eta_0}, \qquad (3.31)$$

where

$$\eta_0 = \frac{\left(z_{1-\alpha} + z_{1-\beta}\right)^2}{\varepsilon^2}. \qquad (3.32)$$

Because the synthesis method considers the variability of the historical trial, there is a bigger variance in the denominator of the test statistic in comparison with the fixed-margin method. As a result, the synthesis method is less powerful.

Example 3.3. Suppose we are going to design a two-arm phase III cardiovascular (CV) disease trial comparing the effect of the test treatment T to an active-control C with 1:1 randomization. The primary endpoint is the rate of the composite endpoint, i.e., death or MI (myocardial infarction) within 30 days. The proportion of the composite endpoint in the historical randomized trial was $\hat{\theta}_C = 0.14$ and $\hat{\theta}_P = 0.16$ for the treatment C ($n_C = 5,000$) and the standard care P ($n_P = 5,000$), respectively. Thus $\delta_{C-P} = 0.14 - 0.16 = -0.02$. The standard error is estimated to be

$$s_e = \sqrt{(0.14(1 - 0.14)/5,000) + 0.16(1 - 0.16)/5,000} = 0.00714.$$

The death rate with treatment T is estimated to be $\hat{\theta}_T = 0.115$. The target power is 90%, and the one-sided significance level is $\alpha = 0.025$. Assume we want to retain 80% of the historical active-control effect, i.e., $\lambda_{NI} = 0.8$ (or about 0.4% more composite events in terms of the fixed NI margin). To calculate the total sample size required for a balanced design ($f_1 = f_2 = 0.5$), we estimate ε from (3.29):

$$\varepsilon = 0.12 - 0.14 + (1 - 0.8)(-0.02) = -0.024.$$

From (3.32), we obtain

$$\eta_0 = (1.96 + 1.28)^2 / (-0.024)^2 = 18,225.$$

Finally, from (3.31), we obtain the total sample size

$$n = \frac{18,225 \left(\frac{0.12(1-0.12)}{0.5} + \frac{0.14(1-0.14)}{0.5} \right)}{1 - (1 - 0.8) \, 0.00714^2 (18,225)} = 10,118.$$

For the superiority design, the total same size would be

$$n = \left(\frac{0.115(1 - 0.115)}{0.5} + \frac{0.14(1 - 0.14)}{0.5} \right) \frac{(1.96 + 1.28)^2}{(0.12 - 0.14)^2} = 11{,}662.$$

2. We now study the hypothesis

$$H_o : \ln \frac{\theta_T}{\theta_C} - \ln \frac{\theta_C}{\theta_P} - \lambda^*_{NI} \leq 0, \tag{3.33}$$

where $\lambda^*_{NI} = \ln \lambda_{NI}$ as given in (3.6). Hypothesis (3.33) is often used for survival problems, where $\frac{\theta_T}{\theta_C}$ represents the hazard rate. The test statistic can again be defined by (3.16), where

$$\hat{\varepsilon} = \ln \frac{\hat{\theta}_T}{\hat{\theta}_C} - \ln \frac{\hat{\theta}_C}{\hat{\theta}_P} - \lambda^*_{NI}. \tag{3.34}$$

The estimated log hazard ratio, $\ln \frac{\hat{\theta}_C}{\hat{\theta}_P}$, is usually obtained from a historical placebo-control trial(s), whereas $\ln \frac{\hat{\theta}_T}{\hat{\theta}_C}$ is obtained from the current NI trial, and

$$\hat{\sigma}^2 = n \left[\text{var}\left(\ln \frac{\hat{\theta}_T}{\hat{\theta}_C} \right) + \text{var}\left(\ln \frac{\hat{\theta}_C}{\hat{\theta}_P} \right) \right], \tag{3.35}$$

where the first and second terms on the right-hand side of the equation are obtained from the current NI and historical trials, respectively. The variance of the log relative risk can be calculated using

$$\sigma_{TC}^2 = \text{var}\left(\ln \frac{\hat{\theta}_T}{\hat{\theta}_C}\right) = \frac{1}{n}\left(\frac{1}{r_T} - \frac{1}{f_T} + \frac{1}{r_C} - \frac{1}{f_C}\right), \qquad (3.36)$$

where r_i and f_i are the response (death) rate and the sample size fraction in group i ($i = T, C$), respectively.

Therefore, with (3.34) and (3.36), the formulations for the p-value (3.24), rejection rules (3.21), power (3.22), and sample size (3.23) are still valid.

Example 3.4. Suppose we are conducting a two-group oncology trial with a 1 year death rate as the primary endpoint (more often it is survival time). Assume that in the historical trial we know $\hat{\theta}_C = 0.4$ and $\hat{\theta}_P = 0.52$, and $\text{var}\left(\ln \frac{\hat{\theta}_C}{\hat{\theta}_P}\right) = 0.0065$. Because a smaller θ_i indicates a better result, λ_{NI}^* should be positive. Assume $\lambda_{NI}^* = 0.4$ or, equivalently, $\lambda_{NI} = e^{0.4} = 1.5$. Given the true rates $\theta_C = 0.4$ and $\theta_P = 0.52$, we know from (3.5) that it can be that $\frac{\theta_T}{\theta_C} = \lambda_{NI}\frac{\theta_C}{\theta_P} = 1.5\frac{0.4}{0.52} \approx 0.85$. This means that the use of $\lambda_{NI}^* = 0.4$ will retain about 85% of the control effect.

From (3.34), we obtain

$$\hat{\varepsilon} = \ln \frac{0.3}{0.4} - \ln \frac{0.4}{0.52} - 0.4 = -0.425,$$

from (3.36), we obtain

$$\hat{\sigma}_{TC}^2 = \frac{1}{n}\left(\frac{1}{0.3(0.5)} - \frac{1}{(0.5)} + \frac{1}{0.4(0.5)} - \frac{1}{(0.5)}\right) = \frac{7.667}{n},$$

and from (3.35) we can obtain $\sigma^2 = n\,(7.667/n + 0.0065) = 7.667 + 0.0065n$. The sample size can be calculated from (3.23):

$$n = \frac{(1.96 + 1.28)^2\,(7.667 + 0.0065n)}{(-0.425)^2} = 445.6 + 0.3778n.$$

Solving for n, we obtain $n=716$ for the noninferiority design. For the superiority design, the sample size would be

$$n = (1.96 + 1.28)^2(7.667) \left/ \left(\ln \frac{0.3}{0.4}\right)^2 \approx 972.\right.$$

We can see that the savings on sample size for the NI trial using (3.33) are dramatic when the event rate is low. When the event rate is high (e.g., 0.3), the savings in sample size are much smaller using (3.33). For high event rates, the method based on (3.27) can be better than the method based on (3.33) in terms of sample size.

3. We now study the hypothesis

$$H_o : \ln \frac{\theta_T}{\theta_C} + \lambda^*_{NI} \ln \frac{\theta_C}{\theta_P} \leq 0. \tag{3.37}$$

The test statistic is given by (3.16), where

$$\hat{\varepsilon} = \ln \frac{\hat{\theta}_T}{\hat{\theta}_C} + \lambda^*_{NI} \ln \frac{\hat{\theta}_C}{\hat{\theta}_P}. \tag{3.38}$$

Here $\ln \frac{\hat{\theta}_C}{\hat{\theta}_P}$ and $\ln \frac{\hat{\theta}_T}{\hat{\theta}_C}$ are the same as previously stated, but the variance is different and is given by

$$\hat{\sigma}^2 = n \left[\text{var} \left(\ln \frac{\hat{\theta}_T}{\hat{\theta}_C} \right) + \lambda^{*2}_{NI} \text{var} \left(\ln \frac{\hat{\theta}_C}{\hat{\theta}_P} \right) \right].$$

Using (3.36), we can obtain

$$\hat{\sigma}^2 = \frac{1}{r_T} - \frac{1}{f_T} + \frac{1}{r_C} - \frac{1}{f_C} + \lambda^{*2}_{NI} \left(\frac{1}{r_C} - \frac{1}{f_C} + \frac{1}{r_P} - \frac{1}{f_P} \right). \tag{3.39}$$

With (3.38) and (3.39), the calculations of p-value (3.24), rejection rules (3.21), power (3.22), and sample size (2.23) are still valid. The can also be formulated in terms of the number of events under, for example, exponential distribution.

As pointed out in the draft FDA guidance (FDA 2010), because of the way the variance of the historical data and the NI data are combined for the synthesis test, the synthesis test is more efficient (it uses a smaller sample size or achieves greater power for the same sample size) than the fixed-margin approach but requires assumptions that may not be appropriate.

3.2.4 Paired Data

Let Y_1 and Y_2 be, respectively, binary response variables of treatments 1 and 2 with the joint distribution $P(Y_1 = i; Y_2 = j) = p_{ij}$ for $i = 0, 1; j = 0, 1$. $\sum_{i=0}^{1} \sum_{j=0}^{1} p_{ij} = 1$. This kind of data is usually displayed in a 2×2 contingency table as in Table 3.1.

Nam and Tango's asymptotic test (Nam 1997; Tango 1998) is given by

$$H_o : p_{01} - p_{10} \geq \delta_{NI} \text{ vs. } H_a : \bar{H}_o. \tag{3.40}$$

Table 3.1 Matched-pair data

	Test		Total
Control	1	0	
1	x_{11}	x_{10}	
0	x_{01}	x_{00}	
Total			n

Define the test statistic in (3.16), where

$$\begin{cases} \hat{\varepsilon} = \hat{p}_{01} - \hat{p}_{10} - \delta_{NI}, \\ \hat{p}_{ij} = x_{ij}/n, \\ \hat{\sigma}^2 = 2\tilde{p}_{10} + \delta_{NI} - \delta_{NI}^2, \end{cases} \tag{3.41}$$

and $\tilde{p}_{10}$ is the restricted MLE of p_{10},

$$\begin{cases} \tilde{p}_{10} = \dfrac{-b + \sqrt{b^2 - 8c}}{4}, \\ b = (2 + \hat{p}_{10} - \hat{p}_{01})\,\delta_{NI} - \hat{p}_{01} - \hat{p}_{10}, \\ c = -\hat{p}_{10}\delta_{NI}\,(1 - \delta_{NI}). \end{cases} \tag{3.42}$$

Nam (1997) proved that under the constraint $p_{01} - p_{10} = \delta_{NI}$, T in (3.16) follows the normal distribution for large n,

$$T \sim N\left(\frac{\sqrt{n}\varepsilon}{\sigma}, 1\right), \tag{3.43}$$

where $\varepsilon = E(\hat{\varepsilon})$ and $\sigma = E(\hat{\sigma})$ can be obtained by replacing $\hat{p}_{ij}$ with p_{ij} ($i = 0, 1; j = 0, 1$) in the corresponding expressions.

Using (3.41) and (3.42), the calculations of the p-value (3.24), the rejection rules (3.21), and power (3.22) are the same, but the sample size calculation requires numerical iterations.

3.3 Three-Arm Design

CHMP (2005) suggested: "A three-armed trial with test, reference and placebo allows some within-trial validation of the choice of noninferiority margin and is therefore associated with fewer difficulties. This is the recommended design and should be used wherever possible."

In the United States, a noninferiority trial with a placebo arm is often considered ethically problematic. However, there are situations when the use of a placebo is permissible. According to Ellenberg and Temple (2000), placebo controls are ethical when delaying or omitting available treatment has no permanent adverse consequences for the patient and as long as patients are fully informed about the alternatives and settings where the available "effective treatment" may not be uniformly accepted as standard treatment and so placebo-control trials are justified. The escape clauses are suggested to be included in the study protocol.

In a three-arm NI trial, we can use the synthesis method and then rewrite the hypothesis test as

$$H_o : \theta_T - \lambda_{NI}\theta_C - (1 - \lambda_{NI})\,\theta_P \leq 0, \text{ and}$$
$$H_a : \theta_T - \lambda_{NI}\theta_C - (1 - \lambda_{NI})\,\theta_P > 0. \tag{3.44}$$

Let the test statistic be

$$T = \frac{\hat{\varepsilon}\sqrt{n}}{\hat{\sigma}}, \tag{3.45}$$

where n is the total sample size,

$$\begin{cases} \hat{\varepsilon} = \hat{\theta}_{NI} - \lambda_{NI}\hat{\theta}_C - (1 - \lambda_{NI})\,\hat{\theta}_P \\ \hat{\sigma} = \sqrt{\dfrac{\hat{\sigma}_T^2}{f_T} + \dfrac{\lambda_{NI}^2\,\hat{\sigma}_C^2}{f_C} + \dfrac{(1 - \lambda_{NI})^2\,\hat{\sigma}_P^2}{f_P}}, \end{cases} \tag{3.46}$$

and f_i is the sample size fraction for the ith group.

T in (3.45) follows a t-distribution with $v = n_T + n_C + n_P - 3$ degrees of freedom under H_0. Thus, noninferiority can be claimed if $T \geq t_{1-\alpha,v}$. Since most NI trials have a large sample size, we can use a normal approximation; therefore, using (3.46), the calculations for the p-value (3.24), the rejection rule (3.21), and power formulation (3.22) are still valid.

However, unlike in the two-arm trial, we now have to reject the hypothesis H_{00} : $\theta_C - \theta_P \leq 0$ first before we test (3.44), as suggested by Pigeot et al. (2003) and Kieser and Friede (2007). Therefore, the sample size and overall power calculations can be obtained using simulations.

There are some dilemmas in three-arm NI trials. For example, what if we failed to reject $H_0 : \theta_C - \theta_P \leq 0$ but rejected $H_0 : \theta_T - \theta_P \leq 0$, and failed to reject $H_0 : \theta_T - \theta_C + \delta_{NI} \leq 0$? Should we claim T superiority to C, or not even claim T is noninferior to C? CHMP's guidance (CHMP 2005) states that when $\theta_C - \theta_P$ is smaller than what was previously estimated, the appropriateness of the predetermined margin is in doubt and modifications may be needed. This inevitably further undermines the validity of the statistical method for the NI design. We will discuss controversies and challenges further in Sect. 3.5.

3.4 The Noninferiority Margin and Regulatory Guidance

3.4.1 ICH Guidance

Different regulatory authorities may have different requirements and recommendations regarding the NI trial in general and the determination of the NI margin. Therefore, it is important to carefully review their guidance documents before designing an NI trial.

According to the ICH E10 guidance, the design and conduct of a noninferiority trial thus involves four critical steps:

1. Determining that historical evidence of sensitivity to drug effects exists. Without this determination, demonstration of efficacy from a showing of noninferiority is not possible and should not be attempted.
2. Designing a trial. Important details of the trial design, e.g., study population, concomitant therapy, endpoints, run-in periods, should adhere closely to the design of the trials used to determine that historical evidence of sensitivity to drug effects exists.
3. Setting a margin. An acceptable noninferiority margin should be defined, taking into account the historical data and relevant clinical and statistical considerations.
4. Conducting the trial. The trial conduct should also adhere closely to that of the historical trials and should be of high quality.

The determination of the noninferiority margin "...should reflect uncertainties in the evidence on which the choice is based, and should be suitably conservative." The guidance states: "In practice, the noninferiority margin chosen usually will be smaller than that suggested by the smallest expected effect size of the active-control because of interest in ensuring some clinically acceptable effect size (or fraction of the control drug effect) was maintained."

3.4.2 FDA Guidance

Conceptually, the NI study design provides two comparisons: (1) a direct comparison of the test drug with the active comparator drug, and (2) an indirect comparison of the test drug with a placebo, based on what is known about how the effect of the active comparator compares with the placebo. For this reason, the determination of the NI margin requires two quantities: (1) $\delta_1 =$ the entire effect of the active-control assumed to be present in the NI study and (2) the minimal clinically meaningful difference δ_2. The NI margin $\delta_{NI} = \min(\delta_1 \ \delta_2)$ is interpreted as the largest clinically acceptable difference (degree of inferiority) of the test drug compared with the active-control, which implies (1) $\delta_{NI} \leq \delta_1$, a condition to rule out "the test drug is worse than the placebo" when the inferiority hypothesis is rejected, and (2) $\delta_{NI} \leq \delta_2$, a condition to rule out "the test drug is inferior to the control by more than a clinically meaningful difference" when the inferiority hypothesis is rejected.

The commonly used method is NI95-H95, in which NI95 means the NI margin is determined by a 95% confidence interval bound (δ_1 = either lower or upper 95% confidence bound of the treatment difference between the active-control and placebo from a historical study), and the NI hypothesis test is also based on a 95% CI. According to the draft FDA guidance (FDA 2010), in this traditional method, there can be flexibility in the CI choice, such as a 90% or even narrower confidence interval, when the circumstances are appropriate to do so (e.g., strong evidence of a class effect, strong biomarker data). It is recognized that use of a fixed margin to define the control response is conservative, as it picks the "worst case" out of a confidence interval that consists of values of effect that are all larger. When the qualities of the historical trials are good and constancy holds well, a narrow confidence interval can be used in determining the NI margin.

The determination of δ_2 is a matter of clinical judgment, which may take into account the actual disease incidence or prevalence and its impact on the practicality of sample sizes that would have to be accrued for a study. According to the draft guidance, there can be flexibility in the δ_2 margin; for example, when:

1. The difference between the active comparator response rate and the spontaneous response rate is large.
2. The primary endpoint does not involve an irreversible outcome such as death.
3. The test product is associated with fewer serious adverse effects than other therapies already available.
4. The test product is in a new pharmacological category and has been shown to be tolerated by patients who do not tolerate therapies that are already available.

The draft guidance indicates that choosing δ_{NI} as 50% of δ_1 has become the usual practice for cardiovascular (CV) outcome studies, whereas in antibiotic trials effect sizes are relatively large, δ_{NI} = 10–15% is common. In large cardiovascular studies, it is unusual to seek retention of more than 50% of δ_1, even if this might be clinically reasonable, because doing so will usually make the study size infeasible.

The guidance allows the NI margin to be determined based on a historical single-arm trial (the active-control arm for the disease being assessed) under circumstances similar to those in which a historically controlled trial can be persuasive (see ICH E10). First, there should be a good estimate of the historical spontaneous cure rate or outcome without treatment. Examination of medical literature and other sources of information may provide data upon which to base these estimates (e.g., historical information on natural history or the results of ineffective therapy). Second, the cure rate of the active-control should be estimated from historical experience, preferably from multiple experiences in various settings, and should be substantially different from the untreated rate.

Since the NI margin is determined (partially) based on clinical judgment, as indicated by the draft guidance, prior information could be characterized in a statistical model or in a Bayesian framework by taking into account such factors as evidence of effects in multiple related indications or on many endpoints. Examples are provided in the appendix of the draft guidance.

Remark. The draft guidance states: "Seeking an NI conclusion in the event of a failed superiority test would almost never be acceptable. It would be very difficult to make a persuasive case for an NI margin based on data analyzed with study results in hand. If it is clear that an NI conclusion is a possibility, the study should be designed as an NI study." If you didn't read this carefully, you may conclude that we can perform the NI test first, followed by a superiority test, without a multiplicity adjustment, but we can't do it the other way around. In fact, the testing sequence is irrelevant as far as the type-I error control is concerned, as long as the NI margin is prespecified before seeing the NI trial data.

Regarding the analysis population, the draft guidance requires performing both ITT and as-treated analyses in NI studies.

The FDA usually requires at least two pivotal studies. However, one NI trial may be sufficient, as the draft guidance states it is common in NI trials for the test drug to be pharmacologically similar to the active-control. (If they were not pharmacologically similar, an add-on study would usually have been more persuasive and more practical.) In that case, the expectation of similar performance (but still requiring confirmation in a trial) might make it possible to accept a single trial and perhaps could also allow less conservative choices in choosing the noninferiority margin. A similar conclusion might be reached when other types of data are available, for example: (1) if there were a very persuasive biomarker confirming similar activity of the test drug and active-control (e.g., tumor response, ACE inhibition, or extent of beta blockage), (2) if the drug has been shown to be effective in closely related clinical settings (e.g., effective as adjunctive therapy with an NI study of monotherapy), and (3) if the drug has been shown to be effective in distinct but related populations (e.g., pediatric versus adult).

3.4.3 CHMP Guidance

CHMP (2005) provides general guidelines on the choice of the noninferiority margin, which include:

1. The selection of the noninferiority margin is based upon a combination of statistical reasoning and clinical judgement.
2. There are many conditions where established effective agents do not consistently demonstrate superiority in placebo controlled trials (e.g. depression or allergic rhinitis). In areas where this lack of sensitivity exists, a noninferiority trial which does not also include a placebo arm is not appropriate. See ICH E10 for a fuller discussion of assay sensitivity.
3. If the performance of the reference product in a trial is very different from what was assumed when defining the noninferiority margin then the chosen margin may no longer be appropriate. The implications of this should be considered at the planning stage.

4. It may be possible to justify a wider noninferiority margin for efficacy if the product has an advantage in some other aspect of its profile. This margin should not, however, be so wide that superiority to placebo is left in doubt.
5. In some extreme situations it may be acceptable to run a superiority trial specifying a significance level greater than 0.05 as an alternative to defining a noninferiority margin (a 15% level of significance has been used as example in the document for demonstrating superiority. This increased alpha must be clearly stated in the protocol and should be discussed with CHMP beforehand regarding the appropriateness for the particular situation).

CHMP (2005) states: "It is not appropriate to define the noninferiority margin as a proportion of the difference between active comparator and placebo. Such ideas were formulated with the aim of ensuring that the test product was superior to (a putative) placebo; however they may not achieve this purpose. If the reference product has a large advantage over placebo this does not mean that large differences are unimportant, it just means that the reference product is very efficacious." However, this is not necessarily the view of the U.S. regulatory authority. A counter argument might be: a patient may consider the two drugs similar in terms of benefit if one prolongs his life for 10 years and the other 9 years and 11 months; however, he will definitely say the two drugs are different in life saving if they prolong life for 3 and 2 months, even though there is a 1 month difference in both situations.

CHMP (2005) also allows a larger NI margin when the test drug can demonstrate advantages on coprimary endpoints. When historical control-placebo trial data are not available and conducting a placebo-control trial is not ethical, such as in oncology settings and some orphan indications, a putative placebo may not be necessary since the treatment benefit over the placebo is generally acceptable. In other cases, it is possible to survey practitioners on the range of differences that they consider to be unimportant and choose the NI margin based upon a summary statistic of the responses.

CHMP (2005) emphasizes: "A judgement must be made regarding whether the difference seen is clinically useful. This judgement is usually made in the context of the safety profile via an assessment of benefit/risk." As we can see, this will be very challenging because it includes a large portion of subjectivity, and sometimes post hoc analyses. While it is necessary, the NI margin also faces challenges in interpretation. For continuous variables, if $\delta_{NI} = \delta_{\min}$ (the minimum clinical difference or the minimum assay detectable level), it can be challenged because it could be that half of the patients showed $\delta = 0$ and the other half showed $\delta = 2\delta_{\min}$, which is important because half of the patients had good responses, even though the average change was $\delta_{\min}$. For binary responses, any percentage always seems meaningful.

During the literature search for determining the NI margin, we should avoid selection bias. Publication bias also should be noted. Constancy is important. We should consider the constancy of trial design and clinical practice over time; pay attention to the changes in standard care, medical practice, the criteria or methods for measuring, entry criteria, the method of diagnosis, concomitant treatments allowed, dosing regime of reference products, endpoints measured, and timing of assessments.

CHMP (2005) states: "It is not appropriate to use effect size (treatment difference divided by standard deviation) as justification for the choice of noninferiority margin. This statistic provides information on how difficult a difference would be to detect, but does not help justify the clinical relevance of the difference, and does not ensure that the test product is superior to placebo." However, it is arguable that we use $\mu\sqrt{n}/\sigma$ instead of $\mu\sqrt{n}$ for the test statistic for superiority. Fleming (2008) and Koch (2008) provide several case studies and insightful discussions on this issue.

3.5 Controversies and Challenges

3.5.1 Assay Sensitivity, Constancy and Biocreep

There are often no or a few historical placebo-control trials available, and therefore the NI margin is difficult to assess precisely. When there are many such historical placebo-control trials available, the variability is often large. Moreover, the constancy does not usually hold exactly due to medical practice change, difference in study populations, and others. The impact due to violating the constancy requirement is difficult to assess.

Biocreep can occur when a test drug is slightly inferior to the comparator from generation to generation. However, the current NI testing method is conservative (see Sect. 3.5.3), and biocreep may not actually happen. Of course, under an extreme situation where all test drugs are inferior or even worse than the placebo, regardless of what hypothesis (superiority or noninferiority) test is used, all the approved drugs will be inferior or worse than placebo (Chang 2007b). We should not be confused by the two different concepts, the type-I error rate and the false discovery rate (FDR). The former is the probability of rejecting the null hypothesis H_o (negative drug) when it is true. The latter (FDR) is the expected proportion of false positive drugs among all the drugs approved (rejecting H_o). Ideally, we want to control FDR below a certain value (e.g., α); however, this is difficult because it depends on both the level of significance of the hypothesis test and the prior distribution of the treatment parameter θs for all test drugs (i.e., the effectiveness of the test drugs).

3.5.2 Conflicting Noninferiority-Superiority Claims

Recall that the noninferiority null hypothesis for T versus C is defined as

$$H_o : \theta_T - \theta_C + \delta_{NI} \leq 0. \tag{3.47}$$

The superiority null hypothesis for C versus T is defined as

$$H_o : \theta_C - \theta_T \leq 0 \tag{3.48}$$

instead of

$$H_o : \theta_C - \theta_T - \delta_{NI} \le 0. \tag{3.49}$$

It is obvious that (3.47) and (3.49) are symmetric in the sense that rejecting (3.47) implies acceptance of (3.49). In other words, if we conclude T is noninferior to C, then C is not superior to T; if T is inferior to C, then C is superior to T. However, (3.47) and (3.48), which are currently used in practice and for drug approval, are consistent. This inconsistency will lead to some contradictory conclusions when the confidence interval for the treatment difference $(T - C)$ lies completely within $(-\delta_{NI}, 0)$. When this happens, we conclude T is not inferior to C based on (3.47) but at the same time have to conclude C is superior to T based on (3.48) because the confidence interval for the difference $(C - T)$ lies completely with $(0, \delta_{NI})$. Note that medical significance has already been considered in NI margin δ_{NI}, as stated in the regulatory guidance.

To give T and C an equal "right" to claim superiority and noninferiority, if there should be a test for superiority/noninferiority for T versus C, then there should be another test for superiority/noninferiority for C versus T and vice versa.

Ideally, to make the superiority testing and noninferiority test symmetric, the null hypothesis for the superiority test should be defined by (3.47) with a larger level of significance. The problem with that is that we will encounter the same challenges for determining δ_{NI}.

3.5.3 Dilemma of Totality Evidence

Suppose we have data from two trials conducted sequentially: a superiority trial for P versus C was conducted first, followed by an NI trial with T versus C. The hypothetical efficacy data are presented in Table 3.2. In the P versus C trial, the p-value $= 0.0227 < \alpha = 0.025$; therefore we claim C is superior to P. In the second NI T versus C trial, the p-value $= 0.0286 > \alpha$; hence we failed to show T is noninferior to C. However, if we consider the totality of the evidence under the constancy assumption (i.e., considering the data from the two trials together), we can find the following:

1. The standard deviation σ_i is the same for all the groups in the two trials.
2. The treatment effect θ_i for the control group is consistent between the two trials.
3. The total sample sizes in the two trials are the same (200) for the control and test groups.
4. The treatment effect is 2 for the control group and 2.8 for the test group.

How can we conclude C is significantly better than P, and T is not even noninferior to C? Don't data show clearly that T is better than, or at least as good as, C? Is there something fundamentally wrong with NI testing?

Furthermore, when $\delta_{NI} > \theta_C - \theta_T > 0$ and the sample size is large enough, we can reject both $H_{os} : \theta_C - \theta_T \le 0$ and $H_{0NI} : \theta_T - \theta_C < -\delta_{NI}$. The first rejection

Table 3.2 Dilemma of totality evidence

Trial	Drug	Effect θ_i	Std dev.	Sample size	P-value
1	Control	2	3.5	100	0.0227
	Placebo	1	3.5	100	
2	Test	2.8	3.5	200	0.0286 (NI)
	Control	2	3.5	100	

Note: One-sided $\alpha = 0.025$, $\delta NI = 0.015 = 50\%$ of the 95% CI lower limit for the treatment difference in trial one

leads to the conclusion that the control is superior to the test drug. On the other hand, the second rejection leads to the conclusion that the test drug is noninferior to the control. These two conclusions are contradictory to each other.

3.5.4 Superiority-Noninferiority Testing

CPMP (2000) states that, in a noninferiority trial, if the null hypothesis is rejected, we can proceed to test the null hypothesis for superiority. No α-adjustment is needed because of the closed test procedure. This argument is supported by, for example, two papers (Dunnett and Gent 1976; Morikawa and Yoshida 1995).

However, Tie-Hua Ng (2007) argues that allowing simultaneous testing of superiority and noninferiority will increase the FDR (false discovery rate or the probability of claiming false superiority) in comparison with the scenario where just one test (either superiority or noninferiority) is allowed. He argues that the compounds that would have been tested for noninferiority will now be tested for superiority and noninferiority simultaneously, and this will increase the probability of false superiority claims. However, he didn't mention the positive side, that the simultaneous testing tends to increase the positive discovery rate (PDR), too. A simple solution to make T and C even is to simultaneously test $H_o : T < C$ and $H_0 : C > T$ so that the chance of a positive claim and the chance of a negative claim increase simultaneously. Readers may refer to Chaps. 10 and 1 for in-depth discussions on type-I error and FDR.

3.5.5 Summary

The NI margin is the most challenging issue in NI design. Especially when the constancy requirements have not been met well, the NI margin is inevitably largely subjective. In some or most cases, a judgment must be made regarding whether the difference seen is clinically useful. This judgment is usually made in the context of the safety profile via an assessment of benefit/risk (CHMP 2005).

There are other methods, such as the modeling approach and the nonparametric approaches, that we have not yet covered. Readers can find the relevant materials in the papers by Siqueira et al. (2008) (with Comments by Brittain and Hu 2009). Wang and her colleagues (2001) discuss group sequential test strategies for superiority and noninferiority hypotheses. However, we will not discuss this issue here. Instead, we will discuss this topic in Chap. 4.

The following questions suggested by D'Agostino (2003) are very helpful in planning an NI trial:

1. Is the disease condition being studied now the same as in the historical studies? Have there been changes in the diagnosis of the disease or curse of the disease?
2. Have there been changes in the standard of care or treatment of the disease condition?
3. Is the same population being studied? Are the new study subjects from similar settings, same age, same gender, etc.?
4. Are the dose and route of administration of the active-control in the historical trials the same as in the current study?
5. Are the outcomes and modes of data collection consistent across studies? Will we allow a retrospective collection of outcomes in the historical controlled studies? If so, what is the effect on our estimate of assay sensitivity?
6. Which historical placebo-control studies do we use? If not all, how do we select those of interest? If some studies showed no significant effect of active-control versus placebo (due to lack of efficacy of the active drug or due to a high placebo effect), then do we include these studies? What are the implications of their inclusion or exclusion?

Wang and her colleagues (2001) discuss group sequential test strategies for superiority and noninferiority hypotheses. However, we will not discuss this issue here. Instead, we will discuss this topic in Chap. 4.

3.6 Exercises

3.1. Suppose we are interested in a trial for evaluating the effect of a test drug on cholesterol in patients with CHD. A two-group parallel design is chosen for the trial with LDL as the primary endpoint. The treatment difference in LDL is estimated to be 5%, with a standard deviation of 0.3. Use at least three different methods to design noninferiority trials and provide justifications for the design you recommended. You can make any assumptions necessary.

3.2. Discuss the Dilemma of Totality Evidence presented in Table 3.2.

3.3. In a noninferiority design, biocreep theoretically can occur. Can biocreep occur with superiority trials, too? If test compounds are randomly drawn from a chemical compound pool with an effective size δ/σ that has the standard normal distribution, study the probability of biocreep using noninferiority trials ($\delta_{NI}=0.02$) and superiority trials ($\delta_{NI} = 0$), respectively. All trials are assumed to have 90% power. What are the probabilities that the first, fifth, and tenth drugs, respectively, are worse than a placebo?

Further Readings and References

Brittain, E., Hu, Z.: Noninferiority trial design and analysis with an ordered three-level categorical endpoint. J. Biopharm. Stat. **19**, 685–699 (2009)

Chan, I.S.F.: Power and sample size determination for noninferiority trials using an exact method. J. Biopharm. Stat. **12**(4), 457–469 (2002)

Chang, M.: Multiple-arm superiority and noninferiority designs with various endpoints. Pharm. Stat. **6**, 43–52 (2007a)

Chang, M.: Adaptive Design Theory and Implementation Using SAS and R. Chapman & Hall/CRC, Boca Raton (2007b)

Chang, M.: Monte Carlo Simulation for the Pharmaceutical Industry. Chapman and Hall/CRC, Raton (2010)

CHMP: Points to consider on switching between superiority and noninferiority. Br. J. Clin. Pharm. **52**, 223–228 (2001)

CHMP: Guideline on the choice of the noninferiority margin, EMEA/EWP/2158/99. London, July 27, 2005 (2005)

Chow, S.C., Shao, J.: On noninferiority margin and statistical tests in active control trials. Stat. Med. **25**, 1101–1113 (2005)

Cook, R.J., Lee, K.A., Li, H.: Noninferiority trial design for recurrent events. Stat. Med. **26**, 4563–4577 (2007)

CPMP: Points to consider on switching between superiority and non-inferiority. www.ema.europa.eu (2000). Accessed 18 May 2010

D'Agostino, R.B.: Editoral, noninferiority trials: Advances in concepts and methodology. Stat. Med. **22**, 165–167 (2003)

D'Agostino, R.B., Massaro, J.M., Sullivan, L.M.: Noninferiority trials: Design concepts and issues-the encounters of academic consultants in statistics. Stat. Med. **22**, 169–186 (2003)

Dunnett, C.W., Gent, M.: An alternative to the use of two-sided tests in clinical trials. Stat. Med. **15**, 1729–1738 (1976)

Dunnett, C.W., Gent, M.: Significant testing to establish equivalence between treatments with special reference to data in the form of 2×2 tables. Biometrics **33**, 593–602 (1977)

Ellenberg, S.S., Temple, R.: Placebo-controlled trials and active controlled trials in the evaluation of new treatment. Part 2: Practical issues and specific cases. Ann. Intern. Med. **133**, 464–470 (2000)

Farrington, C.P., Manning, G.: Test statistics and sample size formulae for comparative binomial trials with null hypothesis of non-zero risk difference or non-unity relative risk. Stat. Med. **9**, 1447–1454 (1990)

FDA: International Conference on Harmonisation. Statistical Principles for Clinical Trials (ICH E 9). Food and Drug Administration, Department of Health and Human Services, Washingtom (1998)

FDA: Guidance for Industry Non-Inferiority Clinical Trials (draft). Food and Drug Administration, Department of Health and Human Services, Washingtom (2010)

Fleming, T.R.: Current issues in noninferiority trials. Stat. Med. **27**, 317–332 (2008)

Hung, H.M., Wang, S.J., O'Neill, R.T.: Issues with statistical risks for testing methods in noninferiority trial without a placebo arm. J. Biopharm. Stat. **17**(2), 201–213 (2007)

Ioannidis, J.P.A.: Why most published research findings are false. PLoS Med. **2**(8), e124 (2005)

Kieser, M., Friede, T.: Planning and analysis of three-arm non-inferiority trials with binary endpoints. Stat. Med. **26**, 253–273 (2007)

Liu, J.P., Hsueh, H.M., Hsieh, E., Chen, J.J.: Tests for equivalence or noninferiority for paired binary data. Stat. Med. **21**, 231–245 (2002)

Koch, G.G.: Commentory, comments on 'Current issues in noninferiority trials'. Stat. Med. **27**, 333–342 (2008)

Kong, L., Kohberger, R.C., Koch, G.G.: Type I error and power in noninferiority/equivalence trials with correlated multiple endpoints: An example from vaccine development trials. J. Biopharm. Stat. **14**, 893–907 (2004)

Koyama, T., Westfall, P.H.: Decision-theoretic views on simultaneous testing of superiority and noninferiority. J. Biopharm. Stat. **15**, 943–955 (2005)

Lu, Y., Jin, H., Genant, H.K.: On the noninferiority of a diagnostic test based on paired observations. Stat. Med. **22**, 3029–3044 (2003)

Morikawa, T., Yoshida, M.: A useful testing strategy in phase III trials: Combined test of superiority and test of equivalence. J. Biopharm. Stat. **5**, 297–306 (1995)

Nam, J.: Establishing equivalence of two treatments and sample size requirements in matched-pairs design. Biometrics **53**, 1422–1430 (1997)

Nam, J., Kwon, D.: Noninferiority tests for clustered matched-pair data. Stat. Med. **28**, 1668–1679 (2009)

Ng, T.H.: Issues of simultaneous tests for noninferiority and superiority, with discussions. J. Biopharm. Stat. **13**, 629–639 (2003)

Ng, T.H.: Simultaneous testing of noninferiority and superiority increases the false discovery rate. J. Biopharm. Stat. **17**, 259–264 (2007)

PAREXEL: Parexel's Bio/Pharmaceutical R&D Statistical Sourcebook 2007/2008. PAREXEL, Waltham (2008)

Pearlman, J.B.: The commercialization of medicine. http://www.google.com (2007). Accessed 10 Sep 2009

Pigeot, I., Schäfer, J., Röhmel, J., Hauschke, D.: Assessing noninferiority of a new treatment in a three-arm clinical trial including a placebo. Stat. Med. **22**, 883–899 (2003)

Rothmann, M., Li, N., Chen, G., Chi1, G.Y.H., Temple, R., Tsou, H.H.: Design and analysis of noninferiority mortality trials in oncology. Stat. Med. **22**, 239–264 (2003)

Shao, J.: Mathematical Statistics. Springer, New York, NY (2003)

Sidik, K.: Exact unconditional tests for testing noninferiority in matched-pairs design. Stat. Med. **22**, 265–278 (2003)

Siqueira, A.L., Whitehead, A., Todd, S.: Active-control trials with binary data: A comparison of methods for testing superiority or noninferiority using the odds ratio, with comments. Stat. Med. **27**, 353–370 (2008)

Snapinn, S., Jiang, Q.: Correction. Stat. Med. **27**, 4855–4856 (2008)

Tang, M.L., Tang, N.S.: Tests of noninferiority via rate difference for three-arm clinical trials with placebo. J. Biopharm. Stat. **14**, 337–347 (2004)

Tango, T.: Equivalence test and confidence interval for the difference in proportions for the paired-sample design. Stat. Med. **17**, 891–908 (1998)

Temple, R.: Active control noninferiority studies: Theory, assay sensitivity, choice of margin. FDA presentation. www.FDA.gov (2002). Accessed 19 Feb 2002

Temple, R., Ellenberg, S.S.: Placebo-controlled trials and active-controlled trials in the evaluation of new treatments. Part 1: Ethical and scientific issues. Ann. Intern. Med. **133**, 455–463 (2000)

Tsong, Y., Chen, W.J.: Noninferiority testing beyond simple two-sample comparison. J. Biopharm. Stat. **17**, 289–308 (2007)

Wang, Y.C., Chen, G., Chi, G.Y.H.: A ratio test in active control non-inferiority trials with time-to-event endpoint. J. Biopharm. Stat. **16**, 151–164 (2006)

Wang, S.J., Hung, H.M., Tsong, Y., Cui, L.: Group sequential test strategies for superiority and noninferiority hypotheses in active controlled clinical trials. Stat. Med. **20**, 1903–1912 (2001)

Wiens, B.L., Heyes, J.F.: Testing for interactions in studies of noninferiority. J. Biopharm. Stat. **13**, 103–115 (2003)

Chapter 4
Adaptive Trial Design

4.1 Concept of Adaptive Trial Design

4.1.1 Reasons for Adaptive Design

The utilization of adaptive trial designs can increase the probability of success, reduce the cost, reduce the time to market, and deliver the right drug to the right patient. Two popular definitions of adaptive design are: (1) Chow and Chang's definition that an adaptive design is a clinical trial design that allows adaptations or modification to aspects of the trial after its initiation without undermining the validity and integrity of the trial (Chow and Chang 2005), and (2) The PhRMA Working Group's definition that adaptive design refers to a clinical trial design that uses accumulating data to decide on how to modify aspects of the study as it continues, without undermining the validity and integrity of the trial (Gallo et al. 2006). Most recently, the FDA released the draft guidance on Adaptive Design for Clinical Drugs and Biologics, where the definition of adaptive trial design is stated as "a study that includes a prospectively planned opportunity for modification of one or more specified aspects of the study design and hypotheses based on analysis of data (usually interim data) from subjects in the study. Analyses of the accumulating study data are performed at prospectively planned timepoints within the study, can be performed in a fully blinded manner or in an unblinded manner, and can occur with or without formal statistical hypothesis-testing."

Commonly used types of adaptive trials include standard group sequential design, sample size reestimation, drop-loser design, adaptive dose-finding study, and response-adaptive randomization (Chang 2007b).

In this chapter, our discussions will focus on the hypothesis-based adaptive designs. There are many different methods for hypothesis-based adaptive designs, for which we are going to present a unified approach using combinations of stagewise p-values. There are four major components of adaptive designs in the frequentist paradigm: (1) type-I error rate or α-control: determination of stopping boundaries, (2) type-II error rate β: calculation of power or sample size, (3) trial monitoring and

M. Chang, *Modern Issues and Methods in Biostatistics*, Statistics for Biology and Health, DOI 10.1007/978-1-4419-9842-2_4, © Springer Science+Business Media, LLC 2011

adaptations: calculation of conditional power and making adaptations (e.g., sample size reestimation, stopping a trial, dropping an inferior arm); and (4) analysis after the completion of a trial: calculations of adjusted p-values, unbiased point estimates, and confidence intervals. The mathematical formulations for these components will be discussed.

4.1.2 Hypothesis-Based Adaptive Design

4.1.2.1 Stopping Boundary

Consider a clinical trial with K stages where at each stage a hypothesis test is performed, followed by some actions that are dependent on the analysis results. Such actions can be early futility or efficacy stopping, sample size reestimation, modification of randomization, or other adaptations. The objective of the trial (e.g., testing the efficacy of the experimental drug) can be formulated using a hypothesis test,

$$H_o \text{ versus } \bar{H}_o, \tag{4.1}$$

where H_o is the null hypothesis (e.g., $H_o : \delta \leq \delta_0$) with δ being the treatment difference and δ_0 a constant; the alternative hypothesis $\bar{H}_o$ is negation of H_o.

Generally, the test statistic T_k at the kth stage can be a function $\eta(p_1, p_2, \ldots, p_k)$ where p_i is the one-sided p-value calculated based on the ith stage subsample and $\eta(p_1, p_2, \ldots, p_k)$ is a strictly increasing function of all p_i ($i = 1, 2, \ldots k$).

The stopping rules are given by

$$\begin{cases} \text{stop for efficacy} & \text{if } T_k \leq \alpha_k, \\ \text{stop for futility} & \text{if } T_k > \beta_k, \\ \text{continue with adaptations} & \text{if } \alpha_k < T_k \leq \beta_k, \end{cases} \tag{4.2}$$

where $\alpha_k < \beta_k$ ($k = 1, \ldots, K - 1$) and $\alpha_K = \beta_K$. For convenience, α_k and β_k are called the efficacy and futility boundaries, respectively.

To reach the kth stage, a trial has to pass through the first to the $(k - 1)$th stages. Therefore, the conditional c.d.f. of T_k is given by

$$\psi_k(t) = \Pr(\alpha_1 < T_1 < \beta_1, \ldots, \alpha_{k-1} < T_{k-1} < \beta_{k-1}, T_k < t)$$

$$= \int_{\alpha_1}^{\beta_1} \cdots \int_{\alpha_{k-1}}^{\beta_{k-1}} \int_{-\infty}^{t} f_{T_1 \ldots T_k} \, dt_k \, dt_{k-1} \ldots dt_1, \tag{4.3}$$

where $f_{T_1 \ldots T_k}$ is the joint p.d.f. of $T_1, \ldots$, and T_k.

4.1.2.2 Type-I Error Control, *p*-value, and Power

When H_0 is true, $\psi_k(t)$ is the stagewise *p*-value p_c if the trial stopped at the kth stage,

$$p_c(t;k) = \psi_k(t|H_0). \qquad (4.4)$$

The stagewise error rate (α spent) π_k at the kth stage is given by

$$\pi_k = \psi_k(\alpha_k|H_0). \qquad (4.5)$$

The stagewise power of rejecting H_o at the kth stage is given by

$$\varpi_k = \psi_k(\alpha_k|H_a). \qquad (4.6)$$

When efficacy is claimed at a certain stage, the trial is stopped. Therefore, the type-I errors at different stages are mutually exclusive. Hence the experiment-wise type-I error rate can be written as

$$\alpha = \sum_{k=1}^{K} \pi_k. \qquad (4.7)$$

Similarly, the power can be written as

$$power = \sum_{k=1}^{K} \varpi_k. \qquad (4.8)$$

Equation 4.5 is the key to determining the stopping boundaries for adaptive designs.

There are several possible definitions of (adjusted) *p*-values. Here we are most interested in the so-called stagewise-ordering *p*-values, defined as

$$p(t;k) = \sum_{i=1}^{k-1} \pi_i + p_c(t;k). \qquad (4.9)$$

The adjusted *p*-value is a measure of overall statistical strength against H_o. The later the H_o is rejected, the larger the adjusted *p*-value is and the weaker the statistical evidence (against H_o) is. A late rejection leading to a larger *p*-value is reasonable because the alpha at earlier stages has been spent. An important characteristic of the adjusted *p*-value is that when the test statistic t is on stopping boundary a_k, p_k must be equal to the alpha spent so far.

4.1.2.3 Selection of Test Statistics

There are many possible forms to choose for the test statistic $\eta(p_1, p_2, \ldots, p_k)$, such as:

1. linear combination (Chang 2007b),

$$T_k = \Sigma_{i=1}^k w_{ki} p_i, \ k = 1, \ldots, K, \text{ where constants } w_{ki} > 0, \tag{4.10}$$

2. product of stagewise p-values (Fisher combination, Bauer and Kohne 1994),

$$T_k = \prod_{i=1}^k p_i, \ k = 1, \ldots, K, \tag{4.11}$$

   and
3. linear combination of inverse-normal stagewise p-values (Lehmacher and Wassmer 1999; Cui et al. 1999; Lan and DeMets 1987)

$$T_k = \Sigma_{i=1}^k w_{ki} \Phi^{-1} (1 - p_i), \ k = 1, \ldots, K, \tag{4.12}$$

where weight, $w_{ki} > 0$, satisfying $\sum_{i=1}^k w_{ki}^2 = 1$, can be a constant or function of data from previous stages and K is the number of analyses planned in the trial. Note that p_k is the naive p-value from the subsample at the kth stage, while $p_c(t; k)$ and $p(t; k)$ are stagewise and stagewise-ordering p-values, respectively.

4.1.2.4 Method for Determining Stopping Boundary

After selection of the test statistic, we can determine the stopping boundaries α_k and β_k by using (4.3) and (4.7) under the null hypothesis (4.1). Once the stopping boundaries are determined, the power and sample size under a particular H_a can be obtained using (4.3) and (4.8) in conjunction with the Monte Carlo method. We can choose one of the following approaches to fully determine the stopping boundaries:

1. *Classical method:* Choose certain types of functions for the boundaries α_k and β_k. The advantage of using a stopping boundary function is that there are only limited parameters in the function to be determined. After the parameters are determined, the stopping boundaries are then fully determined, regardless of the number of stages. The commonly used boundaries are O'Brien and Fleming (1979), Pocock (1977), and Wang and Tsiatis (1987). The Wang-Tsiatis' boundary was originally defined on the standardized z-scale but can equivalently be defined as $\alpha_k = 1 - \Phi(ct_k^\Delta - 0.5)$ on the p-scale, where $t_k = k/K$ or the sample size fraction (information time); c is a constant determined by the significance level α. When the parameter $\Delta = 0$ and 0.5, the Wang-Tsiatis boundary will degenerate to the O'Brien-Fleming and Pocock boundaries, respectively (Chang 2008).

2. *Error-spending method:* Choose certain forms of functions for π_k such that $\Sigma_{k=1}^{K} \pi_k = \alpha$. Traditionally, the cumulative quantity $\pi_k^* = \Sigma_{i=1}^{k} \pi_i$ is called the error-spending function, which can be either a function of stage k or the so-called information time based on the sample size fraction. After the function π_k or equivalently π_k^* is determined, the stopping boundaries α_k and β_k ($k = 1, \ldots, K$) can be determined using (4.3), (4.5), and (4.7).
3. *Nonparametric method:* Choose non-parametric stopping boundaries, i.e., no function is assumed. Instead, use computer simulations to determine the stopping boundaries via a trial and error method. The non-parametric method does not allow for changes to the number and timing of the interim analyses.
4. *Conditional error function method:* One can rewrite the stagewise error rate for a two-stage design as

$$\pi_2 = \psi_2(\alpha_2 | H_o) = \int_{\alpha_1}^{\beta_1} A(p_1)\,dp_1, \qquad (4.13)$$

where $A(p_1)$ is called the conditional error function. For a given α_1 and β_1, by carefully selecting $A(p_1)$, the overall α control can be met (Proschan and Hunsberger 1995). However, $A(p_1)$ cannot be an arbitrary monotonic function of p_1. In fact, when the test statistic (e.g., sum of p-values, Fisher's combination of p-values, or inverse-normal p-values) and constant stopping boundaries are determined, the conditional error function $A(p_1)$ is determined. For example, for the three commonly used adaptive methods, MSP, MPP, and MINP, $A(p_1)$ is given by

$$\begin{cases} A(p_1) = \alpha_2 - p_1 \text{ for MSP}, \\ A(p_1) = \alpha_2/p_1 \text{ for MPP}, \\ A(p_1) = \left(\alpha_2 - \sqrt{n_1}p_1\right)/\sqrt{n_2} \text{ for MINP}, \end{cases} \qquad (4.14)$$

where n_i is the subsample size for the ith stage.

On the other hand, if an arbitrary (monotonic) $A(p_1)$ is chosen for a test statistic (e.g., sum of p-values or inverse-normal p-values), the stopping boundaries α_2 and β_2 may not be constants anymore. Instead, they are usually functions of p_1.
5. *Conditional error method:* In this method, for a given α_1 and β_1, $A(p_1)$ is calculated on the fly or in real time, and only for the observed p_1. Adaptations can be made under the condition that $A(p_1 | H_o)$ is kept unchanged.

Note that α_k and β_k are usually only functions of stage k or information time, but they can be functions of response data from previous stages, i.e., $\alpha_k = \alpha_k(t_1, \ldots, t_{k-1})$ and $\beta_k = \beta_k(t_1, \ldots, t_{k-1})$. In fact using variable transformation of one test statistic to another, the stopping boundaries often change from response-independent to response-dependent. For example, in MSP, we use stopping boundary $p_1 + p_2 \leq \alpha_2$, which implies that $p_1 p_2 \leq \alpha_2 p_2 - p_2^2$. In other words, the MSP stopping boundary at the second stage, $p_1 + p_2 \leq \alpha_2$, is equivalent to the MPP boundary at the second stage, $p_1 p_2 \leq \alpha_2 p_2 - p_2^2$, a response-dependent stopping boundary.

6. *Recursive design method:* Based on Müller and Shäfer's conditional error principle, this method recursively constructs two-stage designs at the time of interim analysis, making the method a simple but very flexible approach to a general K-stage design (Müller and Shäfer 2004; Chang 2007a).

4.2 Adaptive Design Methods

4.2.1 *p-value Weighting Approach*

Chang (2007b) proposed an adaptive design method in which the test statistic is defined as the sum of the stagewise p-values (MSP),

$$T_k = \Sigma_{i=1}^k p_i, \ k = 1, \dots, K, \tag{4.15}$$

where p_i is a stagewise p-value that is calculated based on a subsample (not a cumulative sample) from the ith stage. The type-I error rate at stage k can be expressed as (assume $\beta_i \leq \alpha_{i+1}, i = 1 \dots$)

$$\pi_k = \int_{\alpha_1}^{\beta_1} \int_{\alpha_2-p_1}^{\beta_2} \cdots \int_{\alpha_{k-1}-\Sigma_{i=1}^{k-2} p_i}^{\beta_{k-1}} \int_0^{\alpha_k - \Sigma_{i=1}^{k-1} p_i} \mathrm{d}p_k \mathrm{d}p_{k-1} \cdots \mathrm{d}p_2 \mathrm{d}p_1, \tag{4.16}$$

where for the nonfutility binding rule, let $\beta_i = \alpha_k$, $i = 1 \dots$, i.e.,

$$\pi_k = \int_{\alpha_1}^{\alpha_k} \int_{\max(0,\alpha_2-p_1)}^{\alpha_k} \cdots \int_{\max(0,\alpha_{k-1}-\Sigma_{i=1}^{k-2} p_i)}^{\alpha_K}$$
$$\int_0^{\max(0,\alpha_k - \Sigma_{i=1}^{k-1} p_i)} \mathrm{d}p_k \mathrm{d}p_{k-1} \cdots \mathrm{d}p_2 \mathrm{d}p_1 \tag{4.17}$$

We set up $\alpha_k > \alpha_{k-1}$, and if $p_i > \alpha_k$, then analysis is necessary for stages $i + 1$ to k because there is no chance to reject H_o at these stages.

To control the overall type-I error, it is required that

$$\Sigma_{i=1}^K \pi_i = \alpha. \tag{4.18}$$

Theoretically, (4.17) can be carried out for any k. Here, we provide the analytical forms for $k = 1$–3, which should satisfy most practical needs.

$$\begin{cases} \pi_1 = \alpha_1, \\ \pi_2 = \dfrac{1}{2} (\alpha_2 - \alpha_1)^2, \\ \pi_3 = \alpha_1 \alpha_2 \alpha_3 + \dfrac{1}{3}\alpha_2^3 + \dfrac{1}{6}\alpha_3^3 - \dfrac{1}{2}\alpha_1 \alpha_2^2 - \dfrac{1}{2}\alpha_1 \alpha_3^2 - \dfrac{1}{2}\alpha_2^2 \alpha_3. \end{cases} \tag{4.19}$$

Table 4.1 Stopping
boundaries with MMP

α_1	0.0010	0.0025	0.005	0.010	0.015	0.020
α_2	0.1100	0.1073	0.1025	0.0916	0.0782	0.0600

Note: One-sided $\alpha = 0.025$, $\alpha_2 = \beta_1 = \beta_2$

It might be convenient to define the test statistic as (we refer to this as MMP)

$$T_k = \frac{1}{k}\Sigma_{i=1}^{k}p_i, \ k = 1, \ldots, K, \tag{4.20}$$

so that T_k will be bounded by $[0, 1]$. The stopping boundary corresponding to (4.20) can be obtained by modifying (4.19), where α_k is replaced by $k\alpha_k$ (question for readers: why?); that is,

$$\begin{cases} \pi_1 = \alpha_1, \\ \pi_2 = \frac{1}{2}(2\alpha_2 - \alpha_1)^2, \\ \pi_3 = 6\alpha_1\alpha_2\alpha_3 + \frac{8}{3}\alpha_2^3 + \frac{9}{2}\alpha_3^3 - 2\alpha_1\alpha_2^2 - \frac{9}{2}\alpha_1\alpha_3^2 - 6\alpha_2^2\alpha_3. \end{cases} \tag{4.21}$$

π_i can be viewed as the error spent at the ith stage, which can be predetermined individually or specified as the error-spending function $\pi_k = f(k)$. The stopping boundary can be solved recursively. Specifically, determine π_i $(i = 1, 2, \ldots, K)$; from $\pi_1 = \alpha_1$, solve for α_1; from $\pi_2 = \frac{1}{2}(2\alpha_2 - \alpha_1)^2$, obtain $\alpha_2, \ldots$; and from $\pi_K = \pi_K(\alpha_1, \ldots, \alpha_{K-1})$, obtain α_K.

See Table 4.1 for numerical examples of the stopping boundaries defined by (4.21).

The stagewise-ordering p-value is given by

$$p(t;k) = \begin{cases} t, & k = 1, \\ \alpha_1 + \frac{1}{2}(2t - \alpha_1)^2, & k = 2, \end{cases} \tag{4.22}$$

where $t = p_1$ if the trial stops at stage 1 and $t = \frac{1}{2}(p_1 + p_2)$ if it stops at stage 2.

It is interesting to know that when $p_1 > \alpha_2$, there is no point in continuing the trial because $p_1 + p_2 > p_1 > \alpha_2$, and futility should be claimed. Therefore, statistically it is always a good idea to choose $\beta_1 \le \alpha_2$. However, because the nonbinding futility rule is adopted currently by the regulatory bodies, it is better to use the stopping boundaries with $\beta_1 = \alpha_2$.

The conditional power is the conditional probability of rejecting the null hypothesis during the rest of the trial based on the observed interim data. The conditional power for a two-stage design with MMP is given by

$$cP = 1 - \Phi\left(z_{1-2\alpha_2+p_1} - \frac{\hat{\delta}}{\hat{\sigma}}\sqrt{\frac{n_2}{2}}\right), \ \alpha_1 < p_1 \le \beta_1, \tag{4.23}$$

where $n_2 =$ sample size per group at stage 2; $\hat{\delta}$ and $\hat{\sigma}$ are observed treatment difference and standard deviation, respectively.

To obtain power and conditional power for a general K-stage design using MMP, Monte Carlo simulation can be used (Chang 2007b, 2010).

4.2.2 Fisher Combination Approach

This method is referred to as MPP. The test statistic in this method is based on the product (Fisher's combination) of the stagewise p-values from the subsamples (Bauer and Kohne 1994; Bauer and Rohmel 1995), defined as

$$T_k = \Pi_{i=1}^k p_i, \ k = 1, \dots, K, \tag{4.24}$$

$$\pi_k = \int_{\alpha_1}^{\beta_1} \int_{\alpha_2/p_1}^{\beta_2} \int_{\alpha_3/(p_1 p_2)}^{\beta_3} \cdots \int_{\alpha_{k-1}/(p_1 \cdots p_{k-2})}^{\beta_{k-1}} \int_0^{\alpha_k/(p_1 \cdots p_{k-1})} dp_k \cdots dp_1. \tag{4.25}$$

For a design without a futility boundary, we choose $\beta_1 = 1$. It is interesting to know that when $p_1 < \alpha_2$, there is no point in continuing the trial because $p_1 p_2 < p_1 < \alpha_2$ and efficacy should be claimed. Therefore it is suggested that we should choose $\beta_1 > \alpha_2$ and $\alpha_1 > \alpha_2$. In general, if $p_k \le \max(a_k, \dots \alpha_n)$, stop the trial. In other words, α_k should monotonically decrease in k. The relationships between error spent π_i and stopping boundary α_i at the ith stage are given up to three stages:

$$\begin{cases} \pi_1 = \alpha_1, \\ \pi_2 = \alpha_2 \ln \dfrac{1}{\alpha_1}, \\ \pi_3 = \alpha_3 \left(\ln \alpha_2 - \dfrac{1}{2} \ln \alpha_1 \right) \ln \alpha_1. \end{cases} \tag{4.26}$$

The closed form of π_k for any K-stage design with Fisher's combination is provided by Wassmer (1999). Numerical examples of stopping boundaries for two-stage adaptive designs with MPP are presented in Table 4.2.

The stagewise-ordering p-value for a two-stage design can be obtained using

$$p(t;k) = \begin{cases} t, & k = 1, \\ \alpha_1 - t \ln \alpha_1, & k = 2, \end{cases} \tag{4.27}$$

where $t = p_1$ if the trial stops at stage 1 ($k = 1$) and $t = p_1 p_2$ if the trial stops at stage 2 ($k = 2$).

The conditional power is given by Chang (2007b)

$$cP = 1 - \Phi \left(z_{1 - \frac{\alpha_2}{p_1}} - \frac{\hat{\delta}}{\hat{\sigma}} \sqrt{\frac{n_2}{2}} \right), \ \alpha_1 < p_1 \le \beta_1. \tag{4.28}$$

Table 4.2 Stopping boundaries with MPP

α_1	0.0010	0.0025	0.005	0.010	0.015	0.020
α_2	0.0035	0.0038	0.0038	0.0033	0.0024	0.0013

Note: One-sided $\alpha = 0.025$

4.2.3 *p-value Inversion Approach*

This method is based on inverse-normal p-values (MINP) in which the test statistic at the kth stage, T_k, is a linear combination of the inverse-normal of stagewise p-values. MINP (Lecherman and Wassmer 1999) can be viewed as a general method that includes the standard group sequential design and Cui-Hung-Wang method for sample size reestimation (Cui et al. 1999) as special cases.

Let z_k be the stagewise normal test statistic at the kth stage. In general, $z_i = \Phi^{-1}(1 - p_i)$, where p_i is the stagewise p-value from the ith stage subsample.

In a group sequential design, the test statistic can be expressed as

$$T_k^* = \sum_{i=1}^{k} w_{ki} z_i, \tag{4.29}$$

where the prefixed weights w_{ki} satisfy the equality $\sum_{i=1}^{k} w_{ki}^2 = 1$.

Note that when w_{ki} is fixed, the standard multivariate normal distribution of $\{T_1^*, \dots, T_k^*\}$ will not change regardless of adaptations as long as z_i $(i = 1, \dots, k)$ has the standard normal distribution. To be consistent with the unified formations, in which the test statistic is on the p-scale, we use the transformation $T_k = 1 - \Phi(T_k^*)$ such that

$$T_k = 1 - \Phi\left(\sum_{i=1}^{k} w_{ki} z_i\right), \tag{4.30}$$

where $\Phi = $ the standard normal c.d.f. The corresponding stopping rules for the test statistic (4.30) are given in (4.2).

The stopping boundary and power for MINP can be calculated using numerical integration or computer simulation (see Chap. 9). Table 4.3 gives numerical examples of stopping boundaries for two-stage adaptive designs generated using ExpDesign Studio^{TM}5.0 (www.ctrisoft.net).

The conditional power for a two-stage design with MINP is given by

$$cP = 1 - \Phi\left(\frac{z_{1-\alpha_2} - w_1 z_{1-p_1}}{w_2} - \frac{\hat{\delta}}{\hat{\sigma}}\sqrt{\frac{n_2}{2}}\right), \quad \alpha_1 < p_1 \leq \beta_1, \tag{4.31}$$

where weights satisfy $w_1^2 + w_2^2 = 1$.

Table 4.3 Stopping
boundaries with MINP

α_1	0.0010	0.0025	0.0050	0.0100	0.0150	0.0200
α_2	0.0247	0.0240	0.0226	0.0189	0.0143	0.0087

Note: One-sided $\alpha = .025$, $w_1 = w_2$

4.2.4 Error-Spending Approach

MINPs have fixed weights w_{ki} regardless of the changes in the timing of the interim analyses. For example, if the equal weights for all stages were initially decided, then whether the interim analysis was performed on 10 or 80% of the patients, the weights will not change. Theoretically we can change the weights without peeking at the data, which is exactly the notion of the so-called error-spending method (Lan and DeMets 1987).

If we define the error function as

$$\alpha^*(k) = \sum_{i=1}^{k} \pi_i, \qquad (4.32)$$

then the familywise type-I error is controlled because $\alpha^*(K) = \alpha$.

Because $\pi_k > 0$ is arbitrary as long as $\sum_{k=1}^{K} \pi_k = \alpha$ (or smaller than α), $\alpha^*(k)$ can be any nondecreasing scale function with $\alpha^*(K) = 1$. This is why MSP, MMP, MPP are flexible regarding π_k or $\alpha^*(k)$ selection. These methods are valid if the total number of analyses K is modified but not based on the interim trial results, p_k.

Similarly, an error-spending function can also be used for MINP as long as the timing and the total number of analyses are not dependent on interim results. The MINP can be expanded (i.e., allow the weights w_{ki} to be modified as long as they are not dependent on the interim results from the trial, e.g., $w_{ki} = \sqrt{\frac{n_i}{N_K}}$, where n_i is the subsample size per group from stage i and N_k is the cumulative sample size up to (including) stage k). Historically, the error-spending approach based on MINP with weight $w_{ki} = \sqrt{\frac{n_i}{N_K}}$ was first developed by Lan and DeMets (1987) using a property of a Brownian motion (Wiener process) with the error-spending function

$$\alpha^*(I_k) = \begin{cases} 2\left[1 - \Phi\left(\frac{z_{1-\alpha/2}}{\sqrt{I_k}}\right)\right], & \text{for } 0 < I_k \leq 1, \\ 0, \text{ for } I_k = 0. \end{cases} \qquad (4.33)$$

This error-spending function $\alpha^*(t)$ is an increasing function in information time $I_k = N_k/N_{\max}$ ($N_{\max}$ = the maximum sample size) and satisfies the conditions $\alpha^*(0) = 0$ and $\alpha^*(1) = \alpha$, the one-sided significance level. Note that

$$\sum_{i=1}^{K} \pi_i = \sum_{k=1}^{K} \left[\alpha^*(I_k) - \alpha^*(I_{k-1})\right] = \alpha^*(1) - \alpha^*(0) = \alpha, \qquad (4.34)$$

and thus familywise error is controlled.

Table 4.4 OF-like error-spending stopping boundaries

I_k	0.3	0.4	0.5	0.6	0.7	0.8
α_1	0.00004	0.00039	0.00153	0.00381	0.00738	0.01221
α_2	0.22347	0.02490	0.02454	0.02380	0.02271	0.02142

Note: One-sided $\alpha = .025$. Computed by ExpDesign Studio™5.0

When $\alpha^*(I_k) = \alpha^*(I_{k-1})$, the kth stage interim analysis is used either for futility stopping or modifying the design (such as its randomization) but not for efficacy stopping. Note that (4.33) is an error-spending function very similar to the O'Brien-Fleming stopping boundaries (called OF-like stopping boundary). Other commonly used error-spending functions include the Pocock-like function $\alpha^*(t) = \alpha \ln[1 + (e - 1)t]$ (Kim and DeMets 1992) and power family $\alpha^*(t) = \alpha t^{\theta}, \theta > 0$.

For the two-stage design with OF-like error-spending function (4.33), the stopping boundaries are given in Table 4.4. Please keep in mind that OF-like and O'Brien-Fleming stopping boundaries are two types of stopping boundaries that are very similar but not identical (Proschan et al. 2006; Chang 2008).

We should emphasize that the error-spending method is valid only when the time and the number of interim analyses as well as the weight w_{ki} change are independent of interim analysis results. It is also important to keep in mind that the error-spending function has to be predetermined before the first interim analysis. In other words, the error-spending function should also be independent of interim data. For example, the stopping boundaries in Tables 4.3 and 4.4 are both valid, but we have to predetermine which one to use before we review the interim results.

4.3 Evaluation and Analysis of Adaptive Design

4.3.1 Evaluation Matrix

4.3.1.1 Stopping Probabilities

The stopping probability at each stage is an important property of an adaptive design because it provides the information about time-to-market. The stopping probabilities are also used to calculate the expected samples that measure the average cost or efficiency of the trial design.

There are two types of stopping probabilities: unconditional probability of stopping to claim efficacy (reject H_o) and unconditional probability of stopping to claim futility (accept H_o). The former is called the efficacy stopping probability (ESP), and the latter is called the futility stopping probability (FSP). From (4.3), it is obvious that the ESP at the kth stage is given by

$$ESP_k = \psi_k(\alpha_k) \tag{4.35}$$

and the FSP at the kth stage is given by

$$FSP_k = 1 - \psi_k(\beta_k).$$ (4.36)

4.3.1.2 Expected Duration of an Adaptive Trial

The expected trial duration is definitely an important feature of an adaptive design. The conditionally (on the efficacy claim) expected trial duration is given by

$$\bar{t}_e = \sum_{k=1}^{K} ESP_k \, t_k,$$ (4.37)

where t_k is the time from the first patient in until the kth interim analysis.

The conditionally (on the futility claim) expected trial duration is given by

$$\bar{t}_f = \sum_{k=1}^{K} FSP_k \, t_k.$$ (4.38)

The unconditionally expected trial duration is given by

$$\bar{t} = \sum_{k=1}^{K} (ESP_k + FSP_k) \, t_k.$$ (4.39)

4.3.1.3 Expected Sample Sizes

The expected sample size is a function of the treatment difference and its variability, which are unknowns. Therefore, the expected sample size is really based on hypothetical values of the parameters. For this reason, it is important to calculate the expected sample size under various values of the parameters. The total expected sample size can be expressed as

$$N_{\exp} = \sum_{k=1}^{K} n_k \, (ESP_k + FSP_k) = \sum_{k=1}^{K} n_k \, (1 + \psi_k(\alpha_k) - \psi_k(\beta_k)),$$ (4.40)

where n_k is the sample size at stage k. Equation 4.40 can also be written as

$$N_{\exp} = N_{\max} - \sum_{k=1}^{K} n_k \, (\psi_k(\beta_k) - \psi_k(\alpha_k)),$$ (4.41)

where $N_{\max} = \sum_{k=1}^{K} n_k$ is the maximum sample size.

4.3.1.4 Conditional Power and Futility Index

The conditional power is the conditional probability of rejecting the null hypothesis during the rest of the trial based on the observed interim data so far. The conditional power is commonly used for monitoring an ongoing trial. Similar to the ESP and FSP, conditional power is dependent on the population parameters or treatment effect and its variability. The conditional power at the kth stage is the sum of the probability of rejecting the null hypothesis at stage $k + 1$ through K (K does not have to be predetermined), given the observed data from stages 1 through k,

$$cP_k = \sum_{j=k+1}^{K} \Pr\left(\cap_{i=k+1}^{j-1} (a_i < T_i < \beta_i) \cap T_j \le \alpha_j \,|\, \cap_{i=1}^{k} T_i = t_i \right), \quad (4.42)$$

where t_i is the observed test statistic T_i at the ith stage. For a two-stage design, the conditional power can be expressed as

$$cP_1 = \Pr\left(T_2 \le \alpha_2 | t_1 \right). \quad (4.43)$$

Specific formulations of conditional power for two-stage designs with MSP, MPP, and MINP were provided in earlier sections.

The futility index is defined as the conditional probability of accepting the null hypothesis:

$$FI_k = 1 - cP_k. \quad (4.44)$$

Computer algorithms and programs for calculating the operating characteristics of an adaptive design can be found elsewhere (Chang 2007b, 2010).

4.3.2 Analysis of Adaptive Trial Data

4.3.2.1 Parameter Estimation

Unbiased estimation of parameters is challenging adaptive design. Let's start with a two-stage standard group sequential design. Consider the hypothesis test for mean μ:

$$H_o : \mu \le 0 \text{ versus } H_a : \mu > 0.$$

Let x_{ij} be the independent observations from the jth patient at the kth stage ($k = 1, 2$ and $j = 1, \ldots, n_i$). Assume x_{ij} has the normal distribution $N\left(\mu, \sigma^2\right)$ with known σ. Denote by $\bar{x}_k$ the stagewise sample mean at the kth stage (not based on cumulative data), thus $\bar{x}_1$ and $\bar{x}_2$ are independent. The test statistic at the first stage of the standard group sequential design can be written as $T_1 = \bar{x}_1\sqrt{n_1}/\sigma$, where n_1 is the sample size at the first stage. The stopping rule at the first stage is: stop the trial if $T_1 \ge c_1$ ($p_1 \le \alpha_1$ on the p-scale) and continue otherwise. It is obvious that $T_1 = \bar{x}_1\sqrt{n_1}/\sigma \ge c_1$ implies $x_1 \ge \sigma c_1/\sqrt{n_1}$.

The expectation of the conditional mean at the first stage is

$$\mu_1 = \frac{\int_{\sigma c_1/\sqrt{n_1}}^{\infty} \bar{x}_1 f_{\bar{X}_1}(\bar{x}_1)\, d\bar{x}_1}{\int_{\sigma c_1/\sqrt{n_1}}^{\infty} f_{\bar{X}_1}(\bar{x}_1)\, d\bar{x}_1}. \tag{4.45}$$

The expectation of the conditional mean at the second stage is

$$\mu_2 = \frac{\int_{-\infty}^{\sigma c_1/\sqrt{n_1}} \int_{-\infty}^{\infty} \frac{\bar{x}_1 n_1 + \bar{x}_2 n_2}{n_1 + n_2} f_{\bar{X}_1}(\bar{x}_1) f_{\bar{X}_2}(\bar{x}_2)\, d\bar{x}_1 d\bar{x}_2}{\int_{-\infty}^{\sigma c_1/\sqrt{n_1}} f_{\bar{X}_1}(\bar{x}_1)\, d\bar{x}_1}$$

$$= \frac{\int_{-\infty}^{\sigma c_1/\sqrt{n_1}} \frac{n_1 \bar{x}_1 + n_2 \mu}{n_1 + n_2} f_{\bar{X}_1}(\bar{x}_1)\, d\bar{x}_1}{\int_{-\infty}^{\sigma c_1/\sqrt{n_1}} f_{\bar{X}_1}(\bar{x}_1)\, d\bar{x}_1}. \tag{4.46}$$

For normal distribution $f_{\bar{X}_k}(\bar{x}_1) = N\left(\bar{X}_k; \mu, \sigma^2/n_i\right)$, we have

$$\mu_1 = \frac{1}{1 - \Phi_0(c_*)} \int_{\sigma c_1/\sqrt{n_1}}^{\infty} \bar{x}_1 \frac{1}{\sqrt{2\pi\sigma^2/n_1}} e^{\frac{-(\bar{x}_1 - \mu)^2 n_1}{2\sigma^2}}\, d\bar{x}_1$$

$$= \mu + \frac{\sigma \exp\left(-\frac{c_*^2}{2}\right)}{[1 - \Phi_0(c_*)]\sqrt{2\pi n_1}}, \tag{4.47}$$

where $c_* = c_1 - \mu\sqrt{n_1}/\sigma$.

If n_2 is independent of x_1 (i.e., there is no sample size adjustment), then

$$\mu_2 = \frac{1}{\Phi_0(c_*)} \int_{-\infty}^{\sigma c_1/\sqrt{n_1}} \frac{n_1 \bar{x}_1 + n_2 \mu}{n_1 + n_2} \frac{1}{\sqrt{2\pi/n_1}} e^{\frac{-(\bar{x}_1 - \mu)^2 n_1}{2\sigma^2}}\, d\bar{x}_1$$

$$= \frac{n_1}{n_1 + n_2}\left[\mu - \frac{\sigma}{\Phi_0(c_*)\sqrt{2\pi n_1}} \exp\left(-\frac{c_*^2}{2}\right)\right] + \frac{n_2}{n_1 + n_2}\mu$$

$$= \mu - \frac{n_1 \sigma \exp\left(-\frac{c_*^2}{2}\right)}{(n_1 + n_2)\Phi_0(c_*)\sqrt{2\pi n_1}}. \tag{4.48}$$

From (4.47) to (4.48), the expectation of the conditional mean can be expressed as

$$\mu_{naive} = [1 - \Phi_0(c_*)]\mu_1 + \Phi_0(c_*)\mu_2 = \mu + \frac{n_2}{n_1 + n_2}\frac{\sigma}{\sqrt{2\pi n_1}}\exp\left(-\frac{c_*^2}{2}\right). \tag{4.49}$$

The bias can be calculated as

$$\Delta_{bias} = \mu_{naive} - \mu = \frac{n_2}{n_1 + n_2}\frac{\sigma}{\sqrt{2\pi n_1}}\exp\left(-\frac{c_*^2}{2}\right) < \frac{\sigma}{\sqrt{2\pi n_1}}. \tag{4.50}$$

To calculate the bias, the standard normal c.d.f. can be approximated by

$$\Phi_0(c) = 1 - \frac{(c^2 + 5.575192695c + 12.77436324)\exp\left(-c^2/2\right)}{\sqrt{2\pi}c^3 + 14.38718147c^2 + 31.53531977c + 2(12.77436324)}.$$

$$(4.51)$$

The error of approximation (4.51) is less than 1.9×10^{-5} over $0 \le c < \infty$. The largest error occurs when c ranges from 1.03 to 1.04 (Yun 2009).

In my view, the conditional estimate is more important than the unconditional estimate. The reason is simple: We know from (4.47) to (4.48) that $\bar{x}_1$ is biased upward and $\bar{x}_2$ is biased downward. If the trial stops at stage 1, we should report $\bar{x}_1$ with the adjustment given by (4.47). On the other hand, if the trial stops at stage 2, we should report $\bar{x}_2$ with the adjustment given by (4.48). It doesn't make sense to report x_k with the overall adjustment given by (4.49), especially when the trial stops at stage 2, and adjust x_2 downward using (4.49), knowing that x_2 is already biased downward. Although both the conditional and overall adjustments can provide unbiased estimates, the conditional adjustment makes much more sense.

Equations 4.45–4.50 are valid for MINP, MSP, and MPP because the naive mean is determined by the c_1 (or α_1) and n_1 independent of the definition of the test statistic for the two-stage designs. In other words, for two-stage designs, there are always equivalent stopping boundaries for any two adaptive design methods (MSP, MPP, MINP). However, this conclusion is applicable to a design with more than two stages because such equivalent boundaries don't exist in general.

In general K-stage design, the expectation of the unconditional mean at the nth stage is

$$\mu_n = \frac{\int_{\Omega_1} \cdots \int_{\Omega_{n-1}} \int_{-\infty}^{\infty} \frac{\bar{x}_1 n_1 + \cdots + \bar{x}_n n_n}{n_1 + \cdots + n_n} f_{\bar{X}_1 \cdots \bar{X}_n}(\bar{x}_1, \ldots, \bar{x}_n)\, d\bar{x}_1 \ldots d\bar{x}_n}{\int_{\Omega_1} \cdots \int_{\Omega_{n-1}} \int_{-\infty}^{\infty} f_{\bar{X}_1 \cdots \bar{X}_n}(\bar{x}_1, \ldots, \bar{x}_n)\, d\bar{x}_1 \ldots d\bar{x}_n}, \quad (4.52)$$

where if $x_i \in \Omega_i$, the trial will continue to the $(i+1)$th stage.

For an adaptive design with a sample size adjustment, the calculation of bias is more complicated because sample size at the second stage, n_2, is a function of x_1. Several sample size reestimation rules have been proposed such as the conditional power approach. These rules will lead to different functions of $n_2(x_1)$, and integral (4.46) can only be carried out using numerical methods or simulations.

For a K-stage design, the integral (4.52) may sometimes be easier in p-scale, which may involve the p-value distribution under the alternative hypothesis. The p-value distribution can be easily derived.

Denote by $f^o(t) > 0$ and $f^a(t)$ the distributions of the test statistic T under the null hypothesis H_o and the alternative hypothesis H_a, respectively. The p-value for a one-sided test is defined as $p(t) = \int_t^{\infty} f^o(\tau)\, d\tau$. To derive the distribution of p-value $p(t)$ under H_a, we start with the c.d.f. identity: $F_T(t) = F_P(p(t))$.

Taking the derivative with respect to p (Kokoska and Zwillinger 2000, p. 40), we obtain the p.d.f. of the p-value:

$$P \sim f_P(p) = f^a(t) \frac{1}{|dp(t)/dt|} = \frac{f^a(t)}{f^o(t)}, \tag{4.53}$$

where t is function of p.

When the null hypothesis H_o is true, $f^a(t) = f^o(t)$, p-value P has a uniform distribution in $[0, 1]$.

4.3.2.2 Confidence Interval

The confidence interval calculation is usually complicated for adaptive designs. There are even several different versions of confidence intervals. The so-called repeated confidence interval at the k, RCI_k, consists of all possible values for the parameter for which the null hypothesis will not be rejected given the observed value. When x_{ij} is normally distributed and MINP, the RCI_k can be expressed as

$$(\bar{x} - c_k \sigma_{\bar{x}}, \bar{x} + c_k \sigma_{\bar{x}}),$$

in c_k is the stopping boundary at the kth stage and $\sigma_{\bar{x}}$ is the standard deviation of $\bar{x}$.

A general approach to obtain RCI_k numerically is through Monte Carlo simulations, but we are not going to discuss the simulation details here.

4.3.3 Comparison of Adaptive Design Methods

Different adaptive methods have different stopping boundaries, as shown in Fig. 4.1 for MSP, MPP, and MINP for two-stage adaptive designs. Because of the differences in the stopping boundaries, the same data can lead to different conclusions with different methods. For example, for data point A with $p_1 = 0.025$ and $p_2 = 0.008$, the null hypothesis is rejected by all three methods. However, for data point B with $p_1 = 0.01$ and $p_2 = 0.25$, the null hypothesis is rejected by MPP and MINP but not by MSP. Yet for data point C with $p_1 = 0.07$ and $p_2 = 0.12$, the null hypothesis is rejected by MSP but not by MPP or MINP.

Conditional power is an important feature of an adaptive design. The conditional power curves for different methods (MSP, MPP, and MINP) are constructed based on (4.23), (4.28), and (4.31) with $\alpha_1 = 0.005$ (Fig. 4.2). We know that when a trial is appropriately powered ($\sim 90\%$), the interim p-value is mostly near the target value $\alpha = 0.023$ (one-sided) or smaller. When a trial is underpowered, the interim p-value would be mostly near 0.1. Since an important goal of sample size reestimation is to save the trial when it is underpowered, we should focus on the conditional power when the interim p-value is near 0.1. As we can see from Fig. 4.2, MSP (or equivalently MMP) has higher power near one-sided $p_1 = 0.1$ than MPP

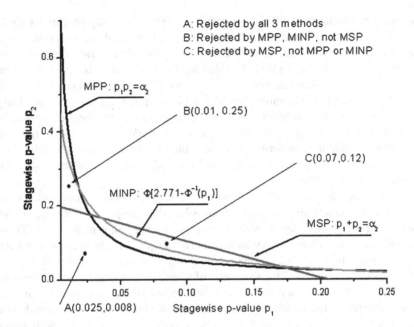

MPP: $p_1 p_2 = \alpha_2$

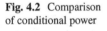

MINP: $\Phi[2.771 - \Phi^{-1}(p_1)]$

Fig. 4.1 Different stopping boundaries at stage 2

Fig. 4.2 Comparison of conditional power

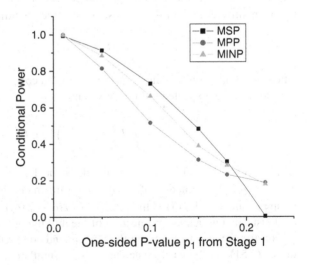

and MINP. For trial results with very large p-values, one-sided $p_1 > 0.18$ (or two-sided $p_1 > 0.36$), which is probably an indication of no or minimal treatment effect, the value of increasing the sample size is in great doubt even though MINP and MPP show a higher conditional power. Also, if the observed treatment effect $\hat{\delta}$ is very small or p-value p_1 is very large, we may be better off starting a new trial than continuing the current trial. Having said that, we may be curious about the reality of underpowered trials. In fact, the recent approval rate for NDAs (new drug applications) submitted to the FDA is about 40%. In contrast, the power for most phase-III trials is about 90%. Considering there are phase-III trials withdrawn by sponsors before they are rejected by the FDA, the failure rate of phase-III clinical trials is realistically more than 60%, which clearly indicates there are plenty of trials that are underpowered due to overestimating the treatment difference or underestimating its variance. The challenge is that we don't know which trials are underpowered, and thus uniformly increasing the sample size across all trials is not a wise practice. This is exactly the reason for introducing an adaptive design with sample size reestimation.

In additional to the conditional power, another commonly used method to compare different adaptive design methods is based on the power of the hypothesis test or equivalently the sample size (maximum or expected sample sizes). These types of criteria are often not very informative for adaptive design because they have not considered the magnitude of treatment difference and reduction in trial duration or time-to-market as well as the flexibility of adaptive designs that allow mitigation of the risks later. A better approach is to use the decision theory discussed in Chap. 2. To illustrate this, let's construct a utility function. We know that the magnitude of a drug effect (e.g., years of survival prolongation) often plays a critical role in terms of the benefit to patients and the profit of the drug maker. Because the true treatment effect (parameter δ for treatment difference) is not known, we use the observed treatment difference $\hat{\delta}$ for the purpose of constructing utility,

$$U = \hat{\delta}^r - C, \tag{4.54}$$

where $r > 0$ is a constant and C is the associated cost, which is often a function of sample size. The expected utility is given by

$$\bar{U} = \int I\left(\alpha - p\left(\hat{\delta}\right)\right) \hat{\delta} \, df\left(\hat{\delta}\right), \tag{4.55}$$

where $I(x)$ is an indication function with value 1 if $x \geq 0$ and 0 otherwise, the p-value $p(\hat{\delta})$ is a function of the observed treatment difference $\hat{\delta}$, α is the level of significance, and $f(\hat{\delta})$ is the p.d.f. of $\hat{\delta}$. $I(\alpha - p(\hat{\delta})) \geq 0$ implies achievement of statistical significance or rejection of the null hypothesis. The constant r should be constructed at least based on the clinical and commercial values. The expected utility (4.51) can be easily calculated using simulations after the cost and r are determined.

In Tables 4.5 and 4.6, we present some typical simulation results, both power and the utility U, respectively, for SSR trials. In the utility comparison, we use $r = 1$ and remove the cost factor by making the expected sample size (cost) the same.

From the tables, we can see that when the trial is underpowered, MSP is better than MPP and MINP in terms of power. MINP always has slightly higher power than MPP. When the power reaches around 70% or higher, MINP is better than

Table 4.5 Comparison of power from MSP (MMP), MPP, and MINP

δ/σ	0.1	0.15	0.2	0.25	0.3	0.35
$\bar{n}$	173	180	180	175	166	153
MSP(MMP)	**0.182**	**0.334**	**0.514**	0.686	0.824	0.915
MPP	0.161	0.308	0.496	0.685	0.835	0.928
MINP	0.161	0.315	0.507	**0.696**	**0.843**	**0.933**

Note: $\bar{n}$ = expected sample size, $\sigma = 1$. Best values are highlighted

Table 4.6 Expected utilities from MSP(MMP), MPP, and MINP

δ/σ	0.1	0.15	0.2	0.25	0.3	0.35
$\bar{n}$	173	180	180	175	166	153
MSP(MMP)	**9.62**	**17.9**	**27.8**	**37.6**	**46.0**	51.7
MPP	7.69	15.2	25.3	36.0	45.3	51.6
MINP	7.90	15.5	25.7	36.5	45.6	**51.8**

Note: $\bar{n}$ = expected sample size, $\sigma = 1$. Best values are highlighted

MSP or MMP (MSP) (Table 4.5). In terms of utility defined by (4.50) with $r = 1$, MMP (MSP) is better until the power reaches about 90% or higher (Table 4.6). The notion of the adaptive design with SSR reminds us to focus on situations where the trial is underpowered. As we discussed earlier, a majority of phase-III trials are underpowered. For this reason, among others, MMP or MSP is recommended for SSR. Keep in mind that the uniformly most powerful test for the classic design may not be applicable in the context of adaptive designs (see Sect. 4.5.2).

4.4 Adaptive Designs in Action

4.4.1 Sample Size Reestimation

Sample size determination is critical in clinical trial designs. It is estimated at about 5,000 patients per NDA on average (Mathieu 2008). The average cost per patient ranges from $20,000 USD to $50,000 USD. A small but adequate sample size will allow sponsors to use their resources efficiently, shorten the trial duration, and deliver the drug to the patients earlier.

From the efficacy point of view, sample size is often determined by the power for the hypothesis test of the primary endpoint. However, the challenge is to estimate precisely the treatment effect and its variability at the time of protocol design. If the effect size of the NME is overestimated or its variability is underestimated, the sample size will be underestimated and consequently the power will be too low to have a reasonable probability of detecting a clinically meaningful difference. On the other hand, if the effect size of the NME is underestimated or its variability is overestimated, the sample size will be overestimated and consequently the power will be unnecessarily higher, which could lead to unnecessary exposure of many patients to a potentially harmful compound when the drug in fact is not effective. The commonly used adaptive design, called sample size reestimation (SSR), emerged to provide a remedy for this problem.

An SSR design refers to an adaptive trial that allows for sample size adjustment or reestimation based on the review of interim analysis results. There are two types of sample size reestimation procedures, based on blinded and unblinded data. In the first scenario, the sample size adjustment is based on the (observed) pooled variance at the interim analysis to recalculate the required sample size, which does not require unblinding the data. In this scenario, the type-I error adjustment is usually negligible. In the second scenario, the effect size and its variability are re-assessed, and the sample size is adjusted based on the unblinded treatment information. The statistical method for the adjustment can be based on the observed effect size or the conditional power.

For a two-stage trial with two parallel groups, the sample size per group for the second stage, n_2, can be calculated based on the target conditional power

$$\begin{cases} n_2 = \dfrac{2\hat{\sigma}^2}{\hat{\delta}^2}\left(z_{1-\alpha_2+p_1}-z_{1-cP}\right)^2, & \text{for MSP,} \\ n_2 = \dfrac{2\hat{\sigma}^2}{\hat{\delta}^2}\left(z_{1-\alpha_2/p_1}-z_{1-cP}\right)^2, & \text{for MPP,} \qquad (4.56) \\ n_2 = \dfrac{2\hat{\sigma}^2}{\hat{\delta}^2}\left(\dfrac{z_{1-\alpha_2}}{w_2}-\dfrac{w_1}{w_2}z_{1-p_1}-z_{1-cP}\right)^2, & \text{for MINP,} \end{cases}$$

where, for the purpose of calculation, $\hat{\delta}$ and $\hat{\sigma}$ are taken to be the observed treatment effect and standard deviation at stage 1, and cP is the target conditional power.

For a general K-stage design, the sample size rule at the kth stage can be based on the observed treatment effect in comparison with the initial assessment:

$$n_j = \left(\frac{\delta}{\bar{\delta}}\right)^2 n_j^0, \; j=k,k+1,\ldots,K, \qquad (4.57)$$

where n_j^0 is the original sample size for the jth stage, δ is the initial assessment for the treatment effect, $\bar{\delta}$ is the updated assessment after interim analyses, given by

$$\bar{\delta} = \frac{\sum_{i=1}^k n_i \hat{\delta}_i}{\sum_{i=1}^k n_i} \text{ for MMP and MPP,} \qquad (4.58)$$

$$\bar{\delta} = \sum_{i=1}^k w_{ki}^2 \hat{\delta}_i \text{ for MINP.} \qquad (4.59)$$

The stagewise p-value p_c given by (4.4) can be calculated using the Monte Carlo method. Specifically, if the trial is stopped at the $\tilde{k}$th stage with $T_{\tilde{k}}=t_{\tilde{k}}$, then the percentage of simulated trials with $T_{\tilde{k}} > t_{\tilde{k}}$ out of all the simulated trials that reach the $\tilde{k}$th is equal to p_c. The stagewise-ordering p-value is given by (4.9), i.e.,

$$p = \sum_{i=1}^{\tilde{k}-1} \pi_i + p_c. \tag{4.60}$$

4.4.2 Adaptive Seamless Design

A seamless design is an adaptive design consisting of multiple treatment groups. At each stage, an interim analysis is performed and the losers (i.e., inferior treatment groups) are dropped based on prespecified criteria. If there is a control arm, it is usually also retained for the purpose of comparison. This type of design can be used in phase-II/III combined trials. A traditional phase-II clinical trial is typically a dose-response study, where the goal is to identify different response characteristics with different doses and select the appropriate dose level (or treatment groups) for the phase-III trials. This type of traditional design is not efficient with respect to time and resources because the phase-II efficacy data are not pooled with data from phase-III trials for the pivotal efficacy analysis. Therefore, it is desirable to combine phases II and III so that the data can be used efficiently. Such a combined study is called an adaptive seamless phase-II/III design, which is one of the most attractive adaptive designs.

For illustration purposes, let's discuss a simple but somewhat conservative approach for a two-stage seamless design (a seamless trial with more stages can be designed similarly). Assume there are m_1 comparisons among M treatment groups at the first stage. These comparisons can be expressed as m_1 null hypotheses:

$$H_{oi}, \ i = 1, \ldots, m_1. \tag{4.61}$$

The corresponding p-values are p_{1i}, $i = 1, \ldots m_1$. With Bonferroni adjustment (if there is a common control group for all the comparisons, the Dunnett method is better), the Bonferroni adjusted p-value is $\tilde{p}_{1i} = m_1 p_{1i}$. Decision rules are described as follows.

At stage 1, (1) if $m_1 p_{1i} \leq \alpha_1$, then reject H_{oi} ($i = 1, \ldots, m_1$); (2) if $m_1 p_{1i} > \beta_1$, then accept H_{oi} ($i = 1, \ldots, m_1$); (3) if $\beta_1 \geq m_1 p_{1 \min} > \alpha_1$, then continue to the second stage and make adaptations (e.g., adjust the sample size and add new arms) if necessary, where $p_{1 \min} = \min\{p_{11}, \ldots, p_{1m_1}\}$.

At stage 2, (1) choose a set of comparisons based on the corresponding p-values $\tilde{p}_{1i}$ or other criteria, such as safety, for the second stage. Assume there are m_2 comparisons at the second stage. (2) Based on the second-stage data, the naive stagewise p-values are calculated as p_{2i} and the Bonferroni adjusted p-value is $\tilde{p}_{2i} = m_2 p_{2i}$.

If MSP is used, the decision rules at stage 2 are: if $\tilde{p}_{1i} + \tilde{p}_{2i} = m_1 p_{1i} + m_2 p_{2i} \leq \alpha_2$, then reject H_{oi} $(i = 1, \ldots, m_2)$; otherwise, don't reject the null. The global null hypothesis can be rejected as long as $m_1 p_{1\,\text{min}} + m_2 p_{2\,\text{min}} \leq \alpha_2$, where $p_{2\,\text{min}} = \{p_{21}, \ldots, p_{2m_2}\}$.

Bauer and Kieser (1999) provided a two-stage method for this purpose, where investigators can terminate the trial entirely or drop a subset of treatment groups for lack of efficacy after the first stage. Shun et al. (2008) developed a simple method using normal approximation.

Let's consider a drop-loser design with three arms: A, B, and C (control). At the first stage, we perform two pairwise comparisons: A versus C and B versus C. The corresponding p-values are denoted by p_{1A} and p_{1B}. If $p_{1A} < p_{1B}$, arm B is dropped; otherwise, arm A is dropped. If we don't drop any arm, the p-values for the two comparisons at the final stage are denoted by p_A and p_B. It is obvious that p_{1A}, p_{1B}, p_A, and p_B are uniformly distributed under the global null that implies all three arms are equally effective. For the drop-loser design, we are interested in the statistic

$$Z^w = I_{AB} Z^A + (1 - I_{AB}) Z^B, \tag{4.62}$$

where $I_{AB} = 1$ if arm B is dropped; otherwise, $I_{AB} = 0$, $Z^A = \Phi(1 - p_A)$, and $Z^B = \Phi(1 - p_B)$.

Shun et al. (2008) found that, under the global null hypothesis, Z^w is approximately normally distributed with mean $E(Z^w) = \sqrt{\frac{\tau}{2\pi}}$ and $\text{var}(Z^w) = 1 - \frac{\tau}{2\pi}$, where the information time for the interim analysis $\tau = \frac{n_1}{n}$ (the sample size fraction at the interim analysis). Therefore they proposed as a test statistic

$$Z^{ws} = \frac{Z^w - \sqrt{\frac{\tau}{2\pi}}}{\sqrt{1 - \frac{\tau}{2\pi}}}, \tag{4.63}$$

which has approximately the standard normal distribution under the global null hypothesis that treatments A, B, and C have the same treatment effect.

The approximate p-value hence can be easily obtained: $p_A = 1 - \Phi(Z^{ws})$. The exact p-value is given by

$$p = p_A + 0.0003130571 \, (4.444461^\tau) - 0.00033. \tag{4.64}$$

Note that we have used the inverse-normal transformation to generalize the Shen-Lan-Soo method to binary and survival endpoints.

4.4.3 Noninferiority-Superiority Adaptive Design

For a standard K-stage group sequential trial, usually either a superiority or noninferiority test is performed at each stage. However, it is often of interest to pharmaceutical companies to perform both superiority (H_S) and noninferiority (H_{NI}) tests in a single trial. Wang et al. (2001) proposed a procedure to test superiority and noninferiority simultaneously in a single adaptive design, where a noninferiority test procedure with a fixed margin was used. Recall that the standard group sequential design is a special case of MINP. The authors proposed two closed test procedures, referred to as GSC S-NI and GSC NI-S, as illustrated in Fig. 4.1. Both procedures control the maximum total type-I error probability for both noninferiority and superiority at the α level. Furthermore, the GSC procedure achieves the power for superiority at the planned level α (i.e., not a reduced power) because of testing superiority and noninferiority simultaneously. The procedures are established on the usual lower limit of the confidence interval, LL_i, for the treatment difference from the ith interim analysis. The fixed noninferiority margin is denoted by δ_{NI} (see Chap. 3, Sect. 3.1.3.1).

The procedure GSC S-NI is described as follows:

1. At stage i, if $LL_i > 0$, then claim superiority and stop the trial; otherwise, continue to step 2.
2. If $LL_i > -\delta_{NI}$, then claim noninferiority; otherwise, the trial continues to stage $i + 1$ (if $i + 1 > K$, conclude noninferiority).

The procedure GSC NI–S is described as follows:

1. At stage i, if $LL_i > -\delta_{NI}$, then claim noninferiority and continue examining for superiority:

   a. If $LL_i > 0$, then claim superiority and stop.
   b. If $LL_i \leq 0$, continue on step 2.

2. If $LL_i > 0$, then claim superiority and stop; otherwise continue to stage $i + 1$ and repeat steps 1 and 2 until loop over all the stages.

These two procedures imply that we can test superiority and noninferiority separately in the sequential trial. Superiority can be claimed regardless of the noninferiority claim as long as the superiority hypothesis H_S is rejected at a stage. Similarly, noninferiority can be claimed regardless of the superiority claim as long as the noninferiority hypothesis H_{NI} is rejected at a stage.

Wang et al. (2001) proved that the previous closed procedures are also valid for a two-stage adaptive design with SSR at the interim analysis using a method equivalent to MINP.

4.5 Adaptive Design Debates

4.5.1 Sufficiency Principle

Jennison and Turnbull (2003), Posch et al. (2003), and Burman and Sonesson (2006) pointed out that the adaptive design using a weighted statistic violates the sufficiency principle because it weighs the same amount of information from different stages

differently. Michael A. Proschan (Burman and Sonesson 2006, discussion) proved
that no test based on the sufficient statistic can maintain a level α irrespective of
whether the prespecified sample size rule is followed.

The "unweighted test" utilizes the distribution of sample size N to choose a
critical level with the desired probability of rejecting the null hypothesis unconditional on N but disregards the observed value of N. Because N is part of the
minimal sufficient statistic, it is not in accordance with the sufficiency principle and
is inefficient (Marianne Frisen, in Burman and Sonesson 2006, discussion).

The key question is: should information (or sufficiency of a statistic) regarding
θ be based on data or data + procedure? The conclusion that each observation
contains the same amount of information is valid in a classic design but not in
an adaptive design because a later observation contains some information from
previous observations due to the dependent sampling procedure. Therefore, an
insufficient statistic in a classic design can become sufficient under an adaptive
design. For example, suppose we want to assess the quantity $\vartheta = \frac{1-R_B}{1-R_A}$, where
R_A and R_B are the true response rates in groups A and B, respectively. In a
classic design with balanced randomization, $\frac{N_A}{N_B}$ is asymptotically approaching 1.
However, in the randomized play-the-winner design, $\frac{N_A}{N_B}$ asymptotically converges
to ϑ. Therefore, the same data $\frac{N_A}{N_B}$ could contain different amounts of information in
different designs.

4.5.2 Minimum Sufficiency Principle and Efficiency

Jennison and Turnbull (2006) raised the question as to when an adaptive design
using nonsufficient statistics can be improved upon by a nonadaptive group
sequential design. Tsiatis and Mehta (2003) have proved that for any SSR adaptive
design there exists a more powerful group sequential design. On the other hand, the
weighted method (or MINP) provides great flexibility, and when the sample size
does not change, it has the same power as the classic group sequential design.

It is really analogous with a two-player game. Player A says to player B: if you
tell me the sample size rule, I can find a group sequential design (with as many
analyses as I want to have) that is more efficient than the adaptive design. Player B
says to player A: if you tell me how many and when you plan the interim analyses, I
can produce an adaptive trial with the same number and timing of the analyses that
is more flexible, and if the sample size does not change, it is identical to the group
sequential design.

4.5.3 Conditionality and Exchangeability Principles

Burman and Sonesson (2006) pointed out that SSR also violates the invariance
and conditionality principles because the weighted test depends on the order
of exchangeable observations. Marianne Frisen (Burman and Sonesson 2006,

discussion) stated similarly: "The 'weighted' test avoids this by forcing a certain error spending. This is done at the cost of violating the conditionality principle. The ordering of the observations is an ancillary statistic for a conclusion about the hypothesis. Thus, by the conditionality principle the test statistic should not depend on the ordering of the realized observations." For a general distribution, not belonging to the exponential family, the weighted test will violate the conditionality principle but not the sufficiency principle (Burman and Sonesson 2006).

If sufficiency and conditionality are important, then the combination of the two is the likelihood principle, which also faces challenges (Robert 1997; Chang 2007a).

4.5.4 Equal Weight Principle

Exchangeable observations should be weighted equally in the test statistic. The equal weight principle views exchangeability from the weight perspective. However, the measurement of the information level is not unique. For example observation x_i, $1/x_i$, or p_i can be counted as the unit of information. The adaptive design method MSP equally weights the evidence (p_i) against H_o from the two stages.

It has been misunderstood that the classic group sequential design equally weights information, but actually it does not because the observations from the first stage have the potential of being used more than once in decision-making (hypothesis-testing); e.g., if $\beta_2 > p_1 > \alpha_1$, the trial continues and the data from the first stage will be combined with data from the second stage to calculate the test statistic for rejecting or accepting the null hypothesis. The patients from the first stage have the chance of "voting twice or more" in the decision process.

4.5.5 Consistency of Stagewise Results

Compared with the classic design, adaptive designs naturally allow for an interim look to check the consistency of results from different stages. If p_1 and p_2 are very different, we may have to look at the reasons, such as baseline difference, gene difference, and others. The question is should we check this consistency for a classic design, too, by splitting the data in different ways?

It is also controversial in adaptive designs (including group sequential designs) that we often reject the null hypothesis with weaker evidence but don't reject the null hypothesis with stronger evidence. For example, in a two-stage group sequential design with the O'Brien-Fleming spending function ($\alpha_1 = 0.0025$ and $\alpha_2 = 0.0238$), we will not reject the null when the p-value $= 0.003 > \alpha_1$ at the interim look but we do reject the null when the p-value $= 0.022 < \alpha_2$. Why don't we reject the null hypothesis when the evidence against the null is stronger (p-value $= 0.003$) and reject H_o when the evidence is much weaker (p-value $= 0.022$)? Let's elaborate on the controversy using the following patient-statistician dilemma.

Suppose you are a patient and a statistician. As a patient, you have to be treated with some drug. As a statistician, you have designed two trials for two NMEs (new molecular entities) for a therapeutic indication with classical and adaptive features, respectively. As a patient, you have specified the criteria for selecting the treatment: rank the two p-values for the efficacy tests from the two NME trials and pick the NME with a smaller associated p-value.

Suppose now that NME 1 with a classical design has tested with 30% improvement ($p = 0.04 < \alpha = 0.05$), statistically significant, whereas NME 2 with an adaptive design has been tested with 50% improvement and the final $p = 0.026$, which is not statistically significant due to the multiple looks at the data. You further examine the sample size and variability of the efficacy data; they are similar between the two groups. The safety, tolerability, cost, and convenience of drug administration are all similar between the two NMEs. As a statistician for the trials, you should recommend NME 1 for treating the disease; as a patient with that disease, you will take NME 2. Since you are the statistician with the disease, what do you do?

4.5.6 Adjusted p-value

Controversies surrounding p-values have been discussed in Chap. 1. Our discussions here focus on the p-value issues that are particular to adaptive design. The type-I error control is not very challenging, and most adaptive designs control the familywise error. However, because hypothesis-testing is primarily based on the concept of repeated experiments, the scope in which the experiment will potentially be repeated is critical. In clinical trials, we virtually never test the same compound for the same indication in a phase-III study repeatedly. For this reason, the implication of control of the experimental error rate α may be totally different from what we initially intended.

The definition, not the calculation, of the p-value is challenging because there are so many options for an adaptive design. Remember that the p-value is the probability of the test statistic under the null hypothesis being more extreme than the critical point. The key lies in how the extreme should be defined. Unlike in a classic design, definitions of extremeness of a test statistic can be defined in many different ways in adaptive designs (e.g., stagewise ordering, sample mean ordering, and likelihood ratio ordering). None of these definitions simultaneously satisfies the concerns raised from statistical, scientific, and ethical perspectives. Similarly, an agreeable definition and calculations of the unbiased point estimate and the confidence interval remain challenging for adaptive designs.

4.5.7 Summary

Adaptive designs violate several commonly accepted statistical principles. The violations on the one hand remind us to adopt the new approaches with extreme caution. On the other hand, the new approaches may suggest that principles of inference only go so far and that new principles may be desirable. Indeed, adaptive designs present great challenges to frequentist statistics and conventional thinking in development. Group sequential designs have been widely used in clinical trials; however, there are many controversial issues with these designs that are only fully realized when we widen the concept to a more general category of adaptive designs.

It is obvious that efficiency in clinical trials is not identical to the power of hypothesis-testing. In clinical trials, the concept of efficiency often includes the power, the time-to-market, and the operational flexibility. Overemphasizing the power can be very misleading when evaluating adaptive designs. This simple fact is often overlooked.

Despite the challenges, adaptive designs have been proved useful in practice and more and more clinical trials have adopted.

4.6 Exercises

4.1. In a two-arm comparative oncology trial, the primary efficacy endpoint is time to progression (TTP). The median of TTP is estimated to be 8 months (hazard rate = 0.08664) for the control group and 10.5 months (hazard rate = 0.06601) for the test group. Assume the trial has a uniform enrollment with an accrual period of 9 months and a total study duration of 24 months. The log-rank test will be used for the analysis. An exponential survival distribution is assumed for the purpose of the sample size calculation. The classic design requires a sample size of 323 subjects per group. Design a group sequential trial using MMP, MPP, and MINP.

4.2. Use each of the adaptive methods (MMP, MPP, and MINP) to design a two-stage trial with a sample size reestimation. Assume the stopping boundary for the first stage $\alpha_1 = 0.01$, the effect size $\delta/\sigma = 0.2$, and power = 40%. The sample size adjustment at the interim analysis is based on (4.52) or (4.53). Compare the six expected sample sizes $\bar{N}$ under the condition $\delta/\sigma = 0.2$ between the two methods. (Hint: Computer simulation programs can be downloaded from www.statisticians. org.)

4.3. In Exercise 4.1, assume the sample size adjustment is based on the following formulation. The sample size per group for the second stage is determined by

$$n_2 = p_1^{\gamma}.$$

Determine the constant γ to minimize the expected sample size $\bar{N}$ under the condition $\delta/\sigma = 0.2$ and $\alpha = 0.01$. (Hint: For a given γ, adjust the maximum sample size N_{max} such that power = 40%.)

4.4. Compare the nine expected sample sizes obtained from Exercises 4.2 and 4.3. Summarize your findings.

4.5. Assume a classic three-arm trial including placebo, low-dose, and high-dose groups. The objective is to prove either the low dose or high dose is effective compared with the placebo at the level $\alpha = 5\%$ using the Dunnett method (see Chap. 1). Calculate the total sample size required for the trial design. Then take an adaptive seamless design using the Shun-Lan-Soo method and compare the sample size against that from the classic design.

4.6. Suppose that in a classic m-group dose-finding trial with a continuous response (variance $\sigma^2 = 1$) the test statistics for pairwise comparisons are defined as

$$Z_i = \frac{\bar{x}_i - \bar{x}_0}{\sqrt{n}},$$

where $\bar{x}_i$ is the mean of the ith group, $i = 0$ for the control group, and n is the sample size per group. Study (analytically or numerically using simulation) the distributions of the following order statistics:

$$Z_{(1)} <, \ldots, < Z_{(m)}.$$

4.7. Do you believe the exchangeability holds between an observation from the first stage and an observation from the second stage of the adaptive design? Why?

Further Readings and References

Bauer, P., Kieser, M.: Combining different phases in development of medical treatments within a single trial. Stat. Med. **18**, 1833–1848 (1999)

Bauer, P., Kohne, K.: Evaluation of experiments with adaptive interim analysis. Biometrics **50**, 1029–1041 (1994)

Bauer, P., Rohmel, J.: An adaptive method for establishing a dose-response relationship. Stat. Med. **14**, 1595–1607 (1995)

Burman, C.F., Sonesson, C.: Are flexible designs sound? (with discussion). Biometrics **62**, 664–683 (2006)

Chang, M.: Adaptive Design Theory and Implementation Using SAS and R. Chapman and Hall/CRC, Boca Raton (2007a)

Chang, M.: Adaptive design method based on sum of p-values. Stat. Med. **26**, 2772–2784 (2007b)

Chang, M., et al.: BIO White Paper: Innovative approaches in drug development. J. Biopharm. Stat. **17**, 775–789 (2007c)

Chang, M.: Classical and Adaptive Designs Using ExpDesign Studio. Wiley, New York (2008)

Chang, M.: Monte Carlo Simulations for the Pharmaceutical Industry: Concepts, Algorithms, and Case Studies. Chapman and Hall/CRC, Boca Raton (2010)

Chang, M., Chow, S.C., Pong, A.: Adaptive design in clinical research – Issues, opportunities, and recommendations. J. Biopharm. Stat. **16**, 299–309 (2006)

Chow, S.C., Chang, M.: Statistical consideration of adaptive methods in clinical development. J. Biopharm. Stat. **15**, 575–591 (2005)

Chow, S.C., Chang, M.: Adaptive Design Methods in Clinical Trials. Chapman and Hall/CRC, Boca Raton (2006)

Cui, L., Hung, H.M.J., Wang, S.J.: Modification of sample-size in group sequential trials. Biometrics **55**, 853–857 (1999)

FDA: Guidance for Industry: Adaptive Design Clinical Trials for Drugs and Biologics (draft). www.fda.org (2010). Accessed 12 Mar 2010

Gallo, P., Chuang-Stein, C., Dragalin, V., Gaydos, B., Krams, M., Pinheiro, J.: Adaptive designs in clinical drug development – an executive summary of the PhRMA Working Group. J. Biopharm. Stat. **16**, 275–283 (2006)

Hu, F., Rosenberger, W.: The Theory of Response-Adaptive Randomization in Clinical Trials. Wiley, Hoboken (2006)

Jennison, C., Turnbull, B.W.: Mid-course sample size modification in clinical trials. Stat. Med. **22**, 971–993 (2003)

Jennison, C., Turnbull, B.W.: Adaptive and non-adaptive group sequential tests. Biometrika **93**, 1–21 (2006)

Kim, K., DeMets, D.L.: Sample size determination for group sequential clinical trials with immediate response. Stat. Med. **11**, 1391–1399 (1992)

Kokoska, S., Zwillinger, D.: Standard Probability and Statistical tables and Formula. Chapman & Hall/CRC, Boca Raton (2000)

Lan, K.K.G., DeMets, D.L.: Group sequential procedures: Calendar versus information time. Stat. Med. **8**, 1191–1198 (1987)

Lehmacher, W., Wassmer, G.: Adaptive sample size calculations in group sequential trials. Biometrics **55**, 1286–1290 (1999)

Ling, X., Hsu, J.: Using the partitioning principle to adaptively design dose-response studies. J. Biopharm. Stat. **16**, 733–743 (2006)

Mathieu, M.P. (ed.): PAREXEL's Bio/Pharma R&D Statistical Sourcebook 2007/2008. PAREXEL. PH (2008)

Müller, H.H., Shäfer, H.: A general ststistical principle of changing a design any time during the course of a trial. Stat. Med. **23**, 2497–2508 (2004)

O'Brien, P.C., Fleming, T.R.: A multiple testing procedure for clinical trials. Biometrika 35, 549–556 (1979)

Pocock, S.J.: Group sequential methods in the design and analysis of clinical trials. Biometrika **64**, 191–199 (1977)

Posch, M., Bauer, P., Brannath, W.: Issues on flexible designs. Stat. Med. **22**, 953–969 (2003)

Proschan, M.A., Hunsberger, S.A.: Designed extension of studies based on conditional power. Biometrics **51**, 1315–1324 (1995)

Proschan, M.A., Lan, K.K.G., Wittes, J.T.: Statistical Monitoring of Clinical Trials, A Uniform Approach. Springer, New York (2006)

Robert, C.P.: The Bayesian Choice. Springer, New York (1997)

Shun, Z., Lan, K.K.G., Soo, Y.: Interim treatment selection using the normal approximation approach in clinical trials. Stat. Med. **27**, 597–618 (2008)

Tsiatis, A.A., Mehta, C.: On the inefficiency of the adaptive design for monitoring clinical trials. Biometrika **90**, 367–378 (2003)

Wang, S.J., Hung, J., Tsong, Y., Cui, L.: Group sequential test strategies for superiority and noninferiority hypotheses in active controlled clinical trials. Stat. Med. **20**, 1903–1912 (2001)

Wang, S.K., Tsiatis, A.A.: Approximately optimal one-parameter boundaries for a sequential trials. Biometrics **43**, 193–200 (1987)

Wassmer, G.: Multistage adaptive test procedures based on Fisher's product criterion. Biom. J. **41**, 279–293 (1999)

Yun, B.I.: Approximation to the cumulative normal distribution using hyperbolic tangent based functions. J. Korean Math. Soc. **46**, 1267–1276 (2009)

Chapter 5
Missing Data Imputation and Analysis

5.1 Missing Data Problems

5.1.1 Missing Data Issue and Its Impact

Missing data are a common occurrence in scientific research and in our daily lives. In a survey, a lack of response constitutes missing data. In clinical trials, missing data can be caused by a patient's refusal to continue in a study, treatment failures, adverse events, or patient relocations.

Missing data will complicate data analysis. In many medical settings, missing data can cause difficulties in estimation, precision, and inference. In clinical trials, missing data can undermine randomization (Little 2010). CHMP's guideline (CHMP 2009) provides advice on how the presence of missing data in a confirmatory clinical trial should be addressed in a regulatory submission. It is stated that the pattern of missing data (including reasons for and timing of the missing data) observed in previous related clinical trials should be taken into account when planning a confirmatory clinical trial.

An analysis that ignores subjects with missing data is called a completer analysis. Completer analyses, on the one hand, can reduce the power of hypothesis-testing due to a reduction in sample size; on the other hand, noncompleters might be more likely to have extreme values (e.g., treatment failure leading to dropout, or extremely good response leading to loss of follow-up). Therefore, the loss of noncompleters could lead to an underestimate of variability, hence artificially narrowing the confidence interval for the treatment effect and artificially increasing the power of the study. Therefore, the overall effect of missing data depends on the situation.

A completer analysis can potentially cause bias if missingness is not at random (i.e., it relates to observed, unobserved or both measurements). Generally, missing data will not be expected to lead to bias in the completer analysis if they are not related to the observed or unobserved measurements (e.g., poor outcomes are no more likely to be missing than good outcomes). However, it is virtually impossible

M. Chang, *Modern Issues and Methods in Biostatistics*, Statistics for Biology and Health, DOI 10.1007/978-1-4419-9842-2_5, © Springer Science+Business Media, LLC 2011

to elucidate whether the relationship between missing values and the unobserved outcome variable is completely absent. Consequently, unbiasedness cannot be firmly asserted in reality.

If subjects with missing data are excluded from the analysis in a clinical trial, it may affect the comparability of the treatment groups and the representativeness of the study sample in relation to the target population (external validity) is questionable.

In this chapter, we study different types of missing data, except censoring survival data, which will be studied in Chap. 6.

5.1.2 Missing Data Taxonomy

5.1.2.1 Syntax Conventions

Let Y_{ij} denote the random variable measured at the jth time point on the ith subject, where $i = 1, \ldots, n$ and $j = 1, \ldots, n_i$. We use vector $\boldsymbol{Y}_i = (Y_{i1}, \ldots, Y_{in_i})'$ to denote the measurements on subject i, where the prime represents the matrix transport. We use an uppercase letter to denote a random variable and a lowercase letter for a corresponding observation. We use superscripts or subscripts, "obs" and "mis", to indicate observed and missing quantities, respectively. Therefore, y_{ij} consists of y_{ij}^{obs} and y_{ij}^{mis}. The indicator $R_{ij} = 1$ if the value of Y_{ij} is observed; otherwise, $R_{ij} = 0$. Let $\boldsymbol{R}_i = (R_{i1}, \ldots, R_{in_i})'$. The mechanism of missingness will be denoted by ϖ_i, and the matrix of covariates for the ith subject is denoted by $X_i = (X_{i1} \ldots, X_{in_i})$.

5.1.2.2 Classification of Missing Mechanisms

According to Rubin (1976) and Little and Rubin (2002), the missing value process can be characterized by way of three different categories in terms of its marginal probability distribution.

1. If the probability of an observation being missing does not depend on observed or unobserved measurements, then the observation is classified as missing completely at random (MCAR). The marginal density for missingness is given by

$$f\left(\boldsymbol{r}_i | \boldsymbol{y}_i, \varpi_i, \boldsymbol{\psi}\right) = f\left(\boldsymbol{r}_i | \varpi_i, \boldsymbol{\psi}\right), \tag{5.1}$$

where $\boldsymbol{\psi}$ is the parameter vector characterizing the mechanism of missingness. MCAR is difficult to find in reality. One may consider a patient moving to another city for nonhealth reasons as MCAR. However, we can reason that if a new oncology drug works well, the patient is more unlikely to move out of the city than otherwise. A car accident may be considered as MCAR, but it could also be caused by one's health condition.

2. If the probability of an observation being missing depends only on observed measurements, then the observation is classified as missing at random (MAR). This assumption implies that the behavior (i.e., distribution) of the post-dropout observations can be predicted from the observed values, and therefore that response can be estimated without bias using exclusively the observed data. Mathematically, the density of MAR is given by

$$f\left(r_i | y_i, \varpi_i, \psi\right) = f\left(r_i | y_i^{obs}, \varpi_i, \psi\right). \tag{5.2}$$

3. When observations are neither MCAR nor MAR, they are classified as missing not at random (MNAR), i.e., the probability of an observation being missing depends on both observed and unobserved measurements. The density of missingness, $f\left(r_i | y_i, \varpi_i, \psi\right)$, cannot be simplified.

Mathematically, there is no way to know whether missing is MACR, MAR, or MNAR. However, we often believe MCAR/MAR can be a good approximation in certain situations.

Ignorability is a property of missingness. Ignorability ensures that ignoring the unobserved data in the analysis will not lead to biased results.

Monotonic missingness is a common and simple pattern of missingness. If the missing data pattern is monotone, then all observations after time point t are missing, where t is the time point when the first missing observation occurs. Sufficient conditions for ignorability are the following two requirements.

1. The joint prior distribution for θ and ψ can factor into independent priors

$$P(\theta, \psi) = P(\theta)P(\psi), \tag{5.3}$$

i.e., the joint distribution is 'distinct.' In this case, the change in one parameter will not cause a change in the other parameter.

2. MAR holds. In other words, the distribution of missingness depends only on the observed data, and all the information about missing data is contained in the observed part of the data. Mathematically, it is characterized as

$$P(R_{ij} | Y, \psi) = P(R_{ij} | Y_{obs}, \psi). \tag{5.4}$$

A commonly used parametric model for missingness is the logistic model that models the continuation probability for subject i, at time j, using

$$p_{ij}(\psi) = P(R_{ij} = 1 | Y_{i1}, \dots, Y_{ij}, \psi) = \frac{\exp(\psi_0 + \psi_1 Y_{i1} + \cdots + \psi_j Y_{ij})}{1 + \exp(\psi_0 + \psi_1 Y_{i1} + \cdots + \psi_j Y_{ij})}. \tag{5.5}$$

For MCAR, $\psi_1 = \cdots = \psi_j = 0$, and for MAR, $\psi_j = 0$.

5.2 Analysis Methods for Missing at Random

5.2.1 Single Imputation Methods

As mentioned earlier, completer analysis often is not preferred. There are several commonly used simple methods that deal with missing data. An example would be the last-observation carry forward (LOCF), which can be used if the outcome for a participant would not change after his dropping out. The LOCF is not unbiased even under the MCAR assumption (Little 2010) and can give the two groups better or worse results. If the timing of two withdrawals is different (e.g., some may withdraw when the drug effect starts to decline, others may withdraw when the efficacy is still at its trough, and others may withdraw from the study due to side-effects) or the baseline covariates differ between the treatment groups, bias can occur. Other kinds of simple implementations, as mentioned in the CHMP guidance (CHMP 2009) are, for e.g., to replace the unobserved measurements by values derived from other sources such as information from the same subject collected before withdrawal, from other subjects with similar baseline characteristics, a predicted value from an empirically developed model, or historical data. Examples of empirically developed models such as unconditional/conditional mean imputation and best/worst case imputation (assigning the worst possible value of the outcome to some dropouts and the best possible value to others) are also mentioned in the guidance.

5.2.2 Generalized Linear Mixed Models

Some statistical approaches to handling missing data do not employ any explicit missing imputation. Generalized estimating equations (GEEs), random-effects approaches, and general linear mixed models (GLMMs) are examples of such models. They are usually valid under MAR assumptions. GLMMs can be used for data with repeated measures. Unlike a general linear model (GLM), in which subjects with missing values are removed from the analysis (i.e., completer analysis), GLMMs utilize all the observed data. GLMs are only valid under MCAR, but GLMMs are valid under MAR.

The general linear mixed model family is given by

$$Y_i = X_i \beta + Z_i \gamma_i + \varepsilon_i, \qquad (5.6)$$

where Y_i is the response vector, X_i is fixed effects with the associated unknown parameter vector β, Z_i is random effects with the associated parameters $\gamma_i \sim N(0, G)$, and the random error term $\varepsilon_i \sim N(0, \Sigma_i)$. It is assumed that γ_i and ε_i are independent.

The fitting of a linear model is usually based on the marginal model that, for subject i, is multivariate normal with mean $X_i\beta$ and covariance $V_i(\alpha) = Z_i G Z_i' + \Sigma_i$. The parameters in α are usually called "variance components." A common approach to estimation and inference is based on maximum likelihood (ML) or likelihood. Assuming independence across subjects, the likelihood takes the form

$$L(\theta) = \prod_{i=1}^{n} \frac{\exp\left[-\frac{1}{2}(Y_i - X_i\beta)' V_i^{-1}(\alpha)(Y_i - X_i\beta)\right]}{(2\pi)^{n_i/2} \sqrt{|V_i(\alpha)|}}. \tag{5.7}$$

After ignoring a constant term, the log-likelihood is given by

$$LL = -\frac{n}{2}\ln|V_i(\alpha)| - \sum_{i=1}^{n}\left[-\frac{1}{2}(Y_i - X_i\beta)' V_i^{-1}(\alpha)(Y_i - X_i\beta)\right]. \tag{5.8}$$

For the linear mixed model case, inference is conventionally based on the marginal model for Y_i, which is obtained from integrating out the random effects. The likelihood contribution for subject i then becomes

$$f_i(y_i|\beta, G, \phi) = \int \prod_{j=1}^{n_j} f_{ij}(y_{ij}|\gamma_i, \beta, \phi) f(\gamma_i|G) \, d\gamma_i. \tag{5.9}$$

Based on (5.9), the likelihood for β, G, and ϕ can be derived as

$$L(\beta, G, \phi) = \prod_{i=1}^{n} f_i(y_i|\beta, G, \phi)$$

$$= \prod_{i=1}^{n} \int \prod_{j=1}^{n_j} f_{ij}(y_{ij}|\gamma_i, \beta, \phi) f(\gamma_i|G) \, d\gamma_i. \tag{5.10}$$

The exponential-family distributions are often used in conditional form,

$$f_i(y_{ij}|\gamma_i, \beta, \phi) = \exp\left(\frac{y_{ij}\theta_{ij} - \psi(\theta_{ij})}{\phi} - c(y_{ij}, \phi)\right), \tag{5.11}$$

with a link function $g(\mu_{ij}) = g(E(Y_{ij}|\gamma_i)) = x_{ij}'\beta + z_{ij}'\gamma_i$, where x_{ij} and z_{ij} are p-dimensional and q-dimensional vectors of known covariate values, vector $\beta = $ unknown fixed regression coefficients, $\phi = $ scale parameter, and θ_{ij} are the canonical parameters. Furthermore, let $f(\gamma_i|G)$ be the density of the $N(0, G)$ distribution for the random effects γ_i. Various covariance structures, such as the compound-symmetric, first-order autoregressive, and unstructured, can be used for G.

The maximization of likelihood (5.10) is challenging because of the presence of n integrals over the high-dimensional random effects. Monte Carlo simulation may be used since the efficiency of Monte Carlo for integrals is independent of dimensionality. Other numerical approximations and quasi-likelihood estimates have also been proposed.

A trial example and SAS program using the mixed model will be illustrated in Sect. 5.4, Example 5.2 and SAS Program 5.4.

5.2.3 Expectation-Maximization Algorithm

The term "expectation-maximization (EM) algorithm" was coined in 1977 (Dempster et al. 1977). The EM algorithm is an iterative algorithm used to calculate maximum likelihood estimates in parametric models in the presence of missing data. After the initial values are chosen, the iteration involves two steps: the expectation or E-step and the maximization or M-step. The condition for the EM algorithm to be valid, in its basic form, is ignorability, and hence MAR.

In the implementation of the EM algorithm, before the E-step and M-step begin, the choice of an initial value of the parameter, $\theta^{(0)}$, is important since this value will affect the speed of convergence. A commonly used value for $\theta^{(0)}$ is the solution from the complete-case (completer) analysis or from some simple method of imputation.

1. The E-step
   Given the parameter values $\theta^{(k)}$ at the kth iteration, the E-step computes the objective function:

   $$Q\left(\theta\,|\theta^{(k)}\right) = \int L\left(\theta\,|y\right) f\left(y_{mis}|y_{obs}, \theta^{(k)}\right) \mathrm{d}y_{mis}$$
   $$= E\left[L\left(\theta\,|y\right)|y_{obs}, \theta^{(k)}\right]. \tag{5.12}$$

2. The M-step
   $\theta^{(k+1)}$ is calculated to maximize the log-likelihood of the imputed data (or the imputed log-likelihood). Formally, $\theta^{(k+1)}$ satisfies

   $$\theta^{(k+1)} = \arg\max_{\theta\in\Theta} Q\left(\theta\,|\theta^{(k)}\right). \tag{5.13}$$

The EM algorithm is guaranteed to be convergent, but the solution can be a local maximum, and the speed of convergence can be slow.

A trial example and SAS program using the mixed model will be illustrated in Sect. 5.4, Example 5.2 and SAS Program 5.5.

5.2.4 Inverse-Probability Weighting Method

5.2.4.1 Univariate Outcome

When data are MAR but not MCAR, a modification of complete-case analysis is to assign a missingness weight to the complete cases so that bias may be reduced. Suppose that in the complete dataset there are ten counts for $y = 1$ but only seven of them are actually observed (70% observed, 30% missing). We weight these observations by the inverse of the proportion of observed (70%), making it equivalent to ten observations for the estimation of the mean. However the proportion being observed is a random variable, so in practice we use the probability of being observed. That is the basic idea behind the inverse-probability weighting (IPW) method.

Consider the simple case in which the intended outcome is Y and the design variables are X (they can also include an auxiliary variable). Define a response indicator, $R = 1$ when Y is observed and $R = 0$ when it is missing. An IPW estimator for the mean of Y can be computed as follows:

1. Specify an appropriate model (e.g., the logistic model) for the missingness $\pi(X, \theta) = P_\theta(R = 1|X)$.
2. Estimate the mean of Y using the weighted average

$$\hat{\mu} = \frac{1}{n} \sum_{i=1}^{n} \frac{R_i Y_i}{\pi\left(X_i, \hat{\theta}\right)}, \tag{5.14}$$

where $R_i = 1$ when Y_i is observed and $R_i = 0$ when Y_i is missing. The estimator (5.14) is obtained by inflating the average of the observed Y by the inverse probability of being observed.

As pointed out by Little (2010) for large samples, this method properly adjusts for bias when the data are MAR, provided the model for $\pi(X, \theta)$ is correctly specified. In finite samples, the method can yield mean estimates that have a high variance when some individual-specific weights are high and π is close to zero. To avoid the high variance, we can lower the limit for the weights, making a trade off between bias and variance.

In addition to the MAR assumption, the IPW method requires that the possible values of the missing responses be the same as those of the observed responses. The IPW method, and generally any method that relies on MAR, is estimating the mean under the condition that everyone remained in treatment in the clinical trial. This is why it is important to collect outcome data after individuals withdraw from treatment.

5.2.4.2 Augmented IPW Estimation Under MAR

IPW can be combined with the GEE method. Hogan et al. (2004) conducted an analysis of repeated binary data from a smoking cessation study. The investigators used IPW to estimate the effect of a behavioral intervention involving supervised exercise on the rate of smoking cessation in women. The publication includes SAS code for fitting the model.

However, IPW with GEE does not make full use of the information in incomplete cases. The augmented IPW GEE procedure remedies this weakness. The procedure is best understood in the simple case in which only the values (Y_{it}) at the last time point, $t = K$, are missing for some subject i, and they are MAR. Suppose one wishes to estimate $\mu = E(Y_K)$, the mean outcome in a particular treatment group in a clinical trial. Let $Z_{iK-} = \{Z_{i1}, \ldots Z_{iK-1}\}$, and let $R_{iK} = 1$ if the ith subject has the observation Y_{iK} at the time point $t = K$, and $R_{iK} = 0$ otherwise. Fit a model $\pi_i(\theta) = P_\theta(R_{iK} = 1 | Z_{iK-})$ as described earlier for the univariate outcome.

The augmented IPW (AIPW) estimator of μ is given by

$$\hat{\mu} = \frac{1}{n}\sum_{i=1}^n \frac{R_{iK}Y_{iK}}{\pi_i(\hat{\theta})} + \frac{1}{n}\sum_{i=1}^n \left\{\frac{R_{iK}}{\pi_i(\hat{\theta})} - 1\right\} g(Z_{iK-}, X_i), \qquad (5.15)$$

where $g(Z_{iK-}, X_i)$ is some function of the observed-data history up to $K - 1$.

The first term is just the IPW estimator of μ. The second (augmentation) term has mean zero, so that $\hat{\mu}$ is still a consistent estimator. However, the variance of $\hat{\mu}$ will depend on the choice of g, where the optimal choice is $E(Y_{iK}|Z_{iK-}, X_i)$, which in practice can be approximated by the regression prediction $\hat{Y}_{iK}$.

5.2.4.3 Imputing Nonmissing Responses

Relevant to the IPW method, Müller et al. (2006) proposed a better estimator (smaller variance) by imputing responses that are not missing.

Let $h(X, Y)$ be a square-integrable function of a random vector (X, Y). We want to estimate its expectation $E[h(X, Y)]$ using the empirical estimator $\frac{1}{n}\sum_{i=1}^n h(x_i, y_i)$. If nothing is known about the distribution of (X, Y), this estimator is efficient. We are interested in the situation where X is always observable but Y is observable only if some indicator R equals one. We assume that R and Y are conditionally independent given X, i.e., Y is MAR. In this case, the empirical estimator is not available unless all R_i are one. Let $\pi(X) = E(R|X) = P(R = 1|X)$. If $\pi(\cdot)$ is known and positive, we could use the estimator $\frac{1}{n}\sum_{i=1}^n \frac{R_i}{\pi(X_i)} h(X_i, Y_i)$. If $\pi(\cdot)$ is unknown, one could replace π by an estimator $\hat{\pi}$, resulting in

$$\frac{1}{n}\sum_{i=1}^n \frac{R_i}{\hat{\pi}(X_i)} h(X_i, Y_i). \qquad (5.16)$$

Surprisingly, even if π is known, replacing π by an estimator can decrease the asymptotic variance. Furthermore, the partially imputed estimator is given by

$$\frac{1}{n} \sum_{i=1}^{n} (R_i h(X_i Y_i) + (1 - R_i) \hat{\chi}(X_i)), \qquad (5.17)$$

where $\hat{\chi}(X_i)$ is an estimator of the conditional expectation,

$$\hat{\chi}(X_i) = E(h(X_i, Y_i)|X_i). \qquad (5.18)$$

An alternative to the partially imputed estimator is the fully imputed estimator

$$\frac{1}{n} \sum_{i=1}^{n} \hat{\chi}(X_i). \qquad (5.19)$$

Müller et al. (2006) show that the fully imputed estimator (5.19) is usually better than the partially imputed estimator (5.17).

5.2.5 Multiple-Imputation Method

Multiple-imputation (MI) methods generate multiple copies of the "complete dataset" by replacing missing values with randomly generated values, using a Bayesian or other method, and analyzing them as complete sets. MI does not model the dropout process but requires a correct specification of the model that relates the distribution of missing responses to the observed data, known as the imputation model.

According to Rubin (1987), MI involves three distinct tasks:

1. The missing values are filled in M times to generate M complete datasets.
2. The M complete datasets are analyzed using the standard procedure.
3. The results from the M analyses are combined into a single inference.

The first step is the key. Consider a Bayesian joint model for the complete data and the missingness

$$\varphi(\theta, Y_{mis}) \propto f(Y_{mis}, Y_{obs}|\theta) \pi(\theta), \qquad (5.20)$$

where $\pi(\theta)$ is the prior of θ. The marginal posterior of θ is given by

$$\pi(\theta|Y_{obs}) = \varphi(\theta) = \int \varphi(\theta, Y_{mis}) \, dY_{mis}. \qquad (5.21)$$

MCMC is often used as a missing-imputation algorithm.

Ignorability is the weakest general condition under which the distribution of missingness does not need to be taken into account when making likelihood-based or Bayesian inferences (Rubin 1987). Without ignorability, MIs would have to be drawn from (5.21).

Because MI uses a Bayesian method to generate missing values, how to have a valid frequentist inference is an interesting topic. Rubin (1976) describes conditions under which the following asymptotic result holds in a frequentist sense, i.e., the test statistic has a t-distribution.

To estimate β, we can use the weighted average of the M estimates,

$$\hat{\beta} = \sum_{m=1}^{M} w_m \hat{\beta}^{(m)}, \tag{5.22}$$

with variance

$$\hat{V} = W + \left(\frac{M+1}{M}\right) B, \tag{5.23}$$

where

$$\begin{cases} W = \sum_{m=1}^{M} w_m \hat{V}^{(m)} \\ B = \sum_{m=1}^{M} w_m \left(\hat{\beta}^{(m)} - \hat{\beta}\right)\left(\hat{\beta}^{(m)} - \hat{\beta}\right)'. \end{cases} \tag{5.24}$$

Under MAR, $w_m = 1/M$. Under MNAR, weight w_m can be calculated using sensitivity methods (Carpenter et al. 2007).

A trial example and SAS program using the multiple-imputation method will be illustrated in Sect. 5.4, Example 5.2 and SAS Program 5.2.

5.2.6 Weighted Generalized Estimating Equations

The GEE model is described as a marginal model for the response Y_{ij} ($j = 1, \ldots, n_i, i = 1, \ldots, n$, and $\Sigma_{i=1}^{n} n_i = N$). The parameter vector β is obtained by solving the system of equations,

$$S(\beta) = \sum_{i=1}^{n} \frac{\partial \mu_i}{\partial \beta'} [V_i(\alpha)]^{-1} (y_i - \mu_i) = 0, \tag{5.25}$$

where the mean $\mu_i = E(Y_i)$ and the marginal covariance matrix

$$V_i(\alpha) = \phi A_i^{1/2} W_i^{-1/2} C_i(\alpha) W_i^{-1/2} A_i^{1/2}, \tag{5.26}$$

in which the variance matrix for repeated measures on subject i is $\phi A_i = \phi \cdot \text{diag}[v(\mu_{i1}), \ldots, v(\mu_{iT})]$, with ϕ being the unknown dispersion parameter and $C_i(\alpha)$ the so-called $n_i \times n_i$ working matrix for the ith subject. If $C_i(\alpha)$ is the true correlation matrix of Y_i, then $V_i(\alpha)$ is the true covariance matrix of Y_i.

With the logistic dropout model (5.5), the weight is given by (e.g., SAS Institute Inc. 2008, p. 1681)

$$\frac{1}{w_i} = (1 - \lambda_{im})^{I(m \leq T)} \prod_{j=2}^{m-1} \lambda_{ij}, \tag{5.27}$$

where $\lambda_{ij} = P\left(r_{ij} = 1 | r_{i,j-1} = 1, X_i, Y_{i,j-1}\right)$, m is the time of dropout for the ith subject $(2 \leq m < T - 1)$, and the indicator $I(m \leq T) = 1$ if $m \leq T$; otherwise $I(m \leq T) = 0$. When the weight matrix W_i is the identity matrix, (5.25) and (5.26) reduce to the estimate for the unweighted GEE.

The dispersion parameter ϕ has to be estimated through iterations, and usually by means of the following Pearson residuals:

$$e_{ij} = \frac{y_{ij} - \mu_{ij}}{\sqrt{v\left(\mu_{ij}\right)/w_{ij}}}. \tag{5.28}$$

Specifically, the dispersion parameter ϕ can be estimated by

$$\hat{\phi} = \frac{1}{N-p} \sum_{i=1}^{n} \sum_{j=1}^{n_i} e_{ij}^2, \tag{5.29}$$

where p is the size of parameter vector $\boldsymbol{\beta}$.

The correlation matrix $C_i(\alpha)$ is dependent on the correlation structure. The following commonly used structures, as well as others, are available in the SAS GENMOD procedure.

1. For the m-independent structure,

$$\text{Corr}\left(Y_{ij}, Y_{i,j+t}\right) = \begin{cases} 1 & \text{for } t = 0, \\ \alpha_t & \text{for } t = 1, 2, \ldots, m, \\ 0 & \text{for } t > m, \end{cases} \tag{5.30}$$

$$\hat{\alpha}_t = \frac{1}{(N - nt - p)\phi} \sum_{i=1}^{n} \sum_{j \leq n_i - t} e_{ij} e_{i,j+t}. \tag{5.31}$$

2. For the exchangeable structure,

$$\text{Corr}\left(Y_{ij}, Y_{ik}\right) = \begin{cases} 1 & \text{for } j = k, \\ \alpha & \text{for } j \neq k, \end{cases} \tag{5.32}$$

$$\hat{\alpha} = \frac{1}{\left(\frac{1}{2} \sum_{i=1}^{n} n_i (n_i - 1) - p\right)\phi} \sum_{i=1}^{n} \sum_{j<k} e_{ij} e_{ik}. \tag{5.33}$$

3. For an unstructured covariance,

$$Corr\left(Y_{ij}, Y_{ik}\right) = \begin{cases} 1 \text{ for } j = k, \\ \alpha_{jk} \text{ for } j \neq k, \end{cases} \tag{5.34}$$

$$\hat{\alpha}_{jk} = \frac{1}{(n-p)\,\phi} \sum_{i=1}^{n} e_{ij}e_{ik}. \tag{5.35}$$

4. For the first-order autoregressive AR(1) structure,

$$\text{Corr}\left(Y_{ij}, Y_{i,j+t}\right) = \alpha^{t} \text{ for } t = 0, 1, \dots, n_i - j, \tag{5.36}$$

$$\hat{\alpha} = \frac{1}{(N-n-p)\,\phi} \sum_{i=1}^{n} \sum_{j \leq n_i - t} e_{ij}e_{i,j+t}. \tag{5.37}$$

The link function g, defined by

$$g\left(\boldsymbol{\mu}_i\right) = \boldsymbol{X}_i\boldsymbol{\beta}, \tag{5.38}$$

can be chosen from various categories. Thus the derivatives are

$$\frac{\partial \boldsymbol{\mu}_i}{\partial \boldsymbol{\beta}'} = \begin{bmatrix} \dfrac{x_{i11}}{g'\left(\mu_{i1}\right)} & \cdots & \dfrac{x_{in_i1}}{g'\left(\mu_{in_i}\right)} \\ \vdots & & \vdots \\ \dfrac{x_{i1p}}{g'\left(\mu_{i1}\right)} & \cdots & \dfrac{x_{in_ip}}{g'\left(\mu_{in_i}\right)} \end{bmatrix}. \tag{5.39}$$

Unlike the classic GLM, GEE uses all data available in pairwise fashion as defined in the estimates for $\hat{\alpha}$ and $\hat{\beta}$.

5.3 Analysis Methods for Missing Not at Random

In many cases, there are a variety of settings for each method, which can lead to different conclusions. Therefore, approaches that investigate different MNAR scenarios, such as pattern-mixture, selection, and shared parameter models, should be explored.

5.3.1 Missing Data Frameworks

The common model-based methods for MNAR are likelihood-based approaches, which can be classified into *selection model*, *pattern-mixture model*, and *shared-parameter model* frameworks by factorization of the full data model (conditional probability density)

$$f\left(y_i, r_i | X_i, \varpi_i, \theta, \psi\right), \tag{5.40}$$

where X_i and ϖ_i denote design matrices for the measurement and missingness mechanisms, respectively. The corresponding parameter vectors are θ and ψ, respectively. For simplicity, we omit X_i and ϖ_i in (5.40), giving simply $f\left(y_i, r_i | \theta, \psi\right)$.

1. The selection model combines a model for the distribution of the complete data with a conditional model for the missingness given the data, i.e., it factorizes the marginal density as

$$f\left(y_i, r_i | \theta, \psi\right) = f\left(y_i | \theta\right) f\left(r_i | y_i, \psi\right), \tag{5.41}$$

where the first factor is the marginal density of the measurement process and the second one is the density of the missingness process, conditional on the outcomes.

In the selection model approach (Diggle and Kenward 1994), the missing-data mechanism was modelled to depend on the missing outcome variable as well as covariates. Gao and Hui (2000) extended the selection model approach from continuous outcomes to binary outcomes. The results from these models tend to be highly sensitive to departures from the assumptions about the shape of the complete-data population.

2. The pattern-mixture model (Little 1993, 1995) factorizes the marginal density as

$$f\left(y_i, r_i | \theta, \psi\right) = f\left(y_i | r_i, \theta\right) f\left(r_i | \psi\right). \tag{5.42}$$

The pattern-mixture model approach models the probability of the missing data and appends it to the joint likelihood for the outcome models conditional on the missing-data status. The pattern-mixture model allows for a different response model (e.g., Bernoulli distribution or logistic regression) for each pattern of missingness. The population of the complete data becomes a mixture of distributions, weighted by the probabilities of the missingness pattern.

3. The shared-parameter model factorizes the marginal density as

$$f\left(y_i, r_i | \theta, \psi, b_i\right) = f\left(y_i | r_i, \theta, b_i\right) f\left(r_i | \psi, b_i\right), \tag{5.43}$$

where parameters b_i for subject-specific latent (or random) effects are included to model certain common latent mechanisms shared by both the measurement and missingness processes.

The notion behind the shared random-effect parameter approach is that there may be some latent quantity underlying a person's susceptibility to two processes (e.g., disease and death). This latent quantity may represent genetic/genomic or environmental risk factors yet to be identified (Lancaster and Intrator 1998; Ten Have et al. 1998).

5.3.2 Selection Model

Let Y_{ij} be measured at time points for the ith subject at time t_{ij}, $i = 1, \ldots, n$, $j = 1, \ldots, n_i$, and $Y_i = (Y_{i1}, \ldots, Y_{in_i})'$. We consider a special type of missingness, the dropout; i.e., once missingness occurs at the jth measuring time, all measurements after that are missing. Suppose a dropout occurs at the occasion $j = D_i$ ($1 < D_i \leq n_i$) for the ith subject, so that the first measurement is always available. We decompose vector Y_i into the observed and missing parts, $Y_i = (Y_i^{obs}, Y_{n_i}^{mis})'$. The likelihood contribution of the ith subject based on the observed data (y_i^{obs}, d_i) is proportional to the marginal density function

$$f(y_i, d_i|\boldsymbol{\theta}, \boldsymbol{\psi}) = \int f(y_i, d_i|\boldsymbol{\theta}, \boldsymbol{\psi}) \, dy_i^{mis} = \int f(y_i|\boldsymbol{\theta}) \, f(d_i|y_i, \boldsymbol{\psi}) \, dy_i^{mis},$$

(5.44)

where we have utilized the selection factorization (5.37).

Let vector $y_{ij-} = (y_{i1}, \ldots, y_{ij-1})$. The Diggle-Kenward model (Diggle and Kenward 1994) for the dropout process allows the conditional probability density to be specified at occasion D_i:

$$f_{ij}(\boldsymbol{\psi}) = \begin{cases} P\left(D_i = j|D_i \geq j, y_{ij-}, y_{ij}, \boldsymbol{\psi}\right), \; j = 2, \\ P\left(D_i = j|D_i \geq j, y_{ij-}, y_{ij}, \boldsymbol{\psi}\right) \times \\ \prod_{k=2}^{j-1}\left[1 - P\left(D_i = k|D_i \geq k, y_{ij-}, y_{ij}, \boldsymbol{\psi}\right)\right], 2 < j \leq n_i, \\ \prod_{k=2}^{n_i}\left[1 - P\left(D_i = k|D_i \geq k, y_{ij-}, y_{ij}, \boldsymbol{\psi}\right)\right], \; j > n_i. \end{cases}$$

(5.45)

A multivariate normal model,

$$Y_i \sim f(Y_i|\boldsymbol{\theta}) = N(X_i\boldsymbol{\beta}, \Sigma_i), i = 1, \ldots, n,$$

(5.46)

is used for the measurement process, where various forms can be chosen for the covariance matrix Σ. Meanwhile, a simplified logistic model from (5.5) for the missing mechanism is,

$$P\left(D_i = j|D_i \geq j, y_{ij-}, y_{ij}, \boldsymbol{\psi}\right) = \frac{\exp(\psi_0 + \psi_1 y_{ij} + \psi_2 y_{ij-1})}{1 + \exp(\psi_0 + \psi_1 y_{ij} + \psi_2 y_{ij-1})}.$$

(5.47)

The likelihood involves marginalization over the unobserved outcomes Y_i^{mis}, which are computationally intensive. Molenberghs and Kenward (2008) provided illustrative examples.

5.3.3 Pattern-Mixture Model

The high sensitivity of the selection model to the misspecification of the measurement process and dropout mechanism has led to growing interest in the pattern-mixture model with the factorization of marginal density for pattern-mixed models (PMMs) given by (5.42). To illustrate the method, let t_i be the index (measurement time, clinic visit) indicating the late measurement for the i th subject. After time t_i, the subject dropped out of the experiment. Here we use $f(y_i|t_i, \theta)$ instead of $f(y_i|r_i, \theta)$ and $f(t_i|\psi)$ instead of $f(r_i|\psi)$. We assume

$$f(y_i|t_i, \theta) = N(\mu(t_i), \Sigma(t_i)). \tag{5.48}$$

A pattern-mixture model is usually overparameterized if there are no restrictions. Different restrictions can be used, such as.,

$$f_i(y_j|y_{j-}, \theta) = \sum_{k=j}^{n_i} \omega_{jk} f_k(y_j|y_{j-}, \theta), \quad j = i+1, \dots, n_i, \tag{5.49}$$

where the weights ω_{jk} satisfy $\sum_{k=j}^{n_i} \omega_{jk} = 1$.

The full density function can be expressed as

$$f_i(y|\theta) = f_i(y^{obs}|\theta) = \prod_{j=1}^{n_i-i-1} \left[\sum_{k=n_i-j}^{n_i} \omega_{n_i-j,k} f_k(y_{n_i-j}|y_{(n_i-j)-}, \theta) \right]. \tag{5.50}$$

Different weights in (5.49) and (5.50) will lead to different models (Yang et al. 2008; Little 1993, 1995; DeGruttola and Tu 1994; Hogan and Laird 1997; Henderson et al. 2000; Vonesh et al. 2006).

There are also various $f(t_i|\psi)$ to choose; an example would be $f(t_i|\psi) = u + vt_i$, where u and v are constants. The likelihood function and MLEs can be constructed using the standard procedures.

5.3.4 Shared-Parameter Models

Recently there have been many discussions of shared-parameter modeling, where the factorization of the marginal density is given as in (5.43).

Gao (2004) proposed a method that models both the probability of disease and the probability of death using shared random-effect parameters. Gao used the Laplace approximation to obtain an approximate likelihood function to avoid high-dimensional integration over the distributions of the random-effect parameters.

Let Y_{ij} be a binary variable denoting disease status ($y_{ij} = 0$ for non-disease, $y_{ij} = 1$ for disease) for the ith subject at the jth assessment, $i = 1, \ldots, n; \, j = 1, \ldots, n_i$. Let D_{ij} be the variable for survival status, with $D_{ij} = 1$ indicating the ith subject died before the jth assessment. Let X_{ij} be the covariates associated with y_{ij} and Z_{ij} the covariates associated with D_{ij}. Let γ_i be an $m \times 1$ vector of unobserved random effects contributing to the probabilities of disease. Let U_{ij} and V_{ij} be the sets of covariates associated with the random effects in the disease model and the death model, respectively.

Gao (2004) starts with a general disease model for the disease outcome by defining the conditional probability of new disease to relate linearly to fixed and random effects by a link function, $\eta(\cdot)$,

$$p_{ij} = \Pr\left(y_{ij} = 1 | y_{ij-1} = 0; X_{ij}, U_{ij}\right) = \eta(X_{ij}\beta + U_{ij}\Sigma^{1/2}\gamma_i), \; j \geq 2, \quad (5.51)$$

where β is the fixed-effect parameter and γ_i in the disease model is the component of $\gamma \sim N(\gamma; 0, I)$, with I being an identity and $\Sigma'\Sigma$ a positive definite covariance matrix.

The mortality model is defined through another link function, $\xi(\cdot)$,

$$\pi_{ij} = \Pr\left(D_{ij} = 1 | D_{ij-1} = 0, Z_{ij}, V_{ij}\right) = \xi\left(Z_{ij}\alpha + V_{ij}\Delta^{1/2}\gamma_i\right), \; j \geq 2, \quad (5.52)$$

where α is the fixed-effect parameter and $\Delta'\Delta$ is a positive definite variance-covariance matrix.

Assuming that y_{ij} and D_{ij} are independent given normally distributed γ_i, the likelihood function of y and D is

$$L = \int f(y|\gamma)g(D|\gamma) \, dN(\gamma; 0, I)$$

$$= \frac{1}{\sqrt{2\pi}} \int \exp\left\{\ln\left[f(y|\gamma)g(D|\gamma)\right] - \frac{1}{2}\gamma'\gamma\right\} d\gamma. \quad (5.53)$$

The derivation of maximum likelihood estimates from the joint likelihood function above usually requires high dimensional integration over the distributions of the random effect parameters. A Monte Carlo method may be used since its efficiency is independent of the dimensionality. Alternatively, Gao (2004) expands $\ln\left[f(y|\gamma)g(D|\gamma)\right] - \frac{1}{2}\gamma'\gamma$ at $\hat{\gamma}_0$ as a second-order Taylor series, where $\hat{\gamma}_0$ maximizes $\ln\left[f(y|\gamma)g(D|\gamma)\right] - \frac{1}{2}\gamma'\gamma$. The approximate log-likelihood function leads to

$$\ln L \approx \ln\left[f(y|\gamma_0)g(D|\gamma_0)\right] - \frac{\hat{\gamma}_0'\hat{\gamma}_0}{2}$$

$$- \frac{1}{2}\ln\left|I - \frac{\partial^2 \ln\left[f(y|\gamma)g(D|\gamma)\right]}{\partial\gamma^2}\right|_{\gamma=\gamma_0}. \quad (5.54)$$

Differently, Yang et al. (2008) propose a shared-parameter model based on a Markov chain, in which y_{ij} is dependent on $y_{i,j-1}$ but independent of $(y_{i1}, \ldots, y_{i,j-2})$. They use a regression-type linear transition model to characterize the process,

$$y_{ij} = x_{ij}\boldsymbol{\beta} + (y_{i,j-1} - x_{i,j-1}\boldsymbol{\beta})\alpha + \xi_i + \varepsilon_{ij}, \tag{5.55}$$

where $\xi_i \overset{iid}{\sim} N(0, \sigma_\xi^2)$ denotes the random intercept for subject i and $\varepsilon_{ij} \overset{iid}{\sim} N(0, \sigma_\varepsilon^2)$ represents the residual errors. Vector $\boldsymbol{\beta}$ contains fixed parameters, such as treatment efficacy, in clinical trials. The parameter α sets up the link between the previous and the current unexplained measurement effects, i.e., between $y_{i,j-1} - x_{i,j-1}\boldsymbol{\beta}$ and $y_{ij} - x_{ij}\boldsymbol{\beta}$.

To model the dropout process, let the indicator variable $r_{ij} = 0$ (or 1) if y_{ij} is observed (or missing due to a dropout). A first-order Markov chain is assumed with a 2×2 matrix of transition probabilities: $P_{lk} = \Pr\left(r_{ij} = k | r_{i,j-1} = l\right)$, $l = 0$ or 1; $k = 0$ or 1. By the definition of dropout, we have $P_{10} = 0$ and $P_{11} = 1$. The transition probabilities P_{00} and P_{01} are modeled by logistic regression:

$$P\left(r_{ij} = k | \xi_i, x_{ij}, r_{i,j-1} = 0\right) = \begin{cases} \dfrac{1}{1 + \exp\left(x_{ij}\boldsymbol{\eta} + \xi_i\gamma\right)} & \text{if } k = 0 \\[2ex] \dfrac{\exp\left(x_{ij}\boldsymbol{\eta} + \xi_i\gamma\right)}{1 + \exp\left(x_{ij}\boldsymbol{\eta} + \xi_i\gamma\right)} & \text{if } k = 1. \end{cases} \tag{5.56}$$

Here the authors use parameters η to calibrate the influence of covariates on the possibility of dropout and γ to indicate whether the dropout process shares the random intercepts with the measurement process. Hence, it tells us whether a dropout is informative.

Based on the measurement and dropout mechanics above, the full likelihood function with parameters $\boldsymbol{\theta} = (\boldsymbol{\beta}', \sigma_\xi^2, \sigma_\varepsilon^2)$ and $\boldsymbol{\varphi} = (\boldsymbol{\eta}, \gamma)'$ can be written as

$$L\left(\boldsymbol{\theta}, \boldsymbol{\varphi}\right) \propto \prod_{i=1}^{n} \int \prod_{j=1}^{d_i-1} p\left(y_{ij} | x_{ij}, y_{i,j-1}, \xi_i, \boldsymbol{\theta}\right) p\left(y_{ij} | x_{ij}, r_{i,j-1}, \xi_i, \boldsymbol{\varphi}\right) p\left(\xi_i\right) \mathrm{d}\xi_i,$$

where $p(\xi_i)$ is the normal p.d.f. of the random intercept ξ_i.

Most models discussed above have been limited to outcome variables, which is clearly not always the case. To include the missing auxiliary variable in the models may not be difficult, but more research needs to be done.

5.4 Analysis Examples Using SAS and SOLAS

For implementing missing data using SAS, we recommend the book by Dmitrienko et al. (2005). Here we give a brief introduction.

Table 5.1 Depression data structure

Patient	Visit	Basval	Change Y	Trt	Ctr
1001	4	25	−7	2	103
1001	5	25	−14	2	103
1001	6	25	−19	2	103
1001	7	25	·	2	103
1002	4	17	−4	1	105
1002	5	17	−8	1	105
1002	6	17	·	1	105
1002	7	17	·	1	105
⋮	⋮		⋮	⋮	⋮

5.4.1 Likelihood Ignorable Analysis

A likelihood ignorable analysis for MAR uses all available information without directly implementing any missing data. The analysis using SAS PROC MIXED is straightforward. The order of the measurements should be correctly specified, which can be done by supplying records with missing data in the input dataset.

Example 5.1. A multicenter depression trial was conducted with the Hamilton Depression Rating Scale as the primary efficacy endpoint. For each patient, a baseline assessment is available and the change from baseline (*Basval*) is denoted by Y. Y is missing when the assessment at postbaseline visit is not available. There are four treatment options (*Trt*). The clinic center is denoted by variable *Ctr*. The data structure is presented in Table 5.1, where a dot represents a missing value.

SAS Program 5.1: MAR Analysis of the Depression Trial

```
Proc mixed data = depression method = ml noitprint ic;
    class Patient Visit Ctr Trt;
    model Y = Trt Ctr Visit Trt*Visit Basval Basval*Visit
    /solution ddfm = satterth;
    repeated visit / subject = patient type = un;
Run;
```

Details about options in Proc Mixed can be found in the SAS User's Guide (SAS Institute 2004).

5.4.2 Multiple-Imputation Method

A multiple-imputation method using SAS involves two steps: implementation and analysis. We illustrate the process with the growth data in Table 5.2.

Example 5.2. The growth data contain growth measurements for girls and boys. For each subject, the distance from the center of the pituitary to the maxillary fissure

Table 5.2 Growth data structure

ID	Sex	Meas8	Meas12	Meas14	Meas10
1	1	26	29.0	31.0	27
2	1	21.5	23.0	26.5	·
3	2	23	24.0	27.5	23.5
4	1	20	26.5	27.0	·
...					

was recorded at ages 8, 10, 12, and 14 years and denoted by variables Meas8, Meas10, Meas12, and Meas14 (Table 5.2). Note that the measurement times are ordered as age = 8, 12, 14, and 10 years because the data at age 10 are incomplete. In this way, a monotone ordering is achieved, which is required for the monotone regression method. The implementation step with SAS PROC MI is presented in SAS Program 5.2.

SAS Program 5.2: Imputation Step

```
Proc mi data = Growth seed = 213 simple Nimpute = 10
    round = 0.1 out = outmi;
    by sex;
    monotone method = reg;
    var Meas8 Meas12 Meas14 Meas10;
Run;
```

To prepare for a standard linear mixed model analysis, we convert the output *outmi* from SAS Program 5.2 to vertical structure using SAS Program 5.3.

SAS Program 5.3: Data Manipulation

```
Proc sort data = outmi;
    by _imputation_ idnr;
Run;
Data outmi2;
    set outmi;
    array y (4) meas8 meas10 meas12 meas14;
    do j = 1 to 4;
    measmi = y(j) ;
    age = 6 + 2*j;
    output;
    end;
Run;
```

The analysis step using the SAS MIXED procedure requires four sets of inputs for the inference task: (1) parameter estimates of the fixed effects (mixbetap), (2) parameter estimates of the variance components (mixalfap), (3) the covariance matrix of the fixed effects (mixbetav), and (4) the covariance matrix of the variance components (mixalfav). An example of a SAS program is presented in SAS Program 5.4.

SAS Program 5.4: Analysis Step Using PROC MIXED

```
Proc mixed data = outmi2 asycov;
   class idnr age sex;
   model measmi = age*sex / noint solution covb;
   repeated age / subject = idnr type = cs;
   by _Imputation_;
   ods output solutionF = mixbetap covb = mixbetav
              covparms = mixalfap asycov = mixalfav;
Run;
```

However, to use PROC MIANALYZE, further data manipulation is required; see SAS Programs 5.17 and 5.18 in the book by Dmitrienko et al. (2005), or the SAS User's Guide for details.

When missingness is nonmonotone, Dmitrienko et al. (2005) suggest generating multiple imputations that render the datasets monotonically missing by including the statement in PROC MI: *mcmc impute = monotone* and then applying a method of choice to the multiple sets of data that are thus completed.

5.4.3 EM Algorithm Using SAS

The MI procedure in SAS provides an EM algorithm for both multivariate normal and categorical data by means of an MCMC imputation method (for general nonmonotone settings). The EM algorithm for the growth data is presented in SAS Program 5.5. PROC MI uses the means and standard deviations from the available cases as the initial estimates for the EM algorithm. The correlations are set equal to zero.

SAS Program 5.5: The EM Algorithm Using PROC MI

```
Proc mi data = Growth seed = 213 simple nimpute = 0;
   em itprint outem = growthem;
   var Meas8 Meas12 Meas14 Meas10;
   by sex;
Run;
```

5.4.4 SOLAS for Missing Data Analysis

SOLAS, developed in conjunction with Prof. Donald Rubin, is a software application that has a user-friendly graphical interface and provides a range of missing-data imputation techniques. The *single-imputation techniques* include the hot deck imputation, in which missing values are replaced with values taken from matching respondents, the last value carried forward, the group means, or the predicted mean from the models. The *predictive-model-based multiple-imputation* methods include the ordinary least-squares regression of imputation for the continuous, integer, and ordinal imputation variables, the discriminant multiple imputation for the nominal imputation variables and the Bayesian imputation method for various types of variables. The *propensity-score-based multiple imputation method* includes an implicit model approach based on propensity scores and an approximate Bayesian bootstrap. The propensity score is the conditional probability of "missingness" given the vector of observed covariates. It also includes a fully configurable logistic regression algorithm.

The Missing Data Pattern in SOLAS^{TM} 3.0 provides a clear overview of the quantity, positioning, and types of missing values in your dataset. By right-clicking on any cell in the matrix, you can identify the variable and observation details. This feature allows you to study the missing-data patterns and helps you to choose the most appropriate imputation techniques. You can also use the Missing Value Pattern to view the monotone and nonmonotone missing values in your dataset.

5.5 Controversies, Challenges, and Recommendations

5.5.1 Comparisons of Different Methods

Single-imputation methods such as the LOCF are simple to implement but they generally do not conform to well-recognized statistical principles for drawing inferences, and often lead to a biased estimate.

Multiple-imputation methods explicitly specify the missing data assumptions and allow one to use large amounts of auxiliary information. They can be relatively straightforward to implement, without special programming needs, and can handle arbitrary patterns of missing data.

The IPW method is simple to implement when the missing values have a monotone pattern, and can be carried out in any software package that allows weighted analyses. The IPW method allows one to include auxiliary variables such as previously observed outcomes. There are potential instabilities with large weights, leading to high variance in finite samples, especially when the missingness model is incorrectly specified. Methods that yield valid inferences when either the outcome regression or the missingness model is correct are said to have a double-robustness property.

Maximum likelihood and Bayesian inference approaches under ignorable missingness provide valid inferences using models that are generally easy to fit with commercial software. Random-effects models can be very useful to simplify a highly multivariate distribution with a few parameters. However, when missingness is not ignorable, the impact is difficult to assess.

It is intuitive to assume a model for the full-data response, as is done in selection models. If MAR is plausible, a likelihood-based selection formulation leads directly to inference based solely on the model for the full-data response, and the inference can be carried out using MLE. However, it may not be intuitive to specify the relationship between nonresponse probability and the outcome of interest, which typically has to be done in the logit or probit scale. Selection models are highly sensitive to parametric assumptions about the full-data distribution. This concern can be alleviated by using semiparametric selection models (Little 2010).

In pattern-mixture models, respondents and nonrespondents have different outcome distributions. The models are explicit in specifying how missing observations are being imputed because the within-pattern models specify the predictive distribution directly. However, pattern-mixture models can present computational difficulties for estimating treatment effects because of the need to average over missing-data patterns; this is particularly true of pattern-mixture specifications involving regression models within each pattern.

5.5.2 How to Implement Missingness

Practically speaking, missing data usually refers to any data points that were intended for collection but were not obtained. Theoretically, any unobserved variable at any time point can be considered a missing value in an analysis, even if the measurement was not intended to be collected at all. In the most general and abstract form, "missing data" can refer to any augmented component of the probabilistic system under consideration, and the inclusion of this component often results in a simpler structure and easier computation (Liu 2003). On the other hand, people may argue that if missing imputation is allowed, one can "make up" any value at any point in time and space, and as many as one wants, in the name of computational convenience.

Regarding the pattern of missingness, in clinical trials missingness is often a mixture of MCAR, MAR, and MNAR because, for example, missingness should not just relate to how one collects and measures the data but also to the behavior of the subject from whom the data are collected. The choice of MAR or MCAR is often simply motivated by mathematical convenience. However, the question is: if we know the missingness is MAR in a practical problem, why do we try to collect it in the first place? The answer may be to increase data points and thus the power for the hypothesis-test. Another argument would be that although MAR is a non-testable assumption, we can get very close to justifying the MAR hypothesis if we include enough variables in the imputation models (Harel and Zhou 2007).

A simple example of MNAR is when the values to be measured are out of the range of the measurement instrument. Another example would be a patient withdrawal due to lack of efficacy or side effects. If the drug is not very effective, causing a large number of dropouts due to ineffectiveness, models based on MAR would not be appropriate.

We may say the true value should be imputed for a missing value; however, the truth is missing and how to impute it is a matter of belief. To elaborate on this, let me share a story with you. When I appeared in court for my first traffic citation,

I argued: "I don't think this is my fault. . . . I've never gotten any citation for a traffic violation in my 13 years driving history." Of course, the judge didn't observe the accident; it is a missing value to her. She replied nicely: "Yes, I know; but everyone has his first time." In this case, who is at fault is unknown or missing. I tried to impute the missingness "longitudinally" by looking back at my own driving history and concluding the missing value should be 0: not my fault. However, the judge imputed the missing value "cross-sectionally" by looking at all the drivers who had 13 years of driving experience and concluded that most of them had traffic violations; therefore it was likely my fault, and the missing value should be 1. Do you think it is fair to make a judgment of me based on other people's behavior?

In clinical trials, the missing imputation faces the same dilemma: should we look for a data pattern within the trial or across different trials, or even in everything happening in the whole world?

Regarding who should perform the data implementation, Harel and Zhou (2007) offer their opinion: Many public-data users differ in their statistical proficiency, computing power, and objectives. Most users only have access to complete-data methodology and software. Database constructors have additional information about the data that can help in modeling the missing values. Therefore, it would be preferable if the missing data modeling was done by the data constructors and not by the users. However, in many cases, that is not possible.

5.5.3 Regulatory Perspective

For clinical trials, the health authority (CHMP 2009) states: "Missing data are a potential source of bias when analyzing clinical trials. . . A critical discussion of the number, timing, pattern, reason for and possible implications of missing values in efficacy and safety assessments should be included in the clinical report as a matter of routine. . . It should be noted that just ignoring missing data is not an acceptable option when planning, conducting or interpreting the analysis of a confirmatory clinical trial. . . The justification for selecting a particular method should not be based primarily on the properties of the method under particular assumptions (for example MAR or MCAR) but on whether it will provide an appropriately conservative estimate for the comparison of primary regulatory interest in the circumstances of the trial under consideration." They believe missing data (completer analyses) violate the strict ITT principle, which requires measurement of all patient outcomes regardless of the protocol adherence. This principle is of critical importance, as confirmatory clinical trials should estimate the effect of the experimental intervention in the population of patients with the greatest external validity.

There are many factors that can affect missingness: (1) the complexity of the measurements, (2) the frequency of measurements, (3) self-reported versus in-clinic measures by clinicians, (4) the nature of the outcome variable, such as modality versus morbidity, (5) the treatment modalities, such as surgical versus medical treatment, (6) frequency of the treatment, (7) the benefit-risk profile of the treatment, (8) duration of the clinical trial (since a longer trial will likely have a larger proportion missing than a shorter trial), (9) the therapeutic indication (missing values are more frequent in those diseases where the adherence of patients to the study protocol is usually low, such as psychiatric disorders, (10) data entry error (some numbers may be easier to missight than others), and (11) the design and conduct of the experiment.

A reduction in missing data can be achieved by favoring clinical trial designs, strengthening data collection, and whenever possible, collecting outcome data after withdrawals. To minimize potential bias, CHMP (2009) recommends that a detailed description of the preplanned methods used for handling missing data and any amendments of that plan and a justification for each amendment should be included in the clinical study report. A critical discussion of the number, timing, pattern, and reasons for and possible implications of missing values in efficacy and safety assessments should be included in the clinical report as a matter of routine. Because of the unpredictability of some problems, the study protocol sometimes allows the possibility of updating the strategy for dealing with missing values in the statistical analysis plan or during the blind review of the data at the end of the trial.

5.5.4 Recommendations for Clinical Trials

At the request of the FDA, the National Research Council convened the Panel on the Handling of Missing Data in Clinical Trials, under the Committee on National Statistics, to prepare "a report with recommendations that would be useful for FDA's development of a guidance for clinical trials on appropriate study designs and follow-up methods to reduce missing data and appropriate statistical methods to address missing data for analysis of results." The panel, chaired by Prof. Rod Little, developed an excellent report, "The prevention and treatment of missing data in clinical trials" (Little 2010). The panel consisted of a group of academic statisticians, but I believe there was some interaction with industry statisticians, as indicated in the acknowledgments. Among many useful suggestions, they recommend the following.

5.5.4.1 Clinical Trial Design

Investigators, sponsors, and regulators should design clinical trials consistent with the goal of maximizing the number of participants who are maintained on the protocol-specified intervention until the outcome data are collected.

The techniques to reduce the occurrence of missingness include (1) adding run-in periods before randomization to identify who can tolerate or respond to the study treatment, (2) using flexible doses (titration), (3) restricting the trial to the target population for whom treatment is indicated, (4) adding the study treatment to a standard treatment, (5) reducing the length of the follow-up period, (6) allowing rescue medication in the event of poor response, and (7) defining outcomes that can be ascertained in a high proportion of participants. Of course, benefits of these options need to be weighed against costs.

5.5.4.2 Clinical Trial Conduct

Trial sponsors should continue to collect information on key outcomes in participants who discontinue their protocol-specified intervention in the course of the study, except in those cases for which a compelling cost-benefit analysis argues otherwise, and this information should be recorded and used in the analysis.

The techniques to limit the amount of missing data include (1) choices of study sites, investigators, participants, study outcomes, time in study and times of measurement, and the nature and frequency of follow-up to limit the amount of missing data, (2) limiting participant burden in other ways, such as making follow-up visits easy in terms of travel and childcare, (3) providing frequent reminders of study visits, (4) training of investigators on the importance of avoiding missing data, (5) providing incentives to investigators and participants to limit dropouts, and (6) monitoring of adherence and in other ways dealing with participants who cannot tolerate or do not adequately respond to treatment.

The panel recommends that study sponsors should explicitly anticipate potential problems of missing data. In particular, the trial protocol should contain a section that addresses missing-data issues, including the anticipated amount of missing data and steps taken in trial design and trial conduct to monitor and limit the impact of missing data.

5.5.4.3 Trial Data Analysis

There is no universal method for handling incomplete data in a clinical trial. Despite differences among the trials, there are common principles that can be applied in a wide variety of settings as suggested by the panel:

1. A basic assumption is that missingness of a particular value hides a true underlying value that is meaningful for analysis.
2. The analysis must be formulated to draw inferences about an appropriate and well-defined causal estimand.
3. Reasons for missing data must be documented as much as possible.
4. The trial designers should decide on a primary set of assumptions about the missing-data mechanism. Those primary assumptions then serve as an anchor point for the sensitivity analyses.
5. The trial sponsors should conduct a statistically valid analysis under the primary missing-data assumptions.
6. The analysts should assess the robustness of the treatment effect inferences by conducting a sensitivity analysis.

Despite efforts to minimize missing data in the design and conduct of clinical trials, the statistical analysis often has to deal with a nontrivial amount of missing data. There is no single correct method for handling missing data. As such, the panel recommends that statistical methods for handling missing data should be specified by clinical trial sponsors in study protocols, and their associated assumptions stated in a way that can be understood by clinicians. Single-imputation methods like last observation carried forward and baseline observation carried forward should not be used as the primary approach to the treatment of missing data unless the assumptions that underlie them are scientifically justified. Sensitivity analyses should be part of the primary reporting of findings from clinical trials. Examining sensitivity to the assumptions about the missing-data mechanism should be a mandatory component of reporting.

5.6 Exercises

5.1. Suppose there are data available from two clinical trials. Trial A is a 2×2 crossover design (one treatment sequence is drugs C and T; the other sequence is drugs T and C) and trial B is a design with two parallel treatment groups (C and T). The statistician wants to combine data from these two clinical trials using the technique for the missing data. He treats trial B as an imaginary 2×2 crossover trial with one group missing the first period and the other group missing the second period. Furthermore, he assumes that the missing data are completely at random (MCAR) because it was not planned to collect the missing data. Discuss his strategy.

5.2. Compare different methods for the missing data analysis under different scenarios, such as percentage of missing data and missing patterns.

Further Readings and References

Carpenter J.R., Kenward, M.G., White, I.R.: Sensitivity analysis after multiple imputation under missing at random: A weighting approach. Stat. Methods Med. Res. **16**, 259–275 (2007)

CHMP: Guideline on missing data in confirmatory clinical trials/1776/99 Rev. 1. www.ema.europa.eu (2009). Accessed 8 Aug 2010

DeGruttola, V., Tu, X.M.: Modeling progression of CD4+ lymphocyte count and its relationship to survival time. Biometrics **50**, 1003–1014 (1994)

Dempster, A.P., Laird, N.M., Rubin, D.B.: Maximum likelihood estimation from incomplete data via the EM algorithm. J. R. Stat. Soc. Ser. B **39**, 1–38 (1977)

Dmitrienko, A., Molenberghs, G., Chuang-Stein, C., Often, W.: Analysis of Clinical Trials Using SAS. SAS Institute, Cary (2005)

Diggle P., Kenward, M.G.: Informative drop-out in longitudinal data analysis. Appl. Stat. **43**, 49–93 (1994)

Gao, S.: A shared random effect parameter approach for longitudinal dementia data with non-ignorable missing data. Stat. Med. **23**, 211–219 (2004)

Gao, S., Hui, S.L.: Estimating the incidence of dementia from two-phase sampling with non-ignorable missing data. Stat. Med. **19**, 1545–554 (2000)

Harel, O., Zhou, X.H.: Multiple imputation: Review of theory, implementation and software. Stat. Med. **26**, 3057–3077 (2007)

Henderson, R., Diggle, P., Dobson, A.: Joint modeling of longitudinal measurements and event time data. Biostatistics **1**, 465–480 (2000)

Hogan, J.W., Laird, N.M.: Model-based approaches to analysing incomplete longitudinal and failure time data. Stat. Med. **16**, 259–272 (1997)

Hogan, J.W., Roy, J., Korkontzelou C.: Biostatistics tutorial: Handling dropout in longitudinal data. Stat. Med. **23**, 1455–1497 (2004)

Horvitz, D.G., Thompson, D.J.: A Generalization of sampling without replacement from a finite universe, J. Am. Stat. Assoc. **47**, 663–685 (1952)

Lancaster, T., Intrator, O.: Panel data with survival: Hospitalization of HIV-positive patients. J. Am. Stat. Assoc. **93**, 46–53 (1998)

Little, R.J.A.: Pattern-mixture models for multivariate incomplete data. J. Am. Stat. Assoc. **88**, 125–134 (1993)

Little, R.J.A.: Modeling the drop-out mechanism in repeated-measure studies. J. Am. Stat. Assoc. **90**, 1112–1121 (1995)

Little, R.J.: Panel on Handling Missing Data in Clinical Trial: The Prevention and Treatment of Missing Data in Clinical Trials. The National Academies Press, Washington (2010)

Little, R.J., Rubin, D.B.: Statistical Analysis with Missing Data, 2nd edn. Wiley, New York (2002)

Liu, J.: Monte Carlo Strategies in Scientific Computing. Springer, New York (2003)

Molenberghs, G., Kenward, M.G.: Missing Data in Clinical Studies. Wiley, Chichester (2008)

Müller, U.U., Schick, A., Wefelmeyer, W.: Imputing responses that are not missing. In: Nikulin, M., Commengs, D., Huber, C. (eds.) Probability, Statistics and Modeling in Public Health. Springer, New York (2006)

Rubin D.B.: Inference and missing data. Biometrika **63**, 581–592 (1976)

Rubin D.B.: Multiple Imputation for Nonresponse in Surveys. Wiley, New York (1987)

SAS Institute: SAS/STAT 9.1 User's Guide, vol. 1–7. SAS Institute, Gary (2004)

SAS Institute Inc.: SAS/STAT 9.2 User's Guide. Cary, NC: SAS Institute Inc. (2008)

Ten Have, T.R., Kunselman, A.R., Pulkstenis, E.P., Landis, J.R. Mixed effect logistic regression models for longitudinal binary response data with informative drop out. Biometrics **54**, 367–383 (1998)

Tsiatis, A.A.: Semiparametric Theory and Missing Data. Springer, New York (2009)

Van Der Laan, M.J., Robins, J.M.: Unified Methods for Censored Longitudinal Data and Causality. Springer, New York (2003)

Vonesh, E.F., Greene, T., Schluchter, M.D.: Shared parameter models for the joint analysis of longitudinal data and event times. Stat. Med. **25**, 143–163 (2006)

Yang, X., Li, J., Shoptaw, S.: Imputation-based strategies for clinical trial longitudinal data with nonignorable missing values. Stat. Med. **27**, 2826–2849 (2008)

Chapter 6
Multivariate and Multistage Survival Data Modeling

6.1 Introduction to Survival Data Modeling

6.1.1 Basic Terms in Survival Analysis

Survival analysis or time-to-event analysis is a branch of statistics dealing with death (failure) or degradation in biological organisms, mechanical or electronic systems, or other areas. This topic is called reliability theory or reliability analysis in engineering, and duration analysis or duration modeling in economics or sociology.

The term lifetime distribution function $F(t)$ is defined as the probability of the event (e.g., death) occurring on or before time t, i.e., $F(t) = P(T \leq t)$. The survival function $S(t)$ is the probability of an individual surviving longer than t, i.e., $S(t) = 1 - F(t)$. Thus the event density is $f(t) = dF(t)/dt$. The hazard function or rate $\lambda(t)$, is defined as the event rate at time t, conditional on survival until time t or later,

$$\lambda(t) \, dt = P(t < T \leq t + dt | T > t) = \frac{f(t) \, dt}{S(t)} = -\frac{S'(t)}{S(t)} dt. \qquad (6.1)$$

Integrating (6.1) with respect to t, we obtain $S(t) = \exp(-\Lambda(t))$, where $\Lambda(t) = \int_0^t \lambda(u) \, du$ is called the cumulative hazard function. From (6.1), we can obtain

$$f(t) = \lambda(t) S(t). \qquad (6.2)$$

The expected future (residual) lifetime at a given time t_0 is defined as $\frac{1}{S(t_0)} \int_0^\infty t \, f(t + t_0) \, dt = \frac{1}{S(t_0)} \int_{t_0}^\infty S(t) \, dt$.

In Chap. 5, we discussed missing-data issues in general. In survival analysis, we usually have a special type of missing data; i.e., censoring. In practice, survival data involve different types of censoring: (1) left-censoring if a data point (time value) is equal to or below a certain value but it is unknown by how much (e.g., missing adverse event start date), (2) right-censoring if a data point is above a certain value

but it is unknown by how much (e.g., lost to follow up), and (3) interval censoring
if a data point is somewhere in an interval between two values. Censoring can occur
at a fixed time point (e.g., prescheduled clinical trial termination) or at a random
time (e.g., early termination). Censoring can be informative or noninformative with
respect to time (treatment/medical intervention). If it is noninformative, the censoring time is statistically independent of the failure time. However, the statistical
independence of the failure time is a necessary but not a sufficient condition for noninformative censoring; there must be no common parameters between survival and
censoring parameters to ensure the censoring is noninformative. Right-censoring is
the most common and can be treated as a competing risk. See Sect. 6.3 for details.

6.1.2 Maximum Likelihood Method

Modeling survival data can be based on a parametric or nonparametric method. Here
we will focus on parametric models. A parametric model can be specified for the
hazard rate $\lambda(t) \geq 0$, survival time $S(t)$, or degradation process (we will discuss
this soon).

The maximum likelihood estimate (MLE) method is commonly used for parameter estimation in survival modeling, which is similar to the MLE for other models,
the only difference being the presence of censoring. Specifically, the likelihood can
be written as

$$L(\theta) = \prod_{t_i \in \Omega_U} P(T = t_i | \theta) \prod_{t_j \in \Omega_L} P(T \leq t_i | \theta) \prod_{t_i \in \Omega_R} P(T > t_i | \theta)$$

$$\cdot \prod_{t_i \in \Omega_I} P(t_{ia} \leq T < t_{ib} | \theta), \tag{6.3}$$

where Ω_U, Ω_L, Ω_R, Ω_I are the sets for uncensored, left-, right-, and interval-
censored data, respectively; $P(T = t_i | \theta) = f(t_i | \theta)$, $P(T \leq t_i | \theta) = 1 - S(t_i | \theta)$,
$P(T > t_i | \theta) = S(t_i | \theta)$, and $P(t_{i,a} < T \leq t_{i,b} | \theta) = S(t_{ia} | \theta) - S(t_{ib} | \theta)$.

The MLE is defined as

$$\hat{\theta}_{mle} = \arg\max L(\theta). \tag{6.4}$$

Under fairly weak conditions (Newey and McFadden 1994, Theorem 3.3), the
maximum likelihood estimator has approximately a normal distribution for a larger
sample size n,

$$\sqrt{n}\left(\hat{\theta}_{mle} - \theta_0\right) \xrightarrow{d} N\left(0, I^{-1}\right),$$

where I is the expected Fisher information matrix given by

$$I = E\left[\nabla_\theta \ln f(x|\theta_0) \nabla_\theta \ln f(x|\theta_0)'\right],$$

where the gradient operator is given by $\nabla_\theta = \sum_i \frac{\partial}{\partial \theta_i}$.

Hougaard (2000) provided two reasons not to use the expected information for survival analysis. He argued that first, for the evaluation, it is necessary to make assumptions on the general censoring pattern, whereas the observed information is based only on the actual observed censoring times. Consequently, the evaluation is only valid under precisely that censoring pattern. Second, for censored data, the expected information is more complicated to evaluate than the observed information because integration is necessary. This is in contrast to many other models, such as nonlinear regression and exponential families, where taking the expectation makes some terms vanish.

6.1.3 Overview of Survival Model

6.1.3.1 Proportion Hazard Model

Proportional hazard models are widely used in practice. Just as the name suggests, a proportional hazard model assumes the hazard is proportional (i.e., independent of time) between any two different groups with covariates $X' = x'_1$ and $X' = x'_2$,

$$h(t) = h_0(t) \exp(X'\beta), \tag{6.5}$$

where X is the vector of observed covariates and β are the corresponding parameters. If the baseline hazard function is specified (e.g., $h_0(t) = \lambda \rho t^{\rho-1}$), (6.5) represents a parametric proportional hazard model; otherwise, (6.5) is the well-known Cox semiparametric proportional hazard model (Cox 1972).

6.1.3.2 Accelerated Failure Time Model

When the proportional hazard assumption does not hold, we may use the accelerated failure time model with a hazard function:

$$h(t) = \exp(X'\beta) h_0(\exp(X'\beta)t). \tag{6.6}$$

Different baseline functions $h_0(\cdot)$ will lead to different parametric models. For the exponential model, $h_0(t) = \lambda$ and $S_0(t) = \exp(-\lambda t)$, where $\lambda > 0$; for the Weibull model, $h_0(t) = \lambda \rho t^{\rho-1}$ and $S_0(t) = \exp(-\lambda t^{\rho})$, where $\lambda, \rho > 0$; for the Gompertz model, $h_0(t) = \lambda \exp(\gamma t)$ and $S_0(t) = \exp(-\lambda \gamma^{-1}(\exp(\gamma t) - 1))$, where $\gamma, \lambda > 0$; and for the loglogistic model, $h_0(t) = \frac{\exp(\alpha)k t^{k-1}}{1+\exp(\alpha)t^k}$ and $S_0(t) = \frac{1}{1+\exp(\alpha)t^k}$, where $\alpha \in \mathbb{R}, k > 0$.

6.1.3.3 Frailty Model

The notion of frailty provides a convenient way to introduce random effects, association and unobserved heterogeneity into models for survival data. In its simplest form, a frailty is an unobserved random factor that modifies the hazard function of an individual or related individuals. The term frailty was coined by Vaupel et al. (1979) in univariate survival models, and the model was substantially promoted for its application to multivariate survival data in a seminal paper by Clayton (1978) on chronic disease incidence in families. The simplest form of frailty model with a (unobserved) scale frailty variable Z can be written as

$$h(t, Z, X) = Z h_0(t) \exp(X'\beta).$$

We will discuss this approach further later.

6.1.3.4 Copula Model

Copula modeling is a general approach to formulating different multivariate distributions. The idea is that a simple transformation can be made of each marginal variable in such a way that each transformed marginal variable has a uniform distribution. Once this is done, the dependence structure can be expressed as a multivariate distribution on the obtained uniforms, and a copula is precisely a multivariate distribution on marginally uniform random variables.

In the context of survival analysis, a copula model is often constructed from marginal survival functions instead of marginal distribution functions. If the arguments of the copula function are univariate survival functions $S_1(t_1) = P(X_1 > t_1)$ and $S_2(t_2) = P(X_2 > t_2)$, the copula function $C(S_1, S_2)$ is a legitimate joint (bivariate) survival function $S(t_1, t_2) = P(X_1 > t_1, X_2 > t_2)$ with marginals S_1 and S_2.

Archimedean copulas are commonly used copulas in survival analysis. Suppose that $\psi : [0, \infty] \to [0, 1]$ is a strictly decreasing convex function such that $\psi(0) = 1$. Then an Archimedean copula can be written as

$$C(S_1, S_2; \theta) = \psi\left(\psi^{-1}(S_1) + \psi^{-1}(S_2)\right), \quad S_1, S_1 \in [0, 1], \qquad (6.7)$$

where θ is the parameter of association. For example, the stable (Gumbel-Hougaard) copula, generated by $\psi^{-1}(s) = (-\ln s)^\theta$, $\theta \geq 1$, can be expressed as

$$S(t_1, t_2; \theta) = \exp\left\{-\left[(-\ln S_1)^\theta + (-\ln S_2)^\theta\right]^{1/\theta}\right\}.$$

Archimedean copulas can be conveniently used for modeling a bivariate survival function with such marginal distributions as Gompertz, Weibull, or even in the semiparametric setup in combination with Kaplan-Meier estimates for the marginal survival functions (Genest and Rivest 1993). All information concerning dependence between the marginals is contained in the association parameter.

6.1.3.5   First-Hitting-Time Model

Many practical problems, such as biomarker or clinical responses, survival time and random vibrations of a bridge, can be modeled using stochastic processes $X(t)$. When the stochastic process reaches a certain level (i.e., $X(t) = ß$) for the first time, it is called first hitting time (FHT). FHT usually indicates a critical state such as a biological inhibition, death, or bridge collapse. The critical value $ß$, called the boundary or threshold, can be a constant or function of time t. Threshold regression refers to the first-hitting-time models with regression structures that accommodate covariate data (Lee and Whitmore 2006).

A very commonly used stochastic process is a Wiener process or Brownian motion, which describes, for example, a particle random motion on the microscope. The macro-behavior (i.e., the average properties for Brownian motion) of the mass is governed by the so-called diffusion equation, which is widely used in science and engineering, the social sciences, and other areas. We will discuss this approach in Sect. 6.3.

6.1.3.6   Multistage Model

A multistage model consists of several stages across a time axis. At each stage, a time-to-event model is applied. In principle, all models mentioned above can be used in multistage models. However, most common multistage models are semi-Markov processes (continuous time, discrete states).

The rationale for using multistage models is that it may not be easy to specify a single model across the entire time course. This is because, for example, the natural course of disease may consist of stages and the time-to-event model is relatively easy to specify for each stage separately. The model within each stage can be the proportional hazard model, frailty model, exponential model, or a combination of them. In principle, a time-dependent hazard model can be approximated by a multistage model with a time-independent hazard rate at each stage, but the number of stages required may be large in order to have the desired precision. The time-independent hazard rate λ does not have to be a constant; it can include covariates (i.e., $\lambda = \lambda(X'\beta)$). The examples to illustrate the method in this chapter will focus on Markov or semi-Markov models because their calculations don't require specific software. However, for more complicated multistage models, a software package is required. The transitional probability matrix for a semi-Markov chain is given by

$$P(t) = e^{At} = I + \sum_{k=1}^{\infty} \frac{A^k t^k}{k!},$$

where $A = \lim_{h \to 0} (P(h) - I)/h$ with I being the identity matrix. We will discuss the multistage approach in Sect. 6.4.

6.1.3.7 Nonparametric Approach

Nelson-Aalen Estimator

Let $Y(t)$ be the number of individuals at risk at (just before) time t and τ_i the occurrence of the ith event. The Nelson-Aalen estimator for the cumulative hazard is given by

$$\hat{\Lambda}(t) = \sum_{\tau_i \le t} \frac{1}{Y(\tau_i)},$$

with variance estimator

$$\hat{\sigma}_\Lambda^2(t) = \sum_{\tau_i \le t} \frac{1}{Y(\tau_i)^2}.$$

The cumulative hazard $\hat{\Lambda}(t)$ approaches to a normal distribution as the sample size approaches infinity. To improve precision, log-transformation can be used.

Kaplan-Meier Estimator

The Kaplan-Meier estimator is given by

$$\hat{S}(t) = \prod_{\tau_k \le t} S(\tau_k | \tau_{k-1}) = \prod_{\tau_i \le t} \left\{ 1 - \frac{1}{Y(\tau_i)} \right\},$$

with variance

$$\hat{\sigma}_S^2(t) = \hat{S}(t)^2 \sum_{\tau_i \le t} \frac{1}{Y(\tau_i)^2}.$$

Alternatively, the variance can be estimated using Greenwood's formulation:

$$\hat{\sigma}_S^2(t) = \hat{S}(t)^2 \sum_{\tau_i \le t} \frac{1}{Y(\tau_i)^2 - Y(\tau_i)}.$$

For a large sample size, $\hat{S}(t)$ has approximately a normal distribution. To improve precision, log-transformation can be used.

Many software packages, such as SAS, R, and STATA, have the built-in capability of performing survival analyses with various models.

6.2 Frailty Model

6.2.1 Univariate Frailty Models

We know an individual's survival time is dependent on his risk factors. If these risk factors are known, they can be included in the analysis by using the proportional hazards model or accelerated failure time model. However, sometimes there are too many covariates to be considered in the model or there are some important unknown or unmeasured covariates. In a proportional hazard model, neglect of a subset of the important covariates leads to biased estimates of both regression coefficients and the hazard rate. To account for such unobserved heterogeneity in the study population, Vaupel et al. (1979) introduced univariate frailty models into survival analysis. The univariate frailty model extends the Cox model such that the hazard of an individual depends in addition on an unobservable random variable Z that acts multiplicatively on the baseline hazard function

$$h(t, Z, X) = Z h_0(t) \exp\left(X'\beta\right), \qquad (6.8)$$

where X is the vector of observed covariates and Z is the unobservable frailty variable, which varies over the population and lowers $(Z < 1)$ or increases $(Z > 1)$ the individual risk. The respective survival function S is given by

$$S(t|Z, X) = \exp\left(-Z \int_0^t h_0(\tau)\, d\tau \, \exp\left(X'\beta\right)\right). \qquad (6.9)$$

$S(t|Z, X)$ may be interpreted as the fraction of individuals surviving at time t after the beginning of follow-up given the vector of observable covariates X and frailty Z. The model has been described at the level of individuals. However, this individual model is not observable. Therefore, it is necessary to consider the model at the population level. The survival function of the total population is the mean of the individual survival functions (6.9). It can be viewed as the survival function of a randomly drawn individual and corresponds to what is actually observed. It is important to note that the observed hazard function will not be similar to the individual hazard rate. What may be observed in the population is the net result for a number of individuals with different Z. The population hazard rate may have a completely different shape than the individual hazard rate (Wienke 2010).

One important issue in frailty models is the choice of the frailty distribution. Examples of frailty distributions are the gamma distribution (Vaupel et al. 1979), a three-parameter distribution (Hougaard 2000), the compound Poisson distribution (Aalen 1992) and the log-normal distribution (McGilchrist and Aisbett 1991).

6.2.2 Multivariate Frailty Models

Multivariate frailty models can be useful when lifetimes in a cluster or recurrent events like infections are considered because in such cases independence between the clustered survival times cannot be assumed. Multivariate models are able to account for dependence between these event times. A general approach is to assume independence among observed data items conditional on a set of unobserved or latent variables (Hougaard 2000); for example, let $S(t_1|Z, X_1)$ and $S(t_2|Z, X_2)$ be the conditional survival functions of two related individuals with different vectors of observed covariates X_1 and X_2, respectively, in (6.9). Integrating out the noise variable Z, the two-dimensional survival function can be written as

$$S(t_1, t_2) = \int_0^\infty S(t_1|z, X_1)\, S(t_2|z, X_2)\, g(z)\, dz, \qquad (6.10)$$

where $g(Z)$ denotes the density of the frailty Z. In the case of twins, $S(t_1, t_2)$ denotes the fraction of twins pairs with twin 1 surviving t_1 and twin 2 surviving t_2.

6.2.3 The Shared Frailty Copula

The shared frailty model is relevant to event times of related subjects (similar organs and repeated measurements). Subjects in a cluster are assumed to share the same frailty Z (Clayton 1978; Hougaard 2000). The survival times are assumed to be conditionally independent with respect to the shared (common) frailty. Conditional on the frailty Z, the hazard function of an individual in a pair is of the form $Z h_0(t) \exp(X'\beta)$, where the value of Z is common to both individuals in the pair and thus is the cause for dependence between survival times within pairs.

$$S(t_1, t_2|Z) = S_1(t_1)^Z S_2(t_2)^Z.$$

In most applications it is assumed that the frailty distribution is a gamma distribution with mean 1 and variance 2. Averaging the conditional survival functions under this assumption, the survival functions can be written as (Wienke 2010)

$$S(t_1, t_2) = \left(S_1(t_1)^{-\sigma^2} + S_2(t_2)^{-\sigma^2} - 1 \right)^{\frac{1}{\sigma^2}}.$$

where $\sigma^2 > 0$ indicates a dependent model and $\sigma^2 > 0$ with $Z = 1$ indicates an independent model.

Shared frailty explains correlations between subjects within clusters. There are a few issues with the model: When covariates are present in a proportional hazard model with gamma-distributed frailty, the dependence parameter and the population heterogeneity are confounded, which implies that the joint distribution can be identified from the marginal distributions (Hougaard 1986). In most cases, a one-dimensional frailty can only induce positive association within the cluster. However, there are some situations in which the survival times for subjects within the same cluster are negatively associated. For example, in the Stanford Heart Transplantation Study, generally the longer an individual must wait for an available heart, the shorter he or she is likely to survive after the transplantation. Therefore, the waiting time and the survival time afterward may be negatively associated. To avoid the above-mentioned limitations of shared frailty models, correlated frailty models were developed (Wienke 2010).

6.2.4 The Correlated Frailty Copula

Correlated frailty models were initially developed for the analysis of bivariate failure time data, in which two associated random variables are used to characterize the frailty effect for each pair. For example, processes of biomarkers 1 and 2 are associated with a joint distribution but don't have a common frailty distribution. These two variables can also be negatively associated, which would induce a negative association between survival times. Assuming gamma-distributed frailties, Yashin and Iachine (1995) used the correlated gamma frailty model, resulting in a bivariate survival distribution of the form:

$$S(t_1, t_2) = \frac{S_1(t_1)^{1-\rho} S_2(t_2)^{1-\rho}}{\left(S_1(t_1)^{-\sigma^2} + S_2(t_2)^{-\sigma^2} - 1\right)^{\frac{\rho}{\sigma^2}}}.$$

Research on applications of correlated frailty models has been done, including a shared log-normal frailty model for the catheter infection (McGilchrist and Aisbett 1991), a shared frailty model with gamma and log-normally distributed frailty for the recurrence of breast cancer (dos Santos et al. 1995), a shared positive stable frailty model for a diabetic retinopathy study (Manatunga and Oakes 1999), and a correlated gamma frailty model to analyze genetic factors involved in mortality due to coronary heart disease in twins (Wienke et al. 2001; Zdravkovic et al. 2002).

6.3 First-Hitting-Time Model

6.3.1 Wiener Process and First Hitting Time

Definition 6.1. A stochastic process $\{X(t), t \geq 0\}$ is said to be a Brownian motion with a drift μ if (1) $X(0) = 0$; (2) $\{X(t), t \geq 0\}$ has stationary and independent increments; and (3) for every $t > 0$, $X(t)$ is normally distributed with mean μt and variance $\sigma^2 t$,

$$X(t) \sim \frac{1}{\sqrt{2\pi\sigma^2 t}} \exp\left(-\frac{(x - \mu t)^2}{2\sigma^2 t}\right). \tag{6.11}$$

The covariance of the Brownian motion is $\text{cov}[X(t), X(s)] = \sigma^2 \min\{s, t\}$. The standard Brownian motion $B(t)$ is the Brownian motion with drift $\mu = 0$ and diffusion $\sigma^2 = 1$. The relationship between the standard Brownian motion and Brownian motion with drift μ and diffusion parameter σ^2 can be expressed as

$$X(t) = \mu t + \sigma B(t). \tag{6.12}$$

The c.d.f. is given by

$$\Pr\{X(t) \le y \mid X(0) = x\} = \Phi\left(\frac{y - x - \mu t}{\sigma\sqrt{t}}\right), \tag{6.13}$$

where $\Phi(\cdot)$ is the c.d.f. of the standard normal distribution.

The first hitting time T is a random variable when $X(t)$ starts from the initial position $X(0) = 0 \in \Omega \backslash \text{ß}$ and reaches a given constant boundary $\text{ß} = b$ of the domain Ω (non-negative values). The FHT for Brownian motion is the inverse normal distribution:

$$T \sim f\left(t \mid \mu, \sigma^2, b\right) = \frac{b}{\sqrt{2\pi\sigma^2 t^3}} e^{-\frac{(b + \mu t)^2}{2\sigma^2 t}}. \tag{6.14}$$

The c.d.f. corresponding to (6.14) is given by

$$F\left(t \mid \mu, \sigma^2, b\right) = \Phi\left[-\frac{(\mu t + b)}{\sqrt{\sigma^2 t}}\right] + e^{-\frac{2b\mu}{\sigma^2}} \Phi\left[\frac{\mu t - b}{\sqrt{\sigma^2 t}}\right]. \tag{6.15}$$

Note that if $\mu > 0$, then the FHT is not certain to occur and the p.d.f. is improper. Specifically, in this case, $P(t = \infty) = 1 - \exp(-2b\mu/\sigma^2)$.

Definition 6.2. In general, an FHT model $<X(t), \text{ß}>$ has two essential components: (1) a parent stochastic process $\{X(t), t \in T, x \in \mathbb{R}\}$ with initial value $X(0) = 0$, where T is the time space and $\mathbb{R}$ is the state space of the process, and (2) a boundary set or threshold ß, where $\text{ß} \subset \mathbb{R}$. Note that ß can be a constant or function vector of time t or a stochastic process.

6.3.2　Covariates and Link Function

In an FHT model, both the parent process $\{X(t)\}$ and boundary ß can have parameters that depend on covariates. As a simple sample, the Wiener process has mean parameter μ and variance parameter σ^2. The boundary ß has parameter x_0,

the initial position. In FHT regression models, these parameters will be connected
to linear combinations of covariates using a suitable regression link function,

$$g\left(\theta\right) = Z\beta', \tag{6.16}$$

where $g\left(\cdot\right)$ is the link function that has the inverse function $g^{-1}\left(\cdot\right)$, θ is the
parameter vector in the FHT model, $Z = (1, Z_1, \ldots, Z_k)$ is the covariate vector
(with a leading unit to include an intercept term), and $\mathbf{fi} = (\beta_0, \beta_1, \ldots, \beta_k)$ is the
associated vector of regression coefficients. The commonly used link functions
include the identity and logistic functions.

There are two different covariates: time-independent (e.g., DNA markers) and
time-dependent covariates (e.g., RNA markers). The use of time-dependent covariates should be taken cautiously since it could be very controversial (see Sect. 6.4).

We can solve (6.16) for θ:

$$\theta = g^{-1}\left(Z\beta'\right). \tag{6.17}$$

6.3.3 Parameter Estimation and Inference

The parameter estimations for FHT models have been dominated by the maximum
likelihood method. Consider a latent health status process characterized by a
Wiener diffusion process. The FHT for such a process follows an inverse Gaussian
distribution. The inverse Gaussian distribution depends on the mean and variance
parameters of the underlying Wiener process (μ and σ^2) and the initial health status
level (x_0), i.e., $\theta = (\mu, \sigma, x_0)$. Let $f(t|\theta)$ and $F(t|\theta)$ be the p.d.f. and c.d.f. of the
FHT distribution, respectively. Using (6.17), we can obtain

$$\begin{cases} f(t|\theta) = f\left(t|g^{-1}\left(Z\beta'\right)\right), \\ F(t|\theta) = F\left(t|g^{-1}\left(Z\beta'\right)\right). \end{cases} \tag{6.18}$$

To form a likelihood function, denote by Z_i $(i = 1, \ldots n_e)$ the realization of
covariate vector Z on the ith subject who had an event at time t_i, and by Z_j
$(j = n_e + 1, \ldots n_e + n_s)$ the realization of covariate vector Z on the jth subject,
who is right-censored at time t_j. Then the likelihood function is given by

$$L\left(\beta\right) = \prod_{i=1}^{n_e} f\left(t_i | g^{-1}\left(Z_i\beta'\right)\right) \prod_{j=n_e+1}^{n_e+n_s} S\left(t_j | g^{-1}\left(Z_j\beta'\right)\right). \tag{6.19}$$

To estimate parameters β, the likelihood or the log-likelihood function can be
used. Numerical gradient methods can be used to find the maximum likelihood
estimates for β. Then the parameter vector θ can be found using (6.17), and the
distribution function $f(t|\theta)$ and $F(t|\theta)$ can be obtained from (6.18).

6.3.4 Applications of First-Hitting-Time Model

Example 6.1. A death can be viewed as the final result of the degradation of an individual's health. If we model an individual's health state using a Wiener process, then death can be viewed as the Wiener process reaching a certain threshold ß. The survival analysis becomes the study of the FHT of the process, which has an inverse normal distribution.

Alternatively, if a gamma process is chosen to model the health state, the survival (FHT) will have an inverse gamma distribution. Singpurwalla (1995) and Lawless and Crowder (2004) consider the gamma process as a model for degradation. The Ornstein-Uhlenbeck process can also be used for modeling the biological process. The FHT for the Ornstein-Uhlenbeck process has the Ricciardi-Sato distribution (Ricciardi and Sato 1988).

Example 6.2. Survival analysis in a clinical trial with treatment switching is a challenge. In randomized oncology trials, a patient's treatment may be switched in the middle of the study because of a progressive disease (PD), which indicates a failure of the initial treatment regimen. In such cases, the total survival time is the sum of two event times: randomization to switching and switching to death. If the test drug is more effective than the control, then the majority of patients in the control group will switch to the test drug and the survival difference between the two treatment groups will be significantly reduced in comparison with the case without treatment switching. This marker-based treatment switch is not random switching but rather response-adaptive switching. Branson and Whitehead (2002) and Shao et al. (2005) proposed different approaches to the problem. Lee et al. (2008) proposed a mixture of Wiener processes for clinical trials with adaptive switching and applied it to an oncology study. It is outlined as follows.

Since the actual or censored survival time can be composed of two intervals, representing the time on the primary therapy and the time on the alternative therapy, the disease may progress at different rates in these two intervals (irrespective of the treatment). We transform survival times from calendar time to the so-called running time, which has the form

$$r = a_1 \tau_1 + \tau_2, \tag{6.20}$$

where τ_1 and τ_2 correspond to time to progression and progression to death, respectively, and a_1 is a scale parameter to be estimated.

The mixture of Wiener processes with FHT used for the modeling is given by

$$\Pr(S > r) = p(1 - F_1(r)) + (1 - p)(1 - F_2(r)). \tag{6.21}$$

The respective lifetime functions $F_j(r)$ ($j = 1, 2$) are the same as (6.15) but expressed in terms of running time r. The parameter p is to be estimated.

6.3.5 *Multivariate Model with Biomarkers*

There are different biomarkers: a pharmacodynamic biomarker informs if a drug has reached its target; a functional response biomarker informs if a drug has affected a target pathway; a pharmacogenomic biomarker (PGx) measures variations in a target; a disease biomarker monitors or predicts disease risk, progression, and improvement; and a surrogate endpoint reflects how a patient feels or physical or mental functions.

Biomarkers, compared with a clinical endpoint such as survival, can often be measured earlier, easier, and more frequently. They are less subject to competing risks and are less confounded by changes in treatment modalities. Among different biomarkers, some are static, such as DNA markers, while others are time-dependent, such as RNA markers. A time-independent biomarker can be treated as a covariate, whereas a time-dependent marker can be treated in multivariate survival models. There are also models that treat a time-dependent variable as a covariate. However, we will show you that the results from such models can be very misleading. The utility of biomarkers in clinical trial designs, especially in adaptive designs, has been discussed in Chang (2007). Here we discuss how to use the biomarker process to assist in tracking the progress of the parent process if the parent process is latent or only infrequently observed. In this way, the marker process forms a basis for a predictive inference about the status of the parent process and its progress toward an FHT. As markers of the parent process, they offer potential insights into the causal forces that are generating the movements of the parent process (Whitmore et al. 1998).

We now introduce the Whitmore-Crowder-Lawless method (Whitmore et al. 1998). Suppose there are the parent survival process, $X(t)$, and a correlated biomarker process, $Y(t)$. They form a two-dimensional Wiener diffusion process $\{X(r), Y(r)\}$ for $r \geq 0$ and the initial condition $\{X(0), Y(0)\} = \{0, 0\}$. Vector $\{X(r), Y(r)\}$ has a bivariate normal distribution with a mean vector $r\mu$, where $\mu = (\mu_x, \mu_y)'$, $\mu_x \geq 0$, and covariance matrix $r\Sigma$ with $\Sigma = \begin{pmatrix} \sigma_{xx} & \sigma_{xy} \\ \sigma_{yx} & \sigma_{yy} \end{pmatrix}$. The correlation coefficient is $\rho = \sigma_{xy}/\sqrt{\sigma_{xx}\sigma_{yy}}$.

The key is to formulate the probability or p.d.f. for the survival and failing subjects. For a survivor at time t, an observed value $Y(t) = y(t)$ for the biomarker constitutes a censored observation of failure time because we know $S > t$. The p.d.f. for survival subjects is given by

$$p_s(y) = \Phi(c_1)\phi(c_2) - e^{\frac{2\mu_x}{\sigma_{xx}}}\Phi\left(c_1 - 2\sqrt{\frac{(1-\rho^2)}{\sigma_{xx}t}}\right)\phi\left(c_2 - \frac{2\sigma_{xy}}{\sigma_{xx}\sqrt{\sigma_{yy}t}}\right),$$

$$(6.22)$$

where ϕ and Φ are, respectively, the standard normal p.d.f. and c.d.f., and

$$\begin{cases} c_1 = \dfrac{1 - \mu_x t - \sigma_{xy} \left(y - \mu_y t \right)}{\sigma_{yy} \sqrt{\sigma_{xx} \left(1 - \rho^2 \right) t}}, \\ c_2 = \dfrac{y - \mu_y t}{\sqrt{\sigma_{yy} t}}. \end{cases} \tag{6.23}$$

For a subject that died at time $S = s$ with an observed value $Y(S) = y(s)$ for the biomarker, the joint p.d.f. is

$$p_f(y, s) = \frac{\exp\left(-\frac{1}{2} W^T \Sigma^{-1} W\right)}{2\pi \sqrt{|\Sigma|} s^2}, \tag{6.24}$$

where

$$W^T = \left(\frac{y - \mu_y s}{\sqrt{s}}, \frac{1 - \mu_x s}{\sqrt{s}} \right). \tag{6.25}$$

The probability of surviving longer than time t is

$$P(S > t) = \int_{-\infty}^{\infty} p_s(y) \, dy. \tag{6.26}$$

Numerical methods can be used to calculate $P(S > t)$.

To carry out maximum likelihood estimation of the parameters, we denote the independent sample observations on failing items by $(\hat{y}_i, \hat{s}_i)$, $i = 1, \ldots, \nu$, and those on surviving items by $\hat{y}_i$, $i = \nu + 1, \ldots, n$. The log-likelihood can then be written as

$$\ln L(\mu, \Sigma) = \sum_{i=1}^{\nu} \ln p_f(\hat{y}_i, \hat{s}_i) + \sum_{i=\nu+1}^{n} \ln p_s(\hat{y}_i). \tag{6.27}$$

The maximum likelihood estimates of the parameters μ and Σ can be found based on (6.27).

From (6.22) through (6.27), we have assumed the threshold for failure is $x = 1$. If failure is defined as $x = a$, then the estimates $\hat{\mu}_x$, $\hat{\sigma}_{xx}$, and $\hat{\sigma}_{xy}$ from (6.20) should be multiplied by a constant a. Other estimates and probabilities are independent of a. Thus no changes are needed.

So far, we have considered a single-marker case. In practice, there is usually more than one relevant marker, while each marker will have a certain degree of correlation with the underlying parent process. We wish to find that the linear combination of the available markers will have the largest possible correlation with the degradation component. Whitmore et al. (1998) extended their method to include a composite marker or a combination of several markers.

Suppose there are k candidate markers available, denoted by $Z(t) = (Z_1(t), \ldots, Z_k(t))$, with the initial condition $Z(0) = 0$. Assume that vector $Z(t)$, together with the degradation component $X(t)$, forms a $k + 1$ dimensional Wiener process. We define the composite marker denoted by $Y(t)$ as

$$Y(t) = \mathbf{Z}(t)\boldsymbol{\beta}' = \sum_{j=1}^{k} Z_j(t)\beta_j, \qquad (6.28)$$

where $\boldsymbol{\beta} = (1, \beta_2, \ldots, \beta_k)$ is a $k \times 1$ vector of coefficients that we wish to estimate. The linear structure of (6.28) assures that the joint process for $Y(t)$ and $X(t)$ retains its bivariate Wiener form. The parameterization is defined by

$$\mu_y = \mu_Z\boldsymbol{\beta}', \; \sigma_{yy} = \boldsymbol{\beta}\Sigma_{ZZ}\boldsymbol{\beta}', \; \sigma_{yy} = \Sigma_{XZ}\boldsymbol{\beta}', \qquad (6.29)$$

where μ_Z and Σ_{ZZ} denote the $k \times 1$ mean vector and $k \times k$ covariance matrix of markers $Z(t)$ and Σ_{XZ} denotes the $1 \times k$ covariate vector of $X(t)$ with $Z(t)$.

The MLEs presented earlier for a single marker can be extended to estimate the optimal composite marker in (6.28). This extension requires rewriting the likelihood function in (6.27) in terms of the new parameterization in (6.29).

6.4 Multistage Model

6.4.1 General Framework of Multistage Model

Multistage models are not only used for longitudinal data but can also be used for multivariate survival analysis if we partition all the possible event scenarios into stages (or states) and build a progressive model. According to Hougaard (2000), a progressive model is a stochastic model in which all states except the initial state have only one possible transition into the state. We consider the time-dependent Markov progressive model in which the probability (density) of transition is usually dependent on the time relative to the previous state but independent of any earlier states. For example, a healthy individual can become a disabled person and then die, as shown in Fig. 6.1. The progressive Markov model says that the transition probability from the state "Disabled" to "Death" is a function of time from "Disabled" but is independent of how healthy he was and how quickly he became a disabled person.

Suppose we have a simple multistage model, as shown in Fig. 6.1, that has three states of an individual: health, disabled, and death. Possible transition directions are indicated by arrows, with a corresponding transition probability $F_i(t)$ and density $f_i(t)$ $(i = 1, 2)$, which are the lifetime and event density functions.

After a multistage model is constructed, we need to formulate the likelihood for the MLE of parameters. Similar to the single stage model discussed in Sect. 6.1, the

Fig. 6.1 Time-dependent
Markov process

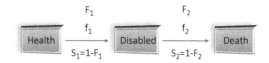

likelihood formulation L (assume the process starting time $t_0 = 0$) can be classified
into the following four different cases:

1. For subject i disabled at time $t = t_{1i}$ and dead at $t = t_{2i}$, the likelihood is
   $l_i = f_1(t_{1i}) f_2(t_{2i} - t_{1i})$.
2. For subject j disabled at time $t = t_{1j}$ and alive (right-censored) at $t = t_{2j}$, the
   likelihood is $l_j = f_1(t_{1j})(1 - F_2(t_{2j} - t_{1j}))$.
3. For subject k disabled before or at time t_{1k} (left-censored) and dead at $t = t_{2k}$,
   the likelihood is $l_k = F_1(t_{1k}) f_2(t_{2k} - t_{1k})$.
4. For subject m disabled before or at time t_{1m} (left-censored) and alive (right-
   censored) at $t = t_{2m}$, the likelihood is $l_m = F_1(t_{1m})(1 - F_2(t_{2m} - t_{1m}))$.

Assume there are n_i subjects in category i. We label the subjects in such a way
that patients 1 to n_1 are in category 1, patients $n_1 + 1$ to $n_1 + n_2$ in category 2,
patients $n_1 + n_2 + 1$ to $n_1 + n_2 + n_3$ in category 3, and patients $n_1 + n_2 + n_3 + 1$ to
$n_1 + n_2 + n_3 + n_4$ in category 4. The likelihood function for the n ($n = n_1 + n_2 +
n_3 + n_4$) observations is given by

$$L = \prod_{i=1}^{n_1} l_i \prod_{j=n_1+1}^{n_1+n_2} l_j \prod_{k=n_1+n_2+1}^{n_1+n_2+n_3} l_k \prod_{m=n_1+n_2+n_3+1}^{n_1+n_2+n_3+n_4} l_m. \tag{6.30}$$

By maximizing L in (6.30), we can obtain the MLE of the parameters.

Example 6.3. In the multistage model in Fig. 6.1, we apply an exponential model
with constant hazard λ_i. The transition probability density is $f_i = \lambda_i \exp(-\lambda_i t)$. It
follows that $F_i = 1 - \exp(-\lambda_i t)$ and $S_i = 1 - F_i(t) = \exp(-\lambda_i t)$. Suppose there
are n_1 observations $(t_{11}, \ldots, t_{1n_1})$ in category 1 and n_2 observations $(t_{21}, \ldots, t_{2n_2})$
in category 2, but no left-censored observations, i.e., $n_3 = n_4 = 0$. The likelihood
function is given by

$$L = \prod_{i=1}^{n_1} \lambda_1 e^{-\lambda_1 t_{1i}} \lambda_2 e^{-\lambda_2(t_{2i}-t_{1i})} \prod_{j=n_1+1}^{n_2} \lambda_1 e^{-\lambda_1 t_{1j}} e^{-\lambda_2(t_{2j}-t_{1j})}. \tag{6.31}$$

The log-likelihood is given by

$$\ln L = (n_1 + n_2) \ln \lambda_1 + n_1 \ln \lambda_2 - \sum_{i=1}^{n_1+n_2} [\lambda_2(t_{2i} - t_{1i}) + \lambda_1 t_{1i}]. \tag{6.32}$$

Fig. 6.2 Effect of treatment switching

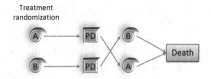

The maximization of $\ln L$ gives

$$\lambda_1 = \frac{n_1 + n_2}{\sum_{i=1}^{n_1+n_2} t_{1i}}; \lambda_2 = \frac{n_1}{\sum_{i=1}^{n_1+n_2} (t_{2i} - t_{1i})}. \tag{6.33}$$

6.4.2 Covariates and Treatment Switching

Covariates such as medical treatment, age, race, and disease status may or may not be time-dependent. In Example 6.4, a progressive disease (PD) is an indication of treatment failure and the patient usually has to switch from the initial treatment to an alternative. Thus, treatment for a patient is a time-dependent variable: before PD with one treatment, after PD with another treatment (Fig. 6.2).

To consider covariates in a multistage model, we can use a link function as defined in (6.16). Then substitute (6.17) into (6.30) and maximize it to obtain MLEs of the parameters $\boldsymbol{\beta}$.

Example 6.4. Suppose patients in a two-group oncology clinical trial are randomized to receive either treatment A or B. If a progressive disease is observed, meaning the patient has developed a resistance to the drug, then the patient will switch the treatment from A to B or B to A (in practice, there are more options, i.e., different combinations of drugs). Let $Z_i(t)$ be a random process for the ith patient. If patient i is on treatment A at time t, then $Z_i(t) = 1$; otherwise, $Z_i(t) = 0$. We use the identity link function

$$\lambda_i(t) = \beta_i(t) Z_i(t). \tag{6.34}$$

Recognizing the different hazard rates before and after PD, we use the piecewise constant hazard

$$\lambda_i(t) = \beta_{i1} Z(t) + \beta_{i2}(1 - Z(t)), i = 1, 2,$$

where $i = 1$ before PD and $i = 2$ after PD. In other words, the hazard rates are β_{11} for treatment A before PD, β_{21} for treatment A after PD, β_{12} for treatment B before PD, and β_{22} for treatment B after PD.

For simplicity we assume PD is always observed immediately (i.e., no censoring on PD). Thus, a typical patient i initially treated with drug A will have the following two possible likelihood functions:

1. PD at time $t = t_{1i}$ and death at $t = t_{2i}$, $l_i = \beta_{11} e^{-\beta_{11} t_{1i}} \beta_{21} e^{-\beta_{21}(t_{2i} - t_{1i})}$, where $i = 1, \ldots, n_1$.

2. PD at time $t = t_{1i}$ and alive (right-censored) at $t = t_{2i}$, $l_i = \beta_{11}e^{-\beta_{11}t_{1i}}$ $e^{-\beta_{21}(t_{2i}-t_{1i})}$, where $i = n_1 + 1, \ldots, n_1 + n_2$.

Similarly, a typical patient i initially treated with drug B will have the following two possible likelihood functions:

1. PD at time $t = t_{1i}$ and death at $t = t_{2i}$, $l_i = \beta_{12}e^{-\beta_{12}t_{1i}}\beta_{22}e^{-\beta_{22}(t_{2i}-t_{1i})}$, where $i = n_1 + n_2 + 1, \ldots, n_1 + n_2 + n_3$.
2. PD at time $t = t_{1i}$ and alive (right-censored) at $t = t_{2i}$, $l_i = \beta_{12}e^{-\beta_{12}t_{1i}}$ $e^{-\beta_{22}(t_{2i}-t_{1i})}$, where $i = n_1 + n_2 + n_3 + 1, \ldots, n_1 + n_2 + n_3 + n_4$.

The likelihood function based on the total $n_1 + n_2 + n_3 + n_4$ observations is the same as (6.30). The log-likelihood function can be given explicitly by

$$\ln L = (n_1 + n_2) \ln \beta_{11} + (n_3 + n_4) \ln \beta_{12} + n_1 \ln \beta_{21} + n_3 \ln \beta_{22}$$
$$- \sum_{i=1}^{n_1+n_2} [\beta_{21}(t_{2i} - t_{1i}) + \beta_{11}t_{1i}]$$
$$- \sum_{i=1+n_1+n_2}^{n_1+n_2+n_3+n_4} [\beta_{22}(t_{2i} - t_{1i}) + \beta_{12}t_{1i}]. \tag{6.35}$$

Letting $\frac{\partial \ln L}{\partial \beta_{jk}} = 0$, we can obtain

$$\begin{cases} \beta_{11} = \dfrac{n_1 + n_2}{\sum_{i=1}^{n_1+n_2} t_{1i}}, \\[2mm] \beta_{12} = \dfrac{n_3 + n_4}{\sum_{i=1+n_1+n_2}^{n_1+n_2+n_3+n_4} t_{1i}}, \\[2mm] \beta_{21} = \dfrac{n_1}{\sum_{i=1}^{n_1+n_2} (t_{2i} - t_{1i})}, \\[2mm] \beta_{22} = \dfrac{n_3}{\sum_{i=1+n_1+n_2}^{n_1+n_2+n_3+n_4} (t_{2i}-t_{1i})}. \end{cases} \tag{6.36}$$

The relative treatment efficacy between the treatment groups can be measured by the hazard ratio:

$$\begin{cases} HR_1 = \dfrac{\beta_{11}}{\beta_{12}}, \text{ before PD}, \\[3mm] HR_2 = \dfrac{\beta_{21}}{\beta_{22}}, \text{ after PD}. \end{cases} \tag{6.37}$$

In practice, cancer drugs are categorized by the number of PDs: newly diagnosed patients usually use first-line drugs, after one PD they use second-line drugs, and so on.

Fig. 6.3 Competing risks

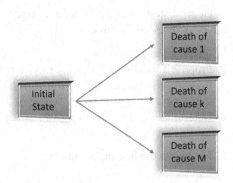

The efficacy should be compared in terms of life saving between the two conditions with and without the new drug B. (1) Without drug B, the patients would be treated with A initially and then treated with some other available drugs. (2) With drug B, the patients will eventually have PD and will be treated with drug B or other drugs. If there are other drugs available (as good as drug B) after the PD, then $HR_1 = \frac{\beta_{11}}{\beta_{12}}$ should be used to measure the survival benefit, which implies that PD is a good surrogate marker for survival.

6.4.3 Latent Process and Competing Risks

Most survival data are gathered under conditions of competing risks, in which two or more causes are competing to determine the observed duration (Fig. 6.3). In a clinical trial, an early withdrawal can be considered as either a censor or a competing risk. Because of the censoring or competing risks, the FHT may not be observable or latent. Latent FHT models are theoretically not necessary, but in practice it is convenient to the concept of latent FHT. An engineer may be interested in how much repair work can be reduced if one or more old machines are replaced with new ones in the production line. Health authorities may be interested in an optimal resource allocation and predicting the survival prolongation by investing resources in different therapeutic areas. Simply investing all government health resources on the treatments of leading causes of death may not be a good idea. Such problems can be dealt with by using the difference in FHT (survival time) between the two models, with and without a certain competing risk. Lee and Whitmore (2006) provided applications of such models in the health and medical field. It is obvious that if the underlying multidimensional Wiener process is correlated, the latent survival times for different causes of death will be dependent. Competing-risk problems are also viewed as cluster survival problems because of the correlation between the risks. A mixed distribution may be required in this case. In what follows, we will discuss independent competing risks. The competing-risks analysis of correlated failure time data or clustered data can be found elsewhere (e.g., Chen et al., 2008).

General steps in building a multistage model with independent competing risks can be outlined as follows:

1. Identify competing risks.
2. Propose a local failure density model $f_k(\boldsymbol{\theta}, t)$.
3. Formulate the lifetime function $F(\boldsymbol{\theta}, t) = \sum_{k=1}^{M} f_k(\boldsymbol{\theta}, t)$ and the survival function $S(\boldsymbol{\theta}, t) = 1 - F(\boldsymbol{\theta}, t)$, where M is the number of competing risks.
4. Determine the link function $g(\boldsymbol{\theta}) = X\boldsymbol{\beta}'$ if any, where X represents covariates; $\boldsymbol{\theta} = g^{-1}\left(X\boldsymbol{\beta}'\right)$.
5. Formulate the likelihood function

$$L = \prod_{i \in \varXi} S\left(g^{-1}\left(X\boldsymbol{\beta}'\right), t_i\right) \prod_{j \notin \varXi} f_{k_j}(\boldsymbol{\theta}, t_j), \tag{6.38}$$

where $\varXi$ is the set of indices for right-censoring observations. Here we have assumed that there is only right-censoring.

6. Obtain the MLE of $\boldsymbol{\beta}'$ by maximizing L. Other parameters of interest can be obtained consequently.

Before we discuss more complicated models, let's study a degenerated case: single-stage competing risks. Denote by f_k the hazard function of the kth cause $(k = 1, \ldots, M)$. Then the total hazard function for the parallel competing-risks model in Fig. 6.3 is $f(u) = \sum_{k=1}^{M} f_k(u)$. In light of (6.2), we assume the hazard density has the form

$$f_k(t) = \lambda_k(t)(1 - F(t)) = \lambda_k S(t), \tag{6.39}$$

where $S(t) = 1 - F(t)$ is the survival function with the lifetime function $F(t) = \int_0^t f(u)\,du$.

Given a subject alive at time t, the probability of dying within the time interval dt due to cause k is given by

$$\lambda_k(t)\,dt = \frac{f_k(t)}{1 - F(t)}dt. \tag{6.40}$$

Summing up (6.40) over all causes and letting $\lambda(t) = \sum_{k=1}^{M} \lambda_k(t)$, we obtain

$$\lambda\,dt = \frac{f(t)}{1 - F(t)}dt = \frac{dF(t)}{1 - F(t)}. \tag{6.41}$$

As shown in Sect. 6.1, the overall survival function derived from (6.41) is

$$S(t) = \exp(-\Lambda(t)) = \exp\left(-\int_0^t \lambda(u)\,du\right). \tag{6.42}$$

From (6.34), we know that $f_{k_j}(t_j) = \lambda_{k_j} S(t_j)$. Substituting this into (6.38) we can obtain the likelihood

$$L = \prod_{i \in \Omega} S(t_i) \prod_{j \notin \Omega} \lambda_{k_j}(t_j) S(t_j). \tag{6.43}$$

The transitional probability from the initial state to the death state due to cause k is given by

$$F_k(t) = \int_0^t \lambda_k(u) S(u) \, du = \int_0^t \lambda_k(u) \exp\left(-\int_0^u \sum_{i=1}^M \lambda_i(v) \, dv\right) du. \tag{6.44}$$

We can see that for each death there is a hazard term, depending only on the actual cause, and an exponential term depending on the integrated hazard for all causes together. It is obvious that $F(t) = \sum_k F_k(t) = 1 - S(t)$.

When all $\lambda_k(t) = \lambda_k, k = 1, \ldots M$, are independent of time, $S(t) = \exp(-\lambda t)$, $\lambda = \sum_{k=1}^M \lambda_k$. Thus, the system acts just like a single risk system with a big hazard (the sum of all individual hazard rates). The transition probability density is given by $f_k(t) = \lambda_k \exp(-\lambda t)$.

To consider the covariates, we can use the identity link function

$$\lambda_k = X_k(t) \boldsymbol{\beta}'(t), \tag{6.45}$$

where X_k represents covariates with corresponding parameters $\boldsymbol{\beta}$. Both of them can be time-dependent or time-independent.

Substituting (6.45) into (6.43), we obtain the likelihood function in terms of parameters $\boldsymbol{\beta}$:

$$L = \prod_{i \in \Omega} \exp\left(-\int_0^{t_i} \sum_{k=1}^M X_k(u) \boldsymbol{\beta}^T(u) \, du\right) \prod_{j \notin \Omega} \lambda_{k_j}(t_j) \exp\left(-\int_0^{t_j} \lambda(u) \, du\right). \tag{6.46}$$

Note that the term $S(t)$ in model (6.39) implies that an individual having a higher risk of dying from one cause will have a higher risk of dying from other causes too. Alternatively, we can remove this constraint and propose as a local model for cause-specific death,

$$f_k(t) = a_k \lambda_k(t) S_k(t) = a_k \lambda_k(t) \exp\left(-\int_0^t \lambda_k(u) \, du\right), \tag{6.47}$$

where α_k is independent of time and $\sum_{k=1}^M a_k = 1$ (see explanation later). Thus a_k can be viewed as a weight.

For the competing-risks model in Fig. 6.3, the total failure density is given by

$$f(t) = \sum_{k=1}^{M} f_k(t) = \sum_{k=1}^{M} \left[a_k \lambda_k(t) \exp\left(-\int_0^t \lambda_k(u)\,du\right)\right]. \tag{6.48}$$

The lifetime function is given by

$$F(t) = \int_0^t f(t)\,dt = \sum_{k=1}^{M} \left[a_k \int_0^t \lambda_k(v)\exp\left(-\int_0^v \lambda_k(u)\,du\right)dv\right]. \tag{6.49}$$

The likelihood function is given by

$$L(a,\beta) = \prod_{i\in\Omega} S\left(g^{-1}\left(X\beta^T\right), t_i\right) \prod_{j\notin\Omega} f_{k_j}\left(g^{-1}\left(X\beta^T\right), t_j\right). \tag{6.50}$$

Because it is usually required that $F(\infty) = 1$ and $F_k(\infty) = 1$ ($k = 1,\ldots,M$), we have

$$\varphi(a) = 1 - \sum_{k=1}^{M} a_k = 0. \tag{6.51}$$

Because of the constraint (6.51), we can use the Lagrange multiple method (Bronshtein et al. 2004) by introducing an extra parameter η. To find MLEs for the parameters, we can solve the equations

$$\frac{\partial(L(a,\beta)+\eta\varphi(a))}{\partial\theta} = 0 \text{ or } \frac{\partial(\ln L(a,\beta)+\eta\varphi(a))}{\partial\theta} = 0, \tag{6.52}$$

where $\theta = (a,\beta,\eta)'$.

A special case is the case with constant hazards λ_k (time-independent) and no covariates. Thus, $f_k = a_k\lambda_k e^{-\lambda_k t}$, $F(t) = \sum_{k=1}^{M} a_k F_k(t)$, $F_k(t) = 1 - e^{-\lambda_k t}$ and $S_k(t) = a_k e^{-\lambda_k t}$.

Let t_i be the time of the ith death and t_j be the censored time for the jth subject. The likelihood is then given by

$$L(a,\lambda) = \prod_{i\notin\Omega} a_{k_i}\lambda_{k_i} e^{-\lambda_{k_i} t_i} \prod_{j\in\Omega} a_{k_j} e^{-\lambda_{k_j} t_j}. \tag{6.53}$$

Let n_k be the number of subjects (alive or dead) associated with cause k among whom n_{kd} subjects died. Then the log-likelihood is given by

$$\ln L(a,\lambda) = \sum_{k=1}^{M} n_k \ln a_k - \sum_{k=1}^{M}\left(\lambda_k \sum_{i=1}^{n_k} t_{ki}\right) + \sum_{k=1}^{M}(n_{kd}\ln\lambda_k), \tag{6.54}$$

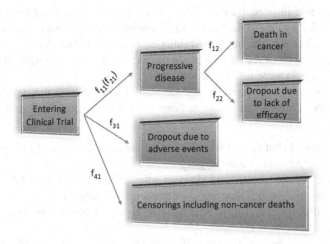

Fig. 6.4 Progressive disease with competing risks

where t_{ki} is the observed time (death or censoring) associated with cause k.
Substituting (6.54) into (6.52), we obtain the MLE of $\boldsymbol{\theta}$:

$$\begin{cases} a_k = \dfrac{n_k}{\sum_{k=1}^M n_k}, \\[2ex] \lambda_k = \dfrac{n_{kd}}{\sum_{i=1}^{n_k} t_{ki}}. \end{cases} \tag{6.55}$$

It can be seen that $a_k = \dfrac{n_k}{\sum_{k=1}^M n_k}$ holds true for general model (6.47), which is consistent with our intuition.

There are many other research studies on competing risks. Among them, Shen and Thall (1998) applied a mixed distribution for multiple nonfatal and fatal competing risks. Chen et al. (2008) studied the competing risks of correlated failure time data.

6.4.4 Competing Risks in Progressive Disease

Suppose that in an oncology clinical trial the patients in the study can be approximately grouped into four categories (Fig. 6.4): (1) progressive disease (PD), then death (D) due to cancer; (2) PD, then dropout due to lack of efficacy (LE); (3) dropout due to adverse events (AE); and (4) dropout due to other reasons. For simplicity, we group other scenarios such as death for other reasons and early withdrawals for other reasons in scenario (4). Scenarios (1), (2), and (3) are considered competing risks because they are likely treatment-related. Scenario (4) is considered non-informative censoring. Here we have generalized the concept of competing risks; i.e., the risks can be a mixture of different events. The reason we can do this is because the likelihood function (joint probability) does not require that all the events be of the same type. In practice, if there are enough patients, we can have more than these four categories.

The complexity of the model is not substantial, even though the steps involved in solving the problem are more tedious. The key is to formulate likelihood functions:

1. A patient with PD at t_{1i} and who died of cancer at t_{2i} has $l_1 = f_{11}(t_{1i}) f_{12}(t_{2i})$. There are n_1 patients in this category.
2. A patient with PD at t_{1i} and dropout after PD at t_{2i} due to LE has $l_2 = f_{11}(t_{1i}) f_{22}(t_{2i} - t_{1i})$. There are n_2 patients in this category.
3. A patient dropout at t_{1i} due to AE has $l_3 = f_{31}(t_i)$. There are n_3 patients in this category.
4. A patient censored at t_{1i} after PD, not because of LE or AE, has $l_4 = (1 - F_{41}(t_{1i}))$, where $F_{41}(t) = \int_0^t f_{41}(u)\, du$. There are n_4 patients in this category.

The likelihood for the patients can be expressed as

$$L = \prod_{i=1}^{n_1} l_1 \prod_{i=1}^{n_2} l_2 \prod_{i=1}^{n_3} l_3 \prod_{i=1}^{n_4} l_4 \qquad (6.56)$$

or

$$L = \prod_{i=1}^{n_1} f_{11}(t_{1i}) f_{12}(t_{2i}) \prod_{i=1}^{n_2} f_{11}(t_{1i}) f_{22}(t_{2i} - t_{1i}) \prod_{i=1}^{n_3} f_{31}(t_i) \prod_{i=1}^{n_4} (1 - F_{41}(t_{1i})).$$
$$(6.57)$$

Since we have used multiple stages, we can choose relatively simple transition probability densities f_{jk}. For example, assume constant λ_{jk} for transition probability densities f_{jk}:

$$f_{jk}(t) = a_{jk} \lambda_{jk} \exp(-\lambda_{jk} t), \qquad (6.58)$$

Again, because of the condition of the transition probabilities at $t = \infty$ (i.e., $\int_0^\infty f_{jk}(t)\, dt = 1$), constants a_k satisfy (through derivations similar to the previous MLE derivations)

$$a_{j1} = \frac{n_j}{n_1 + n_2 + n_3 + n_4}, j = 1, 2, 3, 4. \qquad (6.59)$$

Therefore, we have

$$F_{jk}(t) = \int_0^t f_{jk}(u)\, du = a_{jk}(1 - \exp(-\lambda_{jk} t)). \qquad (6.60)$$

Using the identity link function, $\lambda_{jk} = X\boldsymbol{\beta}'_{jk}$, where X represents covariates. We assume a_{jk} is covariate-independent such that

$$f_{jk}\left(t; a_{jk}, \boldsymbol{\beta}_{jk}\right) = a_{jk} X \boldsymbol{\beta}'_{jk} \exp\left(-X\boldsymbol{\beta}'_{jk}t\right), \tag{6.61}$$

$$F_{jk}\left(t; a_{jk}, \boldsymbol{\beta}_{jk}\right) = a_{jk}\left(1 - \exp\left(-X\boldsymbol{\beta}'_{jk}t\right)\right). \tag{6.62}$$

Substituting (6.61) and (6.62) into (6.57) and then taking derivatives with respect to vector $\boldsymbol{\beta}'_{jk}$, the MLEs of the parameters can be found using numerical methods.

Other transition probability densities can also be used, such as the Weibull distribution with $S(t) = \exp(-\lambda t^{\gamma})$ or $f(t) = \lambda \gamma t^{\gamma-1} \exp(-\lambda t^{\gamma})$, Gompertz distribution with hazard $\lambda(t) = \lambda w^t$, $S(t) = \exp(-\int_0^t \lambda w^u du) = \exp(\frac{\lambda}{1+t}w^{t+1}) - \exp(\lambda w)$, and $f(t) = -\frac{dS(t)}{dt}$, where the positive constant w can be $< 1, = 1$, and > 1. We can also construct the transition probability using the FHT distribution given by (6.14) or (6.15). The simplest case is probably the model with constant transition probability density (rate), which leads to a homogeneous Markov process or finite-state continuous time Markov chains. However, such an oversimplified model is not very practical in survival analysis, though it is useful elsewhere.

6.4.5 Longitudinal Multivariate Model

Unlike in Sect. 6.3.5, where we modeled the correlation between parent and marker processes, we are going to model the correlation of the hitting times between parent and marker processes directly, which will greatly simplify the problem.

For the problem presented in Fig. 6.5, with one primary disease process $X_1(t)$, a disease marker process $X_2(t)$, and a (composite) PGx marker process $X_3(t)$, we can specify the joint transition probability densities

$$f_{ij}(t_1, t_2, t_3), \tag{6.63}$$

or more explicitly

$$f_{ij}(t_{11}, t_{12}, t_{21}, t_{22}, t_{31}, t_{32}). \tag{6.64}$$

We then can obtain the conditional "survival" probability

$$S_{ij}^c = \int f_{ij}(\boldsymbol{u}|t_{km}) d\boldsymbol{u}, \quad i = 1, 2, 3; j = 1, 2, \tag{6.65}$$

where the integration is carried out with respect to all censored variables. For example, if $X_1(t)$ is right-censored at $t = t_{12}$, $X_2(t)$ is left-censored at $t = t_{21}$,

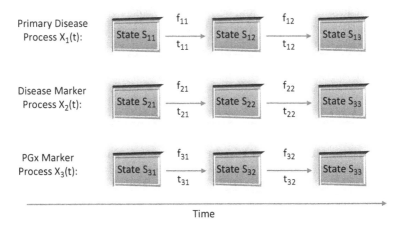

Fig. 6.5 Longitudinal multivariate model

and $X_3(t)$ has no censoring, the conditional "survival" probability is given by

$$S_{ij}^c = \int_0^{t_{21}} \int_{t_{12}}^{\infty} f_{ij}(t_{11}, u_{12}, u_{21}, t_{22}, t_{31}, t_{32})\, du_{12} du_{21}, \quad i = 1, 2, 3; j = 1, 2,$$
(6.66)

where we have assumed that t_{21} imposes no constraint on the upper limit of t_{12}; otherwise, the upper limit ∞ should change to the upper limit imposed by t_{21}.

The contribution of this individual likelihood to the overall likelihood function is S_{ij}^c, whereas for an individual without censoring, the contribution is $f_{ij}(t_{11}, t_{12}, t_{21}, t_{22}, t_{31}, t_{32})$. Therefore the likelihood function is

$$L = \prod_{\Omega} S_{ij}^c \prod_{\bar{\Omega}} f_{ij},$$
(6.67)

where Ω is the censoring set and $\bar{\Omega}$ is the noncensoring set.

The consideration of covariates using the link function and MLE of parameters is similar to what we discussed earlier. If there are a larger number of markers, it is difficult to construct valid joint transition probability densities. Therefore we can use composite markers, as suggested by Whitmore et al. (1998) in Sect. 6.3.5.

6.5 Challenges and Controversies

One of the main challenges in multivariate models is the construction of the transition probabilities. Alternatively, we may use time-dependent covariates if we are only interested in the primary or parent process. However, regression with time-dependent covariates has controversies, as discussed below.

Table 6.1 Responses in clinical endpoint (CE) and biomarker

Subject Id		1	2	3	4	5	6	7
Treatment A	CE	1	2	3	4	5	6	7
	Biomarker	1	2	3	4	5	6	7
Subject Id		8	9	10	11	12	13	14
Treatment B	CE	1	2	3	4	5	6	7
	Biomarker	3	4	5	6	7	8	9

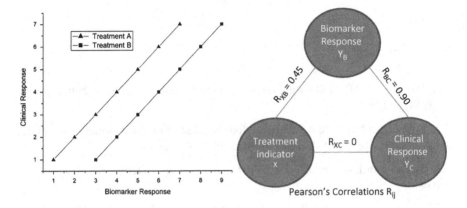

Fig. 6.6 Correlation $\neq$ prediction

Suppose we have data from a hypothetical trial as shown in Table 6.1. There are seven subjects in each treatment group (A or B), and every subject was measured for clinical and biomarker responses. We first calculate Pearson's correlations between the variables: the treatment, biomarker, and clinical endpoint. The results are presented in Fig. 6.6. We can see that the correlations between them are not transitive. In other words, a correlation between treatment and the biomarker (R_{XB}) and a correlation between the biomarker and the clinical endpoint (R_{BC}) do not ensure a correlation (R_{XC}) between treatment and the clinical endpoint (Fig. 6.6).

The results in Table 6.1 show that Pearson's correlation between the biomarker and the clinical endpoint is 1 (perfect correlation) in both treatment groups. If the data from the two groups are pooled, the correlation between the biomarker and the clinical endpoint is still high, about 0.9. The average response with the clinical endpoint is 4 for each group, which indicates that there is no treatment effect. On the other hand, the average biomarker response is 6 for the test group and 4 for the control group, which indicates that the drug has effects on the biomarker.

Given the data, what we would typically do is fit a regression model with the data in which the dependent variable is the clinical endpoint (Y_C) and the independent variables (predictors) are the biomarker (Y_B) and the treatment (X). After model fitting with the data in Table 6.1, we can obtain

$$Y_T = Y_B - 2X. \tag{6.68}$$

This model fits the data well based on the model-fitting p-value and R^2. Specifically, R^2 is equal to 1. The p-values for the model and all parameters are equal to 0. The coefficient 2 in model (6.68) is the separation between the two lines. Based on (6.68), we would conclude that both the biomarker and the treatment affect the clinical endpoint. However, if the population is well represented by the data, the treatment has no effect on the clinical endpoint at all. In fact, the biomarker predicts the response in the clinical endpoint, but it does not predict the treatment effect on the clinical endpoint, i.e., it is a prognostic marker.

6.6 Exercises

6.1. Prove the FHT for Brownian motion is the inverse normal distribution given by (6.14) and (6.15).

6.2. Suppose in Example 6.3 there are four (instead of two) categories of patients, as specified in Sect. 6.3.1. Derive the MLEs of λ_1, λ_2, λ_3, and λ_4.

6.3. Suppose in Example 6.3 $\lambda_1 = a_1 t$ and $\lambda_2 = a_2 t$. Derive the MLEs of a_1 and a_2.

6.4. Suppose in Example 6.3 $\lambda_1 = \lambda_{01}\omega_1^t$ and $\lambda_2 = \lambda_{02}\omega_2^t$. Derive the MLEs of the parameters.

6.5. Study the bias of the estimators λ_1 and λ_2 given by (6.33).

6.6. Study the bias of the estimators defined by (6.36).

6.7. Study the competing risk problem presented in Fig. 6.3, assuming the death for each cause follows the Gompertz model with a hazard rate of $\lambda(t) = \lambda\omega^t$.

6.8. Discuss the challenges presented in Table 6.1 and Fig. 6.6.

Further Readings and References

Aalen, O.O.: Modeling heterogeneity in survival analysis by the compound Poisson distribution. Ann. Appl. Probab. **4**(2), 951–972 (1992)

Aalen, O.O., Gjessing, H.K.: Survival models based on the Ornstein–Uhlenbeck process. Lifetime Data Anal. **10**, 407–423 (2004)

Aalen, O., Borgan, O., Gjessing, H.: Survival and Event History Analysis. Springer, New York (2010)

Alonso, A., Molenberghs, G., Geys, H., Buyse, M., Vangeneugden, T.: A unifying approach for surrogate marker validation based on Prentice's criteria. Stat. Med. **25**, 205–221 (2006)

Branson, M., Whitehead, W.: Estimating a treatment effect in survival studies in which patients switch treatment. Stat. Med. **21**, 2449–2463 (2002)

Bronshtein, I.N., Semendyayev, K.A, Musiol, G., Muehlig, H., Mühlig, H.: Handbook of Mathematics. Springer, New Nork (2004)

Chang, M.: Adaptive Design Theory and Implementation Using SAS and R. Chapman & Hall/CRC, Boca Raton (2007)

Chen, B.E., Kramer, J.L., Greene, M.H., Rosenberg, P.S.: Competing risks analysis of correlated failure time data. Biometrics **64**, 172–179 (2008)

Clayton, D.G.: A model for association in bivariate life tables and its application in epidemiological studies of familial tendency in chronic disease incidence. Biometrika **65**, 141–151 (1978)

Cox, D.R.: Regression models and life-tables. J. R. Stat. Soc. B **34**, 187–220 (1972)

Crowder, M.J.: Classical Competing Risks. Chapman & Hall/CRC, Boca Raton (2001)

Genest, C., Rivest, L.P.: Statistical inference procedures for bivariate Archimedean copulas. J. Am. Stat. Assoc. **88**, 1034–1043 (1993)

De Gruttola, V.G., Clax, P., DeMets, D.L., Downing, G.J., Ellenberg, S.S., Friedman, L., Gail, M.H., Prentice, R., Wittes, J., Zeger, S.L.: Considerations in the evaluation of surrogate endpoints in clinical trials: Summary of a National Institutes of Health workshop. Control. Clin. Trials **22**, 485–502 (2001)

dos Santos, D.M., Davies, R.B., Francis, B.: Nonparametric hazard versus nonparametric frailty distribution in modelling recurrence of breast cancer. J. Stat. Plan. Infer. **47**, 111–127 (1995)

Duchateau, L., Janssen, P.: The Frailty Model. Springer, New York (2008)

Hosmer, D.W., Lemeshow, S., May, S.: Applied Survival Analysis: Regression Modeling of Time to Event Data. Wiley, Hoboken (2008)

Hougaard, P.: Survival models for heterogeneous populations derived from stable distributions. Biometrika **73**, 671–678 (1986)

Hougaard, P.: Analysis of multivariate survival data. Springer, New York (2000)

Lawless, J., Crowder, M.: Covariates and random effects in a gamma process model with application to degradation and failure. Lifetime Data Anal. **10**, 213–227 (2004)

Lee, M.L.T., DeGruttola, V., Schoenfeld, D.: A model for markers and latent health status. J. R. Stat. Soc. Ser. B **62**, 747–762 (2000)

Lee, M.L.T., Chang, M., Whitmore, G.A.: A Threshold regression mixture model for assessing treatment efficacy in a multiple myeloma clinical trial. J. Biopharm. Stat. **18**, 1136–1149 (2008)

Lee, M.L.T., Whitmore, G.A.: Threshold regression for survival analysis: Modeling event times by a stochastic process reaching a boundary. Stat. Sci. **21**(4), 501–513 (2006)

Manatunga, A.K., Oakes, D.: Parametric analysis of matched pair survival data. Lifetime Data Anal. **5**, 371–387 (1999)

Marubini, E., Valsecchi, M.G.: Analysing Survival Data from Clinical Trials and Observational Studies. Wiley-Interscience, New York (2004)

McGilchrist, C.A., Aisbett, C.W.: Regression with frailty in survival analysis. Biometrics **47**, 461–466 (1991)

Molenberghs, G., Buyse, M., Burzykowski, T.: The history of surrogate endpoint validation. In: Burzykowski, T., Molenberghs, G., Buyse M. (eds.) The Evaluation of Surrogate Endpoint. Springer, New York (2005)

Newey, W.K., McFadden, D.: Large sample estimation and hypothesis testing. In: Engle, R., McFadden, D. (eds.) Handbook of Econometrics, vol. IV, Chap. 36, pp. 2111–2245. Elsevier Science, Amsterdam (1994)

Peace, K.E. (ed.): Design and Analysis of Clinical Trials with Time-to-Event Endpoints. Chapman and Hall/CRC, Boca Raton (2009)

Ricciardi, M., Sato, S.: First-passage-time density and moments of the Ornstein–Uhlenbeck process. J. Appl. Probab. **25**, 43–57 (1988)

Shao, J., Chang, M., Chow, S.C.: Statistical inference for cancer trials with treatment switching. Stat. Med. **24**, 1783–1790 (2005)

Shen, Y., Thall, P.: Parametric likelihoods for multiple non-fatal competing risks and death. Stat. Med. **17** 999–1015 (1998)

Singpurwalla, N.D.: Survival in dynamic environments. Stat. Sci. **10**, 86–103 (1995)

Singpurwalla, N.D.: Reliability and Risk, a Bayesian Perspective. Wiley, West Sussex (2006)

Tsiatis, A.A., Degruttola, V., Wulfsohn, M.S.: Modeling the relationship of survival to longitudinal data measured with error. Applications to survival and CD4 counts in patients with AIDS. J. Am. Stat. Assoc. **90**, 27–41 (1995)

Van Der Laan, M.J., Robins, J.M.: Unified Methods for Censored Longitudinal Data and Causality. Springer, New York (2003)

Vaupel, J.W., Manton, K.G., Stallard, E.: The impact of heterogeneity in individual frailty on the dynamics of mortality. Demography **16**, 439–454 (1979)

Weir, C.J., Walley, R.J.: Statistical evaluation of biomarkers as surrogate endpoints: A literature review. Stat. Med. **25**, 183–203 (2006)

Whitmore, G.A.: First-passage-time models for duration data: Regression structures and competing risks. The Statistician **35**, 207–219 (1986)

Whitmore, G.A., Crowder, M.J., Lawkess, J.F.: Failure inference from a marker process based on a bivariate Wiener model. Lifetime Data Anal. **4**, 229–251 (1998)

Wienke, A.: Frailty Models in Survival Analysis. Chapman and Hall/CRC, Boca Raton (2010)

Wienke, A., Holm, N., Skytthe, A., Yashin, A.I.: The heritability of mortality due to heart diseases: A correlated frailty model applied to Danish twins. Twin Res. **4**, 266–274 (2001)

Williamson, P.R., Kolamunnage-Dona, R., Philipson, P., Marson, A.G.: Joint modeling of longitudinal and competing risks data. Stat. Med. **27**, 6426–6438 (2008)

Yashin, A.I., Iachine, I.A.: Genetic analysis of durations: Correlated frailty model applied to survival of Danish twins. Genet. Epidemiol. **12**, 529–538 (1995)

Zdravkovic, S., Wienke, A., Pedersen, N.L., Marenberg, M.E., Yashin, A.I., de Faire, U.: Heritability of death from coronary heart disease: A 36-year follow-up of 20,966 Swedish twins. J. Intern. Med. **252**, 247–254 (2002)

Chapter 7
Meta-Analysis

7.1 Concept of Meta-Analysis

7.1.1 The Art and Science of Meta-Analysis

Meta-analysis is a statistical technique of performing integrated analyses by combining results of several independent studies to answer specific questions. In fact, any time we make a decision we have actually performed, often implicitly, a meta-analysis in our mind. This kind of meta-analysis varies from individual to individual. The analyses we are going to discuss are formal, explicit, and retrospective analyses, but may be more subjective than prospective analyses that are planned before the experiment data are available.

Meta-analyses are undertaken for a variety of reasons. A large number of them are undertaken with the broad aim of summarizing existing evidence. On the other hand, many meta-analyses are undertaken to inform specific decisions and may be extended to incorporate economic considerations in a decision analysis framework (Sutton and Higgins 2008). Well-conducted meta-analyses allow a more objective appraisal of the evidence than traditional narrative reviews, provide a more precise estimate of a treatment effect, and may explain heterogeneity between the results of individual studies. Poorly conducted meta-analyses, on the other hand, may be biased due to exclusion of relevant studies, inclusion of inadequate studies, or the use of inappropriate models.

Meta-analysis is not only a science but also an art because of the great heterogeneity among studies: differences in interventions, place and time of the experiments, study design, evaluation method, and endpoint. Sometimes very different results or conclusions can be reached with different methods. For this reason, we should conduct meta-analysis in a cohesive way and avoid ad hoc approaches as much as we can. The QUOROM statement (Moher et al. 1999) offers guidelines for reporting meta-analyses of randomized controlled trials.

Since the development of the QUOROM statement, there have been several conceptual, methodological, and practical advances regarding the conduct and reporting

Table 7.1 2×2 contingency table

	Failure/death	Success/survival
Drug A	a	b
Drug B	c	d

of systematic reviews and meta-analyses. Also, reviews of published systematic reviews have found that key information about these studies is often poorly reported. Realizing these issues, an international group that included experienced authors and methodologists developed PRISMA (Preferred Reporting Items for Systematic reviews and Meta-Analyses) as an evolution of the original QUOROM guideline for systematic reviews and meta-analyses of evaluations of health care interventions (Liberati et al. 2009).

The PRISMA Statement consists of a 27-item checklist and a four-phase flow diagram. The checklist includes items deemed essential for transparent reporting of a systematic review. In the Explanation and Elaboration document, the meaning and rationale for each checklist item are explained, including an example of good reporting and, where possible, references to relevant empirical studies and methodological literature (www.prisma-statement.org).

There are a large number of recent publications on meta-analysis. For an introduction to meta-analysis of controlled clinical trials, see the book by Whitehead (2002). For the step-by-step practical guidance to meta-analysis, see the introductory book by Borenstein et al. (2009), which has minimal statistical background.

In this chapter, we will review many different methods for meta-analysis. The core methods are based on the normality assumption. The methods are equally applicable to several different types of data such as the mean for continuous variables or the risk ratio or hazard ratio for binary variables under the large-sample assumption. Therefore, it is helpful to review different study endpoints and see how they can form (approximately) a normal distribution.

7.1.2 Study Endpoints

There are three common endpoints: binary/categorical/ordinal, continuous, and survival. For binary data, we often present them in a 2×2 table as shown in Table 7.1.

7.1.2.1 Odds Ratio

The term odds ratio is defined as

$$OR = \frac{ad}{bc}. \tag{7.1}$$

When the cell frequencies a, b, c, and d are the expected values, OR is a population parameter. When a, b, c, and d are observed values, (7.1) is an estimation of the parameter. The same interpretations are applicable to (7.2)–(7.8).

The log odds ratio is given by

$$\ln OR = \ln a + \ln d - \ln b - \ln c. \tag{7.2}$$

For a large sample size, $\ln OR$ is approximately a normal distribution with a variance of (Fleiss 1993)

$$\text{var}\,(\ln OR) = \frac{1}{a} + \frac{1}{b} + \frac{1}{c} + \frac{1}{d}. \tag{7.3}$$

When there is a zero cell, we usually add 0.5 to each cell as an approximation.

7.1.2.2 Relative – Risk

The risk ratio or relative risk (RR) is defined as the ratio between the probability $(a/(a+b))$ of an event in the treatment group and the probability $(c/(c+d))$ of an event in the control group,

$$RR = \frac{a(c+d)}{c(a+b)}. \tag{7.4}$$

The variance of $\ln RR$ is given by

$$\text{var}\,(\ln RR) = \frac{1}{a} - \frac{1}{a+b} + \frac{1}{c} - \frac{1}{c+d}. \tag{7.5}$$

7.1.2.3 Risk Difference

The risk difference (RD) or rate (proportion) difference is defined by

$$RD = \frac{a}{a+b} - \frac{c}{c+d}. \tag{7.6}$$

For a large sample size, RD has approximately a normal distribution with variance

$$\text{var}\,(RD) = \frac{a\,(b-a)}{(a+b)^3} + \frac{c\,(d-c)}{(c+d)^3}. \tag{7.7}$$

7.1.2.4 Number Needed to Treat (NNT)

Another commonly used measure in clinical trials is the number needed to treat (NNT), which is the reciprocal of the risk difference,

$$NNT = \left(\frac{a}{a+b} - \frac{c}{c+d} \right)^{-1}. \tag{7.8}$$

The interpretation of NNT can be the number of patients that need to be treated using the new treatment rather than placebo to prevent one additional adverse outcome.

7.1.2.5 Ordinal Endpoint

For an endpoint with more than two categories, we can collapse them into two categories and use the methods for the binary endpoint for the meta-analysis. This approach is also applied when there is a mixture of a different number of categories among the trials.

7.1.2.6 Continuous Endpoint

For continuous variables $x_i \overset{iid}{\sim} N\left(\theta_x, \sigma^2\right)$, $y_i \overset{iid}{\sim} N\left(\theta_y, \sigma^2\right)$, $(i = 1, \dots, n)$, the mean difference, defined by

$$\bar{x} - \bar{y} = \frac{1}{n_1} \sum_{i=1}^{n_1} x_i - \frac{1}{n_2} \sum_{i=1}^{n_2} y_i, \tag{7.9}$$

has approximately a normal distribution for a large sample with mean θ and variance $\sigma^2(\frac{1}{n_1} + \frac{1}{n_2})$.

Since different measurement scales or instruments may be used in different experiments under meta-analysis (e.g., some may range from 0 to 100, others may range from 0 to 1), to make them comparable a standard index may be created such as the standard mean, which is defined as mean divided by the standard deviation. We may also rescale them to, for example, 0–1. However, if they measure different things, scaling could be more problematic and could invalidate the meta-analysis.

7.1.2.7 Survival Endpoint

Denote the hazard rate by λ_i for group i; the hazard ratio (HR) is defined as

$$HR = \frac{\lambda_1}{\lambda_2}. \tag{7.10}$$

For a larger sample size, the observed $\ln HR$ has approximately a normal distribution.

7.1.3 Basic Methods

The basic, widely applicable, meta-analysis method is a weighted average of point estimates (one from each study), with weights w_i based on the within-study and/or between-study variances of the parameter estimates $\hat{\theta}_i$ (e.g., the treatment difference). The commonly used models are fixed-effect and random-effect models. A fixed-effect meta-analysis usually takes the inverse variances of the estimates as weights, and interpretation relies on an assumption of a common effect underlying every study. A random-effect meta-analysis incorporates the underlying among-study variation of effects into the weights. Both methods can be extended to incorporate study-level covariates. The fixed-effect methods are classic or relatively standardized, don't have much recent development, and are criticized for not being able to take the between-study variation or covariates into consideration.

For both the fixed-effect and the mixed-effect models, the parameter estimate is given by

$$\hat{\theta} = \frac{1}{\sum_{i=1}^{K} w_i} \sum_{i=1}^{K} w_i \hat{\theta}_i, \qquad (7.11)$$

and

$$\mathrm{var}\left(\hat{\theta}\right) = \frac{1}{\left(\sum_{i=1}^{K} w_i\right)^2} \sum_{i=1}^{K} w_i^2 \sigma_{\theta_i}^2. \qquad (7.12)$$

The difference between the fixed-effect and random-effect models is in weight w_i. For the fixed-effect model, we have $w_i = 1/\sigma_{\theta_i}^2$, where $\sigma_{\theta_i}^2$ is within study variance. For the random-effect model, we have $w_i = 1/(\sigma_{\theta_i}^2 + \sigma^2)$, where σ^2 is between-study variance. The parameter can be mean, $\ln OR$, $\ln RR$, or $\ln RD$.

The test statistic for testing $H_o : \theta \leq 0$ is defined as

$$T = \frac{\hat{\theta}}{\sqrt{\mathrm{var}\left(\hat{\theta}\right)}}, \qquad (7.13)$$

which usually has approximately the standard normal distribution under the condition $\theta = 0$.

The two-sided $100(1 - \alpha)\%$ confidence interval can be constructed as

$$CI = \left(\hat{\theta} - z_{1-\alpha/2}\sqrt{\mathrm{var}\left(\hat{\theta}\right)}, \hat{\theta} + z_{1-\alpha/2}\sqrt{\mathrm{var}\left(\hat{\theta}\right)}\right). \qquad (7.14)$$

7.2 Subject-Based Meta-Analysis

Meta-analyses can be based on individual patient data (IPD) or subject-based. Collecting individual patient data from original study investigators is widely regarded as the ideal approach to meta-analysis. However, IPD is usually available only for some of the patients. A systematic review with individual patient data meta-analysis to evaluate diagnostic tests is provided by Khan et al. (2003). Tobias et al. (2004) investigated meta-analysis based on individual patient data in epidemiological studies. IPD random-effect models have been developed for continuous, binary, survival, and ordinal outcome variables (Higgins et al. 2001; Turner et al. 2000; Tudor et al. 2005). The majority of meta-analyses use simple fixed-effect pooling after obtaining an effect size from each study dataset, with only a small proportion considering among-study heterogeneity and adopting a random-effect approach (Sutton and Higgins 2008).

If IPD are available, the model for meta-analysis can be similar to the model for each individual study but includes the additional factor, study, in the model (Whitehead 1997).

7.3 Study-Based Meta-Analysis

The study-based model is based on summary data from each individual study. The simplest study-based model is a fixed-effect model, which assumes the true effect is the same for all studies. In other words, a fixed-effect model concerns the true treatment effect for the overall population, whose characteristics are shared by subpopulations in the meta-analysis. A random-effect model, however, allows the true effect to vary across studies, with the mean true effect as the parameter of interest. The introduction of parameters for the subpopulation allows a distributional link between parameters for the subpopulations and the parameter for the overall population.

7.3.1 The Fixed-Effect Model

$$\hat{\theta}_i = \theta + \varepsilon_i. \tag{7.15}$$

The most intuitive way to combine individual studies into a meta-analysis is the weighting method. Let $\hat{\theta}_i$ ($i = 1, \ldots K$) be the mean of the ith independent study with variance $\sigma_{\theta_i}^2$ and sample size n_i per group (two-group design). The population parameter θ can be estimated by (7.11) and the variance estimated by (7.12).

In principle, weight w_i can be, for example, $1/n_i$ (ethically justified), $1/\sigma_{\theta_i}$, or $1/\sigma_{\theta_i}^2$. Under a homogeneous variance, $\sigma_i = \sigma$ (standard deviation for the individual patient; note $\hat{\sigma}_{\theta_i} = \hat{\sigma}\sqrt{2/n_i}$). The three weights will not lead to identical results. We will discuss weights further in Sect. 7.6. We will also examine the meaning of θ.

The most commonly used method for estimating the weight is probably MLE. Under the normality assumption with a fixed-effect model, we have

$$\hat{\theta}_i \overset{ind}{\sim} N\left(\theta, \sigma_{\theta_i}^2\right), \tag{7.16}$$

where $\sigma_{\theta_i} = \hat{\sigma}_{\theta_i}$ is assumed known.

The log-likelihood is given by

$$LL = -\sum_{i=1}^{K} \frac{\left(\theta - \hat{\theta}_i\right)^2}{2\sigma_{\theta_i}^2} + \ln \sigma_{\theta_i} + \text{constant.} \tag{7.17}$$

To maximize LL, take $\frac{\partial LL}{\partial \theta} = 0$, which leads to the MLE (7.11) of θ with

$$w_i = \frac{1}{\sigma_{\theta_i}^2}. \tag{7.18}$$

Substituting (7.18) into (7.12), we obtain

$$\text{var}\left(\hat{\theta}\right) = \frac{1}{\sum_{i=1}^{K} w_i}. \tag{7.19}$$

Therefore, we have

$$\hat{\theta} \sim N\left(\theta, \frac{1}{\sum_{i=1}^{K} w_i}\right). \tag{7.20}$$

Using (7.20), constructing the CI of θ and performing the hypothesis test are straightforward tasks.

The result (7.20) is robust even when the normality does not hold well. In such a case, (7.17) becomes an approximation.

When the normality does not hold, (7.17) can be viewed as a Taylor second-order expansion,

$$LL = -\sum_{i=1}^{K} \frac{\left(\theta - \hat{\theta}_i\right)^2}{2\sigma_{\theta_i}^2} + C_i + O\left(\frac{\theta - \hat{\theta}_i}{\sigma_{\theta_i}}\right)^3,$$

where C_i is not dependent on θ_i.

As we have discussed in Sect. 7.1, θ can be the mean, $\ln OR$, $\ln RD$, $\ln RR$, or $\ln HR$. Under the large-sample assumption, they all have normal distributions. With the given variances, the application of the inverse-variance weighting method is straightforward.

Table 7.2 Outcomes from two studies of Alzheimer's disease

		Selegiline			Placebo		
Trial	Rating scale	No. of patients	Std. mean	Std. dev.	No. of patients	Std. mean	Std. dev.
1	GBS	9	−.0203	.1733	9	.0172	.1783
2	BDS	15	.0016	.0076	15	.0027	.0129

Deeks (2002) empirically investigated four summary statistics: odds ratios (OR), risk differences (RD) and risk ratio of beneficial outcomes (RR(B)), and risk ratio of harmful outcomes (RR(H)). Based on a sample of 551 systematic reviews, he concluded that the RR and OR models are on average more consistent than RD. From a second sample of 114 meta-analyses, evidence indicates that for interventions aimed at preventing an undesirable event, the greatest absolute benefits are observed in trials with the highest baseline event rates, corresponding to the model of constant RR(H). Deeks concludes that selection of a summary statistic solely based on identification of the best-fitting model by comparing tests of heterogeneity is problematic, principally due to low numbers of trials, and suggests that the choice of a summary statistic should be guided by both empirical evidence and a clinically informed debate as to which model is likely to be closest to the expected pattern of treatment benefit across baseline risks.

Example 7.1. The outcomes from two studies of Alzheimer's disease are presented in Table 7.5 of Exercise 7.1. For illustration purposes, we perform a meta-analysis that just includes the first two trials. The Gottfries-Brane-Steen (GBS) score ranges from 0 to 36. The Blessed Dementia Scale (BDS) ranges from 0 to 84. A lower value means good. Because of the different scales, we rescale them into a range of 0–1. To do that, we divide the GBS scores by 36 and BDS scores by 84. The resulting outcomes are presented in Table 7.2.

The mean difference is $\hat{\theta}_1 = -0.0375$, with variance $\sigma^2_{\theta_1} = \frac{0.1733^2 + 0.1783^2}{2(9-1)} = 0.0039$ for trial 1. Similarly, $\hat{\theta}_2 = -0.0011$ and $\sigma^2_{\theta_2} = \frac{0.0076^2 + 0.0129^2}{2(15-1)} = 0.000008$ for trial 2. $\sum_{i=1}^{K} w_i = 125,260$. The estimated mean of the Selegiline effect on the standard rating scale is calculated from (7.11): $\hat{\theta} = (\frac{-0.0375}{0.0039} + \frac{-0.0011}{0.000008})\frac{1}{125260} = -0.00117$. From (7.12) or (7.19), we have $\text{var}(\hat{\theta}) = \frac{1}{125260} = 0.00000798$. The test statistic from (7.13) is $T = -0.00117/\sqrt{0.00000798} = -0.41418$. The p-value obtained from the standard c.d.f. is $p = 0.3394$. The two-sided 95% confidence interval is given by $-0.00117 \pm 196\sqrt{0.0798}$.

To interpret the difference $\hat{\theta}$ in a particular rating scale, we can multiply $\hat{\theta}$ by the scale factor. For example, $\hat{\theta} = -0.00117$ on the standardized scale is equivalent to $\hat{\theta} = -0.00117(84) = -0.09828$ on the Blessed Dementia Scale. Of course, the interpretation of meta-analysis results can be controversial.

Table 7.3 Cases of pre-eclampsia in nine diuretics trials

Trail	Cases/total Treated	Control	Odds Ratio	ln OR	Variance (ln OR)
1	14/131	14/136	1.04	0.04	0.16
2	21/385	17/134	0.40	−0.92	0.12

Example 7.2. The outcomes of nine clinical trials that examine the effect of taking diuretics during pregnancy on the risk of pre-eclampsia are summarized in Table 7.6 in Exercise 7.2. For illustration purposes, we perform a meta-analysis that just includes the first two trials. The OR, ln OR, and var(ln OR) in Table 7.3 are calculated using (7.1)–(7.3).

The variance can be obtained from (7.19), $\text{var}(\hat{\theta}) = (\frac{1}{0.16} + \frac{1}{0.12})^{-1} = 0.06857$. The log odds ratio can be obtained from (7.11), $\hat{\theta} = 0.06857(\frac{0.04}{0.16} + \frac{-0.92}{0.12}) = -0.5086$. The test statistic $T = \frac{-0.5086}{\sqrt{0.06857}} = -1.9423$, and p-value $p = 0.026$. The 95% confidence interval is $0.06857 \pm 1.96\sqrt{0.06857}$.

7.3.1.1 Mantel-Haenszel Method

In addition to the weighting method, the Mantel and Haenszel (1959) method for combining odds ratios from different strata can be used directly for meta-analyses.

The pooled estimate for the OR is given by

$$OR_{MH} = \frac{\sum_{i=1}^{K} \frac{a_i d_i}{n_i}}{\sum_{i=1}^{K} \frac{b_i c_i}{n_i}}. \tag{7.21}$$

The ln OR_{MH} has approximately a normal distribution with a variance (Robins et al. 1986) of

$$\text{var}(\ln OR_{MH}) = \frac{\sum_{i=1}^{K} P_i R_i}{2\left(\sum_{i=1}^{K} R_i\right)^2} + \frac{\sum_{i=1}^{K}(P_i S_i + Q_i R_i)}{2\sum_{i=1}^{K} R_i \sum_{i=1}^{K} S_i} + \frac{\sum_{i=1}^{K} Q_i S_i}{2\left(\sum_{i=1}^{K} S_i\right)^2}, \tag{7.22}$$

where $P_i = (a_i + d_i)/n_i$, $Q_i = (b_i + c_i)/n_i$, $R_i = a_i d_i/n_i$, and $S_i = b_i c_i/n_i$.

Engels et al. (2000) summarized methods for pooling risk differences and odds ratios. For ordinal endpoints, when individual patient data are available, we can use the proportional odds model for ordinal data; when only study-level data are available, we can collapse the ordinal data into binary data. This approach is also applicable when the studies in the meta-analysis have different numbers of categories.

7.3.2   Assessing Heterogeneity

The termed "heterogeneity" here refers to the differences across studies in populations, exposures/interventions, outcomes, design, and/or conduct. A forest plot can be useful for a visual assessment of consistency of results across studies.

Traditionally, a chi-square test is undertaken to determine whether there is statistically significant evidence against a null hypothesis of no heterogeneity. Cochran's heterogeneity statistic, Q, is calculated using the inverse variance weights w_i as

$$Q = \sum_{i=1}^{K} w_i \left(\hat{\theta}_i - \hat{\theta}\right)^2, \tag{7.23}$$

where $\hat{\theta}_i$ is the $\ln OR$, $\ln RR$, or RD in each trial and $\hat{\theta}$ is the common $\ln OR$, $\ln RR$, or RD estimated from the meta-analysis.

7.3.3   Random-Effect Model

The random-effect model can be specified as

$$\hat{\theta}_i = \theta + \mu_i + \varepsilon_i, \tag{7.24}$$

$$\hat{\theta}_i | \theta_i, \sigma_{\theta_i} \overset{ind}{\sim} N\left(\theta_i, \sigma_{\theta_i}^2\right), \tag{7.25}$$

and

$$\theta_i = N\left(\theta, \tau^2\right). \tag{7.26}$$

But for now we use the restricted maximum likelihood (REML). This is a method for estimating variance components in GLM using the marginal distribution for $\boldsymbol{\theta} = \{\theta_1, \dots, \theta_K\}$. The log-likelihood to be maximized is

$$LL\left(\theta, \tau^2 | \theta_1, \dots \theta_K, \sigma_{\theta_1}^2, \dots, \sigma_{\theta_K}^2\right)$$

$$\propto \sum_{i=1}^{K} \left[\ln\left(\tau^2 + \sigma_{\theta_i}^2\right) + \frac{\left(\hat{\theta} - \hat{\theta}_i\right)^2}{\tau^2 + \sigma_{\theta_i}^2} \right] + \ln \sum_{i=1}^{K} \frac{1}{\tau^2 + \sigma_{\theta_i}^2}. \tag{7.27}$$

The REML of τ^2 is the solution to (Normand 1999)

$$\hat{\tau}^2 = \frac{\sum_{i=1}^{K} \left[w_i^2\left(\hat{\tau}\right) \left(\frac{K}{K-1} \left(\hat{\theta}_i - \hat{\theta}\right)^2 - \sigma_{\theta_i}^2 \right) \right]}{\sum_{i=1}^{K} w_i^2\left(\hat{\tau}\right)}. \tag{7.28}$$

The estimator for the population mean is then calculated as

$$\hat{\theta} = \frac{\sum_{i=1}^{K} w_i\,(\hat{\tau})\,\hat{\theta}_i}{\sum_{i=1}^{K} w_i\,(\hat{\tau})},$$

(7.29)

where

$$w_i\,(\hat{\tau}) = \frac{1}{\hat{\tau}^2 + \sigma_{\theta_i}^2}.$$

(7.30)

The inferences are made using

$$\hat{\theta} \sim N\left(\theta, \frac{1}{\sum_{i=1}^{K} w_i\,(\hat{\tau})}\right).$$

(7.31)

This method is available in the SAS Mixed procedure (Normand 1999; Whitehead 1997).

The iteration procedure (7.28)–(7.29) is not convenient. A noniterative procedure for $\hat{\tau}^2$ can be obtained by using the method of moments and equating Q_w to its expected value (DerSimonian and Laird 1986; Borenstein et al. 2009),

$$\hat{\tau}^2 = \frac{Q - (K - 1)}{\sum_{i=1}^{K} \frac{1}{\sigma_{\theta_i}^2} - \left[\sum_{i=1}^{K} \frac{1}{\sigma_{\theta_i}^2}\right]^{-1} \sum_{i=1}^{K} \frac{1}{\sigma_{\theta_i}^4}},$$

(7.32)

where Q is given by (7.23).

Example 7.3. In Example 7.2, we have used a fixed-effect model. We now use the random-effect model for the same problem. Since $\hat{\theta} = -0.5086$ from Example 7.2, we can obtain Q from (7.23): $Q = (0.04 - (-0.5086))^2/0.16 + (-0.92 - (-0.5086))^2/0.12 = 3.29$ and $\hat{\tau}^2$ from (7.31): $\hat{\tau}^2 = \frac{3.29-(2-1)}{14.583-(108.51)/14.583} = 0.321$. From (7.30), we obtain $w_1\,(\hat{\tau}) = 1/(0.321+0.16) = 2.08$ and $w_2\,(\hat{\tau}) = 1/(0.321+0.12) = 2.27$. From (7.29), $\hat{\theta} = (2.08(0.04) + (2.27)(-0.92))/(2.08 + 2.27) = -0.461$. The test statistic $T = \hat{\theta}/\sqrt{\sum_{i=1}^{K} w_i\,(\hat{\tau})} = -0.461/\sqrt{2.08 + 2.27} = -0.221$, and p-value $p = 0.4125$. This p-value is much bigger than the p-value from the fixed-effect model ($p = 0.026$) because of the among-study variability included in the random-effect model. The 95% confidence interval is $-0.461 \pm 1.96\sqrt{2.08 + 2.27} = -0.461 \pm 4.0879$.

The parameter estimation in the random-effect model is sensitive to the estimation of among-study variance, which is poor when there are only a few studies. Brockwell and Gordon (2001) show that the DerSimonian and Laird method does not adequately reflect the error associated with parameter estimation, especially when the number of studies is small. Several different methods have been proposed including the profile likelihood method, the nonparametric maximum likelihood, and Bayesian models (Chap. 10 of this book; Smith et al. 1995).

7.3.3.1 Profile Likelihood Method

When an estimate problem usually involves more than one parameter, we can use the profile likelihood method (PLM). In PLM, the maximization proceeds in a stepwise fashion based on the number of parameters. A profile likelihood function can be used to find the global maximum and to construct a confidence interval for a parameter. For the moment, the profile likelihood function is defined as

$$L_\theta(\theta_0) = L(\theta_0; \hat{\tau}^2(\theta_0)),$$ (7.33)

where $\hat{\tau}^2(\theta_0)$ satisfies

$$\hat{\tau}^2(\theta_0) = \sum_i \left[\frac{(y_i - \theta_0)^2 - \hat{\sigma}_i^2}{\left(\hat{\sigma}_{\theta_i}^2 + \hat{\tau}^2(\theta_0)\right)^2} \right] \left[\sum_i \frac{1}{\left(\hat{\sigma}_{\theta_i}^2 + \hat{\tau}^2(\theta_0)\right)^2} \right]^{-1}.$$ (7.34)

Clearly $\hat{\tau}^2(\theta_0)$ is not assumed fixed for all θ_0.

An approximate $(1 - \alpha)100\%$ confidence interval for θ is then given by values of θ_0 that satisfy

$$\ln(L_\theta(\theta_0)) > \ln(L(\hat{\theta}_{ML}, \hat{\tau}^2_{ML})) - \frac{1}{2}C_{1-\alpha}(\chi_1^2),$$ (7.35)

where $C_\gamma(\chi_1^2)$ is the γ-quantile of the χ_1^2-distribution and $\hat{\theta}_{ML}$ is the maximum likelihood estimate; i.e., the solution of $L(\hat{\theta}_{ML}) = L(\hat{\theta}_{ML}, \hat{\tau}^2_{ML}) = 0$ (Brockwell and Gordon 2001). After $\hat{\theta}_{ML}$ is found, the minimum and maximum values of θ_0 can be found through iterations based on (7.35) and (7.33).

Brockwell and Gordon (2001) compared several fixed-effect and random-effect models as well as the profile likelihood method using simulations. They found that the random-effect methods generally perform better than the fixed-effect methods, with respect to coverage probabilities. However, particularly when the number of studies is modest (fewer than 20), the commonly used DerSimonian and Laird method has a coverage probability considerably below 0.95. This suggests that the error associated with the estimation of τ^2 is not adequate. The profile likelihood method usually produces the highest coverage probabilities. The coverage probabilities for small k were considerably closer to 0.95 than for the two other random-effect methods.

7.3.4 Mixture Model for Relative Risk

Kuhnert and Böhning (2007) compare three statistical models (approximate likelihood, multilevel, and profile likelihood) used to estimate the relative risk. The three models can be derived through the general mixture model as described below.

We express the treatment effect in a two-group (T = treatment, C = Control) study as the relative risk $\theta_i = \frac{p_i^T}{p_i^C}$, which can be estimated as $\frac{x_i^T n_i^C}{x_i^C n_i^T}$. Here x_i^T and x_i^C are the number of events in the treatment and control groups, respectively; n_i^C and n_i^T are the number of subjects in the treatment and control groups, respectively. To model the cluster (study) structure, we can use the nonparametric mixture distribution:

$$f(x_i|\boldsymbol{\theta},\boldsymbol{q}) = \sum_{j=1}^{m} f(x_i|\theta_j)q_j, \tag{7.36}$$

where $f(x_i|\theta_j)$ is a parametric density, called the mixture kernel, x_i contains the data for trial i, $\boldsymbol{\theta} = (\theta_1,\ldots,\theta_m)$, $\boldsymbol{q} = (q_1,..,q_m)$, $q_j > 0$, and $\sum_{j=1}^{m} q_j = 1$, with m being the number of components or clusters. For the homogeneous model, $m = 1$; usually $m < K$ (the number of studies).

The three different models can be derived from the mixture model using three different kernels.

Let δ_{ij} be the latent indicator variable δ_{ij}, defined as 1 if trial i belongs to component j and 0 otherwise. The unconditional joint density of (x_i, δ_{ij}) is given by

$$\prod_{j=1}^{m} \left[q_j\, f\left(x_i|\theta_j\right)\right]^{\delta_{ij}}, \tag{7.37}$$

where the product in (7.37) is taken over all components. The full-sample log-likelihood becomes

$$\sum_{i=1}^{K}\sum_{j=1}^{m} \delta_{ij} \ln\left[q_j\, f\left(x_i|\theta_j\right)\right] = \sum_{i=1}^{K}\sum_{j=1}^{m} \delta_{ij} \ln\left[q_j\right] + \sum_{i=1}^{K}\sum_{j=1}^{m} \delta_{ij} \ln\left[f\left(x_i|\theta_j\right)\right]. \tag{7.38}$$

An advantage is that in (7.38) the qs and θs can be maximized separately. In the EM algorithm, the unobserved indicator δ_{ij} is replaced by its expected value, conditional on current values of θ_j and q_j ($j = 1,\ldots,m$), leading to the E-step (DerSimonian and Laird 1986; Kuhnert and Böhning 2007):

$$e_{ij} = \frac{q_j\, f\left(x_i|\theta_j\right)}{\sum_{t=1}^{m} q_t\, f\left(x_i|\theta_t\right)}. \tag{7.39}$$

Replace e_{ij} for δ_{ij} in (7.38) and maximize the expected log-likelihood in q_i, leading to the M-step that is specified for the three different models as follows.

7.3.4.1 Approximate Likelihood Model

The logarithmic relative risk, $\phi_i = \ln(\theta_i)$, can be estimated as

$$\hat{\phi}_i = \ln\left(\frac{x_i^T}{n_i^T}\right) - \ln\left(\frac{x_i^C}{n_i^C}\right).$$

Assume $\hat{\phi}_i$ has approximately a normal distribution with unknown mean θ_i and known standard deviation σ_i.

Therefore, the associated kernel $f(x_i|\theta_j)$ in the mixture model is the normal density, written as

$$f(x_i|\theta_j) = f\left(\hat{\phi}_i|\theta_j\right) \approx \frac{1}{\sqrt{2\pi}\hat{\sigma}_i} \exp\left(-\frac{\left(\hat{\phi}_i - \ln(\theta_j)\right)^2}{2\hat{\sigma}_i^2}\right). \tag{7.40}$$

The log-likelihood can be written as

$$\sum_{i=1}^{K}\sum_{j=1}^{m} e_{ij} \ln\left[f\left(x_i|\theta_j\right)\right] = \sum_{i=1}^{K}\sum_{j=1}^{m} \frac{-e_{ij}\left(x_i - \ln(\theta_i)\right)}{2\hat{\sigma}_i^2}. \tag{7.41}$$

Thus the MLE in the M-step is given by

$$\hat{\theta}_j = \exp\left(\frac{\sum_{i=1}^{K} e_{ij}x_i/\hat{\sigma}_i^2}{\sum_{i=1}^{K} e_{ij}/\hat{\sigma}_i^2}\right). \tag{7.42}$$

7.3.4.2 The Multilevel Model

The ML model captures the hierarchical structure of the data used in the meta-analysis. The first level (within study) can be modeled by means of the log-linear regression:

$$\begin{cases} p_i^C = e^{\alpha_i}, \\ p_i^T = e^{\alpha_i+\beta_i}, \end{cases} \tag{7.43}$$

where α_i is in this case the baseline parameter and $\beta_i = \phi_i = \ln(p_i^T/p_i^C)$. Let $x_i = \left(x_i^T, n_i^T, x_i^C, n_i^C\right)$. Under the assumption that the observations have a Poisson distribution, the likelihood for trial i is given as

$$f\left(x_i|p_i^C, p_i^T\right) = \left[e^{-n_i^T p_i^T}\frac{\left(n_i^T p_i^T\right)^{x_i^T}}{x_i^T!}\right] \times \left[e^{-n_i^C p_i^C}\frac{\left(n_i^C p_i^C\right)^{x_i^C}}{x_i^C!}\right]. \tag{7.44}$$

Substituting (7.43) into (7.44), we obtain the likelihood for the ith trial:

$$f\left(x_i|\alpha_i, \beta_i\right) = e^{-n_i^T e^{\alpha_i+\beta_i}}\frac{\left(n_i^T e^{\alpha_i+\beta_i}\right)^{x_i^T}}{x_i^T!} \times e^{-n_i^C e^{\alpha_i}}\frac{\left(n_i^C e^{\alpha_i}\right)^{x_i^C}}{x_i^C!}. \tag{7.45}$$

The log-likelihood function is given by (omitting the terms not involving the parameters α_j, β_j, and θ_i)

$$\sum_{i=1}^{K}\sum_{j=1}^{m} e_{ij} \ln\left[f\left(x_i | \alpha_j, \beta_j\right)\right] = \sum_{i=1}^{K}\sum_{j=1}^{m} e_{ij}\left(x_i^C \alpha_j - n_i^C \exp\left(\alpha_i\right)\right.$$

$$\left. + x_i^T\left(\alpha_j + \beta_j\right) - n_i^T \exp\left(\alpha_i + \beta_i\right)\right). \quad (7.46)$$

The MLEs in the M-step are given by

$$
\begin{cases}
\hat{\alpha}_j = \ln\left(\dfrac{\sum_{i=1}^{K} e_{ij} x_i^C}{\sum_{i=1}^{K} e_{ij} n_i^C}\right), \\[2ex]
\hat{\beta}_j = \ln\left(\dfrac{\sum_{i=1}^{K} e_{ij} x_i^T \sum_{i=1}^{K} e_{ij0} n_i^C}{\sum_{i=1}^{K} e_{ij} n_i^T \sum_{i=1}^{K} e_{ij} x_i^C}\right), \\[2ex]
\hat{\theta}_j = \dfrac{\sum_{i=1}^{K} e_{ij} x_i^T \sum_{i=1}^{K} e_{ij} n_i^C}{\sum_{i=1}^{K} e_{ij} n_i^T \sum_{i=1}^{K} e_{ij} x_i^C}.
\end{cases}
\quad (7.47)
$$

The effect parameter $\hat{\beta}_j$ is the log relative risk.

7.3.4.3 Profile Likelihood Model

The profile likelihood (PL) model is usually complex and sometimes only exists in an iterative form. Fortunately, in our case, a simple PL model will do the job. The joint density function $f\left(x_i | p_i^C, p_i^T\right)$ is the same as (7.44). Substituting p_i^T with $\theta_i p_i^C$ in (7.44), we obtain

$$f\left(x_i | p_i^C, \theta_i\right) = \left[e^{-n_i^T \theta_i p_i^C} \frac{\left(n_i^T \theta_i p_i^C\right)^{x_i^T}}{x_i^T!}\right]\left[e^{-n_i^C p_i^C} \frac{\left(n_i^C p_i^C\right)^{x_i^C}}{x_i^C!}\right]. \quad (7.48)$$

To follow the PL approach, we replace p_i^C with its profile maximum likelihood estimator (PMLE). The PMLE, denoted by $\tilde{p}_i^C$, can be obtained by taking the derivative of $f\left(x_i | p_i^C, \theta_i\right)$ with respect to p_i^C and setting the result to 0, which leads to

$$\tilde{p}_i^C = \frac{x_i^T + x_i^C}{n_i^T \theta_i + n_i^C}. \quad (7.49)$$

The PMLE $\tilde{p}_i^C$ replaces p_i^C in (7.48), and the resulting outcome is denoted by $f(x_i | p_i^C = \tilde{p}_i^C, \theta_i)$.

Thus in the M-step, we obtain the MLE of θ_i by maximizing the following log-likelihood using numerical methods and Monte Carlo simulations:

$$\hat{\theta}_i = \underset{\theta_i}{\arg\max} \sum_{i=1}^{K}\sum_{j=1}^{m} e_{ij} \ln\left[f\left(x_i | p_i^C = \tilde{p}_i^C, \theta_i\right)\right]. \quad (7.50)$$

Kuhnert and Böhning (2007) develop the implementation algorithms and analyze 22 trials to prevent respiratory tract infections and show that by using the multilevel approach in the case of baseline heterogeneity, the number of clusters or components is considerably overestimated. They conclude that the profile likelihood can be considered a clear alternative to the approximate likelihood model. In the case of strong baseline heterogeneity, the profile likelihood method shows superior behavior when compared with the multilevel model.

7.4 Meta-Analysis in Complex Settings

7.4.1 Individual and Aggregate Data Mixtures

A simple way to deal with the mixture of IPD and AD is to reduce IPD to AD and then apply standard AD meta-analysis techniques. However, a better and more complex approach is to include both patient-level and study-level parameters. The model can use a dummy variable to distinguish IPD trials from AD trials and to constrain which parameters the AD trials estimate. Riley and colleagues (2008a) show that this is important when assessing how patient-level covariates modify the treatment effect, as aggregate-level relationships across trials are subject to ecological bias and confounding. Thus they develop models to separate within-trial and across-trial treatment-covariate interactions; this ensures that only IPD trials estimate the former, while both IPD and AD trials estimate the latter in addition to the pooled treatment effect and any between-study heterogeneities.

For each IPD trial, there are patient responses, y_{ij}, and their residual variances, σ_i^2. However, for each AD trial, there is only one "patient" with the response $\hat{\theta}_i$ and variance $V(\hat{\theta}_i)$. A dummy variable, D_i, is defined to distinguish between responses from IPD trials ($D_i = 1$) and responses from AD trials ($D_i = 0$). This ensures that only the IPD trials estimate their trial effect, θ_i, and their residual variance, σ_i^2, but allows both the IPD trials and the AD trials to estimate the pooled treatment effect, θ, and the between-study variance, τ^2. The model can be expressed as follows:

$$\begin{cases} y_{ij}^* = D_i\phi_i + \theta_i x_{ij} + \varepsilon_{ij}^*, \\ \theta_i = \theta + u_i, \\ u_i \sim N(0, \tau^2), \\ \varepsilon_{ij}^* \sim N(0, V_i^*). \end{cases} \tag{7.51}$$

For each IPD trial, $y_{ij}^* = y_{ij}$ and $V_i^* = \sigma_i^2$; for each AD trial, there is only one response ($j = 1$), and we set $x_{i1} = 1$, $y_{i1}^* = \hat{\theta}_i$, and $V_i^* = V(\hat{\theta}_i)$, with the latter assumed to be known. The necessary SAS code is available from the authors on request. This model can also have covariates included.

Fig. 7.1 Data mixture in meta-analysis

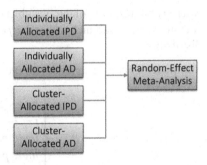

Sutton et al. (2008) propose a (random-effect) meta-analysis model that synthesizes individual-level and aggregate-level binary outcome data while exploring the effects of binary covariates also available in a combination of individual participant and aggregate-level data. Their model also involves a mixture of cluster and individual participant allocated designs. The Bayesian model uses Markov chain Monte Carlo (MCMC) to estimate parameters. Both models, with and without covariates, are studied.

Here are four different categories of two-arm studies that are included in the model: (1) IPD individually allocated studies; (2) IPD cluster-allocated studies; (3) AD individually allocated studies; and (4) AD cluster-allocated studies (often analyzed by ignoring clustering). Each of these study/datatype combinations is modeled separately in the analysis, but each contributes to one overall meta-analysis, as outlined schematically in Fig. 7.1. The model includes four submodels and one parent model.

The model includes four submodels and one parent model.

Submodel One: The model for individually allocated IPD studies is

$$\begin{cases} Y_{ij} \sim \text{Ber}(p_{ij}), \\ \text{logit}(p_{ij}) = \mu_j + \theta_j trt_{ij}, \\ \mu_j \sim N(0, 10^6), \end{cases} \tag{7.52}$$

where Y_{ij} = binary response of the ith subject in the jth noncluster-allocated IPD study, p_{ij} = probability of response, Ber = Bernoulli, and trt = treatment.

Submodel Two: The model for cluster-allocated IPD studies is given by

$$\begin{cases} Y_{ikj} \sim \text{Ber}(p_{ikj}), \\ logit(p_{ikj}) = \mu_{kj} + \theta_j trt_{ikj}, \\ \mu_{kj} \sim N(\psi_j, \tau_{cj}^2), \\ \psi_j \sim N(0, 10^6), \\ \tau_{cj} \sim U(0, 0.1), \end{cases} \tag{7.53}$$

where Y_{ikj} = response of the ith subject in the kth cluster of the jth cluster-allocated IPD study, τ_{cj}^2 = variance within the jth cluster, $\theta_j = \ln OR$, and $U\,(\cdot,\cdot)$ = uniform distribution.

Submodel Three: The model for individually allocated AD studies is

$$\begin{cases} r_{Cj} \sim Bin(p_{Cj}, n_{Cj}), \\ r_{Tj} \sim Bin(p_{Tj}, n_{Tj}), \\ logit(p_{Cj}) = \lambda_j, \\ logit(p_{Tj}) = \lambda_j + \theta_j, \\ \lambda_j \sim N(0, 10^6), \end{cases} \tag{7.54}$$

where r_{ij} = the number of events in the ith arm (the subscripts $i = C$ = control, $i = T$ = test) out of n_{ij} subjects.

Submodel Four: The model for cluster-allocated AD studies is

$$\begin{cases} \delta_j = 1 + (m_j - 1)\rho_j, \\ \tilde{\sigma}_j^2 = \sigma_j^2 \delta_j, \\ T_j \sim N(\theta_j, \tilde{\sigma}_j^2), \end{cases} \tag{7.55}$$

where δ_j is called the design effect, m_j = the average cluster size, ρ_j is the intraclass correlation coefficient in the jth study, and $\tilde{\sigma}_j^2$ = adjusted variance in the jth study.

This submodel combines AD cluster-allocated studies assuming the reported analysis (data source) ignored the effect of clustering. Since this will result in these studies being given more weight in the analysis than they should, an attempt has been made to adjust this by inflating the variances of the treatment effects. The proposed adjustment is simply multiplying a factor of δ_j, as defined in (7.55).

Parent Model: The model for combining all estimates of the intervention effect from the four data sources is

$$\begin{cases} \theta_j \sim N(\theta, \tau^2), \\ \theta \sim N(0, 10^6), \\ \tau \sim U(0, 0.1). \end{cases} \tag{7.56}$$

This part of the model specifies a random effect to be placed across all $\ln(OR)$ estimates, the θ_js, from submodels 1–4 (i.e., they are specified as exchangeable). These intervention effects are assumed to be normally distributed with mean θ and variance τ^2. Both parameters are given vague prior distributions. This is the standard random-effect model for combining treatment effects commonly used in meta-analysis.

The WinBug software package can be used for the simulation. The posterior θ and τ^2 are the outcomes for the overall treatment effect $\ln OR$ and its variance, respectively.

7.4.2 *Mixture of Matched and Unmatched Pairs*

It is not uncommon that a meta-analysis involves a mixture of clustered and unclustered measures. Chang (2011) developed a simple method to analyze the mixture of matched and unmatched pairs, which is outlined as follows.

Let x_{ts} be the response of the sth subject in treatment group t, $s = 1, \ldots, n_1$ for paired data, and $s = 1, \ldots, n_{t2}$ for unpaired data.

For paired data, let the treatment difference $\hat{\delta}_p = \frac{1}{n_1} \sum_{i=1}^{n_1} (x_{2i} - x_{1i})$; for unpaired data, the treatment difference is estimated by $\hat{\delta}_u = \frac{1}{n_{12}} \sum_{i=1}^{n_{12}} x_{2i} - \frac{1}{n_{22}} \sum_{i=1}^{n_{22}} x_{1i}$.

We now propose the estimator for the treatment difference using a linear combination of δ_p and δ_u,

$$\hat{\delta} = w_p \hat{\delta}_p + w_u \hat{\delta}_u.$$

where the prefixed weight $w_p + w_u = 1$. Therefore, given the unbiased estimators $\hat{\delta}_p$ and $\hat{\delta}_u$ of the treatment difference δ, $\hat{\delta}$ will also be an unbiased estimator of δ:

$$E\hat{\delta} = w_p E\hat{\delta}_p + w_u E\hat{\delta}_u = \delta.$$

The variance of $\hat{\delta}$ is given by

$$\sigma_{\hat{\delta}}^2 = w_p^2 \sigma_{\hat{\delta}_p}^2 + \left(1 - w_p\right)^2 \sigma_{\hat{\delta}_u}^2.$$

The variance can also be expressed as a function of the common variance $\left(\sigma_x^2\right)$ of x_{ij},

$$\sigma_{\hat{\delta}}^2 = 2w_p^2 \left(1 - \rho\right) \frac{\sigma_x^2}{n_1} + \left(1 - w_p\right)^2 \left(\frac{1}{n_{12}} + \frac{1}{n_{22}}\right) \sigma_x^2,$$

where ρ is the correlation coefficient between the matched observations.

The weights w_p and w_u can be chosen such that the variance is minimized. This can be accomplished by letting

$$\frac{\partial \sigma_{\hat{\delta}}^2}{\partial w_p} = 0,$$

which leads to

$$w_p = \frac{1}{1 + 2\left(1 - \rho\right) \frac{n_{12} n_{22}}{n_1 (n_{12} + n_{22})}}.$$

When $n_{12} = n_{22} = n_2$, the weight becomes

$$w_p = \frac{1}{1 + \left(1 - \rho\right) \frac{n_2}{n_1}}.$$

It is helpful to look into some special cases: (1) for paired data only, $n_2 = 0$, and thus $w_p = 1$ and $w_u = 0$; (2) for independent data, $n_1 = 0$, and thus $w_p = 0$ and $w_u = 1$; (3) when $\rho > 0$, $w_p > n_1/(n_1 + n_2)$, when $\rho < 0$, $w_p < n_1/(n_1 + n_2)$, and as $\rho \to 0$, $w_p \to n_1/(n_1 + n_2)$.

Usually, ρ is determined independent of the current data. However, if ρ is (approximately) independent of $\hat{\delta}_u$ and $\hat{\delta}_p$, it can be estimated from the data.

For hypothesis test

$$H_o : \delta \leq 0 \text{ versus } H_a : \delta > 0,$$

we can define the test statistic as

$$T = \frac{\hat{\delta}}{\hat{\sigma}_\delta} \sim N\,(\delta, 1)\,.$$

When $\delta = 0$, T has the standard normal distribution: $T \sim N\,(0, 1)$. The two-sided $(1 - \alpha)100\%$ confidence interval for treatment difference δ is given by

$$w_p\delta_p + \left(1 - w_p\right)\delta_u \pm z_{1-\alpha/2}\left[w_p^2\sigma_{\delta_p}^2 + \left(1 - w_p\right)^2\sigma_{\delta_u}^2\right].$$

7.4.3   p-value Combination Approaches

To deal with a situation such as a mixture of endpoints (continuous, binary, categorical), study populations, interventions, assessment methods, and even differences in study design and conduct, we can use methods of p-value combinations.

Let $T_k = \sum_{i=1}^k p_i$, where p_k are independent variables with uniform distributions on $[0,1]$. We can prove (Sadooghi-Alvandi et al. 2009) that the p.d.f. of T_k is given by

$$f_k(x) = \begin{cases} \frac{1}{(k-1)!} \sum_{i=0}^k (-1)^i \binom{k}{i} (x - i)^{k-1}\,I\,(x > i) & \text{for } 0 \leq x \leq k, \\ 0, \text{ otherwise,} \end{cases} \tag{7.57}$$

where the indicator function $I\,(x > i)$ is defined as 1 if $x > i$ and 0 otherwise. As $k \to \infty$, T_k approaches the normal distribution $N\,(k/2, k/12)$.

The overall "treatment effect" can be estimated by $\sum w_i\hat{\theta}_i$, where the w_is are predetermined weights.

Theorem 7.1. *Let T_n be the product of n independent, uniform $[0,1]$ random variables p_i $(i = 1, \ldots, n)$:*

$$T_n = \prod_{i=1}^n p_i\,. \tag{7.58}$$

Then the c.d.f. of T_n is given by

$$F_n(x) = x \sum_{i=0}^{n-1} \frac{(-\ln x)^i}{i!}, \tag{7.59}$$

where $0 < x \le 1$ and $F_n(0) = 0$.

Proof. (Feller 1957) Let $Y_i = -\ln p_i$ for $1 \le i \le n$ such that Y_i are mutually independent and exponentially distributed because

$$\Pr(Y_i \ge t) = \Pr\left(p_i \le e^{-t}\right) = e^{-t}.$$

Therefore, $Z = Y_1 + \ldots, + Y_n$ is the sum of independent, exponential random variables and has an Erlang distribution with the p.d.f. given by (Kokoska and Zwillinger 2000),

$$f(z) = \frac{z^{n-1}e^{-z}}{(n-1)!},$$

and the c.d.f. given by

$$G_n(z) = 1 - e^{-z} \sum_{i=0}^{n-1} \frac{z^i}{i!}, \quad z > 0. \tag{7.60}$$

Since $T_n = e^{-Z}$ and $e^{-Z} < x$ if and only if $Z > -\ln x$, the c.d.f. of T_n is given by $1 - G_n(-\ln x)$. Substituting $-\ln x$ for z in (7.60) proves the theorem.

7.4.4 Cumulative Meta-Analysis

7.4.4.1 Sequential Approaches and Statistical Power

Cumulative meta-analysis typically refers to the retrospective undertaking of a series of meta-analyses, each one repeated upon the inclusion of an additional study. For instance, an infinitely updated cumulative meta-analysis with a constant rejection boundary would eventually yield a statistically significant finding even under the null hypothesis (Sutton and Higgins 2008). Researchers who use sequential methods for cumulative meta-analyses include Pogue and Yusuf (1997), and Whitehead (1997), among others. Since the studies are often conducted at different times with different protocols, the heterogeneity among studies is generally not ignorable. The estimation of the between-study variation is particularly problematic in the earlier stage of the cumulative meta-analyses when the number of studies is small. Lan et al. (2003) proposed a method based on the Law of the Iterated Logarithm and by using a penalty factor for the test statistic to account for multiple tests. Their method can account for estimation of heterogeneity in the treatment effects across studies.

Definition 7.1. The Law of Iterated Logarithm: If $\{X_n\}$ are independent, identically distributed random variables with mean zeros and unit variances, let $Z_n = (X_1 + \ldots + X_n)/\sqrt{n}$. Then

$$P\left(\limsup_{n\to\infty} \frac{Z_n}{\sqrt{\ln(\ln n)}} = \sqrt{2}\right) = 1. \tag{7.61}$$

The asymptotically bounded property of statistic $\frac{Z_n}{\sqrt{\ln(\ln n)}}$ can be used to construct the sequential tests for the meta-analysis. For the fixed-effect model, Lan et al. simply pooled the data from different studies and proposed the following test statistic for the hypothesis-testing $H_o : \theta \leq 0$ for two independent two-arm trials at the kth meta-analysis,

$$Z_k^* = \frac{Z_k}{\sqrt{\varsigma \ln\left(\ln \sum_{i=1}^{k} w_i\right)}}, \tag{7.62}$$

where Z_k is the classical test statistic based on cumulative data from all first k trials, $w_i = \frac{1}{\sigma_{\hat\theta_i}^2}$ is the inverse variance of $\hat\theta_i$, and ς can be determined through simulation.

For one-sided α-level testing, the rejection rule is to reject H_o if $Z_k^* \geq z_{1-\alpha}$ and otherwise retain H_o. For $\alpha = 0.025$, the simulation results of Lan et al. suggest that $\varsigma = 1.5$ is a good choice for practical use with sample size $n_i \geq 20$ for the ith trial and number of analyses $K \leq 25$. For $n_i \geq 300$, $\varsigma = 1$ is sufficient to control the familywise type-I error. In general, when K increases or n_i is reduced, ς should increase.

The penalty factor $\sqrt{\varsigma \ln(\ln \sum_{i=1}^{k} w_i)}$ is used in the test statistic due to multiple-testing. Alternatively, we can keep Z_k unchanged and adjust the critical value $z_{1-\alpha}$ by multiplying the same factor, which becomes a sort of error-spending approach in adaptive designs.

For the mixed-effect model, (7.62) still holds but the weight w_i is modified to

$$w_i^* = \frac{1}{\sigma_{\theta_i}^2 + \tau^2}, \tag{7.63}$$

where τ^2 can be the DerSimonian-Larid estimate (7.32).

The precision of estimating the between-study availability τ^2 is largely dependent on the number of studies in the meta-analysis; therefore, in the first several analyses in the sequential meta-analysis, τ^2 cannot be precisely estimated and causes some unstable conditions. Equation (7.62) is stable because the w_i or the τ^2 is within the ln function and the square root, which makes the dominator much less sensitive to the change of the between-study variability τ^2. An alternative is to use the Bayesian prior for τ^2 as proposed in Chap. 10.

7.5 Graphical Presentations

In a traditional forest plot (Fig. 7.2), a collection of confidence intervals from studies can be visually misleading: the eye is drawn to the longer CI bars, and thus less informative studies will draw more attention. Therefore, it is helpful to use proportional symbols for point estimates to reduce this distortion. Sometimes color can also be added.

7.5.1 Funnel Plots

Funnel plots (Fig. 7.3) are another way to visualize the results from meta-analyses. A funnel plot is a scatterplot of treatment effects against a precision measure or "study size." A funnel plot can be used visually to "detect" bias or systematic heterogeneity. Light and Pillemer (1984) state: "If all studies come from a single underlying population, this graph should look like a funnel, with the effect sizes homing in on the true underlying value as n increases. If there is publication bias there should be a bite out of the funnel." A symmetric funnel shape indicates that

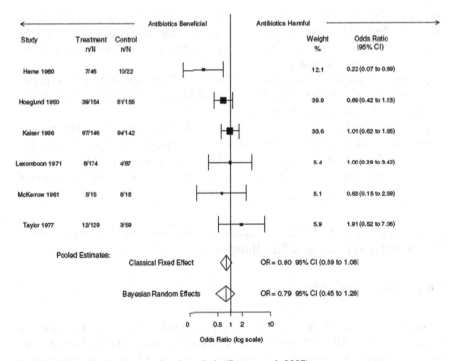

Fig. 7.2 Forest plot with proportional symbols (Sutton et al. 2007)

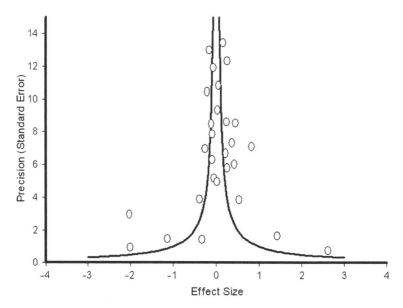

Fig. 7.3 Funnel plot of precision by effect size

publication bias is unlikely. An asymmetric funnel plot indicates a relationship between effect and sample size. Such a relationship leads to doubts over the appropriateness of a simple meta-analysis and suggests that there needs to be investigation of possible causes.

A variety of choices of measures of "study size" or "precision" are available, including total sample size, standard error of the treatment effect, and inverse variance of the treatment effect (weight).

Caution should be taken with the funnel plot: the visual effect of the funnel plot can be dramatically affected by the scales used on the axis; if high-precision studies really are different from low-precision studies with respect to effect size (e.g., due to different populations examined), a funnel plot may give the wrong impression of publication bias.

7.6 Controversies and Challenges

7.6.1 Inclusion of Studies

There are several challenges when selecting the individual studies to be included in the meta-analyses. This is because meta-analyses have different objectives, and individual studies differ in many ways: different study populations, drug competitors, efficacy endpoint definition, measuring method and timepoint, experiment design (e.g., parallel or crossover), information included in the publication (e.g., mean, standard deviation, CI, standard error, sample size, p-value), and general quality in trial conduct, analysis, and reporting. Thus, determining the set of studies to be included in the meta-analysis study is an art and a science. There is little consensus on the best practice, but the proposed alternatives include (1) restricting those studies meta-analyzed to only those of the best quality, either as a primary or sensitivity analysis, but this approach may be result in too few studies to allow meta-analysis to draw sensible conclusions; (2) down-weighting studies based on a quantitative assessment of quality, but the weight selection is subjective (Tritchler 1999); (3) exploring the effect of components of quality via meta-regression (Jüni et al. 1999); and (4) using "assay sensitivity" as an inclusion criterion for meta-analysis (Gelfand et al. 2006).

7.6.2 Inclusion, Analysis, and Reporting Bias

The issue of publication and related biases is always a concern in the scientific community, especially with meta-analysis, since if statistically significant or "positive" results are more likely to be published, a meta-analysis based on the resulting literature will be biased. In other words, if individual studies have a global "positive-bias" trend, meta-analyses have a global "positive-bias" on top of the "positive-bias" trend; i.e., more bias. On the other hand, if all studies have a "positive-bias" with the exception of this one, then this study will have a relatively "negative bias." The funnel plot is used to explore the potential bias. However, a symmetric funnel plot doesn't ensure nonbias, especially when the size is small. Similarly, an asymmetric funnel plot does not guarantee bias is present.

It is controversial as to whether adjustment for publication bias should be encouraged. Despite some disagreement, many authors have considered their adjustment methods as a form of sensitivity analysis. Jackson (2006) investigates how publication bias affects the estimation of the among-study heterogeneity parameter in a random-effect meta-analysis model, Sutton et al. (2002) allow different levels of publication bias across studies of different designs, and Bennett et al. (2004) uses capture–recapture methods across electronic databases in order to estimate the number of missing studies (Sutton and Higgins 2008).

One relevant and interesting controversy is that if we repeatedly investigate the reporting bias, what is the false positive discovery (false bias) rate (see Chap. 1)? Remember the studies that have "identified" reporting bias are much easier to publish and draw more attention than research studies that have no bias findings. This recursive nature of reporting bias makes the issue very complicated.

One practical limitation of carrying out an IPD regression analysis is that it relies on datasets for all studies in the meta-analysis that are available. Study designs often involve many aspects. Even if the data are available, simply performing the analysis

Table 7.4 Meta analysis versus mega-analysis

	Control		Test		
Trail	Deaths/patients	Risk	Deaths/groups	Risk	Risk ratio
A	20/100	0.20	40/100	0.40	$0.2/0.4 = 0.50$
B	40/400	0.10	20/100	0.20	$0.1/0.2 = 0.50$
Total	60/500	0.12	60/200	0.30	$0.12/0.3 = 0.40$

on the final dataset without fully understanding the design aspects is problematic for the validity and interpretation of meta-analysis results.

There are recent research studies that are not well covered in this chapter. Examples would be meta-analysis using a binary surrogate endpoint to predict the effect of intervention on the true endpoint (Baker 2006), meta-analysis for a crossover design (Curtin et al. 2002), meta-analysis for matched-pair and unmatched data (Sutton et al. 2000), and meta-analyses for survival endpoint (Parmar et al. 1998; Moodie et al. 2004; Fiocco et al. 2009).

7.6.3 Inconsistency in Weight Selection

The controversies in weight selection in meta-parameter estimation can be illustrated as follows. Suppose we split the data from a trial into two parts as if they were from two smaller "trials." We then perform a meta-analysis based on these two smaller "trials" and estimate the parameter θ by $\hat{\theta}_{meta} = \frac{1}{\sqrt{w_1+w_2}}(w_1\theta_1 + w_2\theta_2)$, where $w_i = 1/\sigma_{\theta_i}^2 = \frac{n_i}{\sigma_i^2}$. However, the data are actually a single trial, and thus the parameter is usually estimated by $\hat{\theta} = \frac{1}{\sqrt{w_1+w_2}}(w_1\theta_1 + w_2\theta_2)$, where $w_i = n_i$, the sample size of the ith artificially divided trial. The two estimates $\hat{\theta}_{meta}$ and $\hat{\theta}$ for the same parameter θ are usually different. Furthermore, using the inverse variance weight $w_i = 1/\sigma_{\theta_i}^2$, the outcomes from different patients weigh differently if the variance σ_i^2 is different among the trials. This creates an ethical controversy; i.e., violating the principle of "one person one vote."

Here we actually discuss the controversies between the meta-analysis and the so-called mega-analysis. In a mega-analysis, all data from different trials are lumped together to obtain one estimate, treating patients from different trials as if they were from the same trial and ignoring the treatment difference between the trials. This controversy can also be illustrated in the following example for the binary endpoint (Table 7.4). The trials (A and B) both have two parallel treatment groups (control and test). In both trials, the risk ratio is 50%. However, the sample size is different in the two trials, which leads to different risk ratios for the meta-analysis (50%) and mega-analysis (40%).

7.7 Exercises

7.1. The outcomes of seven studies of Alzheimer's Disease are presented in Table 7.5. Different scales were used for these studies (Whitehead 1997, p. 221). The ranges of the different rating scales are GBS (0–36), BDS (0–84), NOSIE (0–320), DS (1–7), and PIADL (0–24). Perform meta-analyses using the fixed-effect and random-effect models, and generate the forest plot.

7.2. The outcomes of nine clinical trials that examine the effect of taking diuretics during pregnancy on the risk of pre-eclampsia are summarized in Table 7.6 (Thompson and Pocock 1991). Fill in the numbers in the empty cells, perform a meta-analysis, and generate the forest and funnel plots.

7.3. Suppose there are six cancer studies. Their outcomes are presented in Table 7.7 (Whitehead 1997, p. 239). Perform a meta-analysis using a p-value combination method.

7.4. Develop a model for meta-analysis when the outcomes are the mixture of continuous and binary variables.

Table 7.5 Results from seven studies of Alzheimer's disease

		Selegiline			Placebo		
Trial	Rating scale	No. of patients	Mean	Std. dev.	No. of patients	Mean	Std. dev.
1	GBS	9	−0.73	6.24	9	0.62	6.42
2	BDS	15	0.13	0.64	15	0.23	1.08
3	NOSIE	79	−0.84	6.28	77	0.43	6.64
4	BDS	59	−1.90	3.47	49	1.04	3.52
5	BDS	62	−2.02	2.44	46	0.63	2.59
6	DS	172	−0.02	0.89	169	0.01	0.89
7	PIADL	25	0.88	2.82	24	0.08	2.83

Table 7.6 Cases of pre-eclampsia in nine diuretics trials

	Cases/total		Odds		Variance
Trail	Treated	Control	ratio	ln OR	(ln OR)
1	14/131	14/136	1.04	0.04	0.16
2	21/385	17/134	0.40	−0.92	0.12
3	14/57	24/48	0.33	−1.12	0.18
4	6/38	18/40			
5	12/1011	35/760			
6	138/1370	175/1336			
7	15/506	20/524			
8	6/108	2/103			
9	65/153	40/102			

Table 7.7 Outcomes from six cancer studies

Study	1	2	3	4	5	6
ln OR	−0.329	−0.385	−0.216	−0.220	−0.225	0.125
p-value	0.048	0.029	0.216	0.063	0.115	0.898

7.5. Repeated measures are often present in clinical trials, e.g., the primary efficacy endpoint is measured twice at different timepoints. Develop a model for meta-analysis with repeated-measures data.

7.6. Conduct three sets of sequential/cumulative meta-analyses using the data in Tables 7.3–7.5.

Further Readings and References

Baker, S.G.: A simple meta-analytic approach for using a binary surrogate endpoint to predict the effect of intervention on true endpoint. Biostatistics **7**, 58–70 (2006)

Baujat, B., Mahe, C., Pignon, J.P., Hill, C.: A graphical method for exploring heterogeneity in meta-analyses: Application to a meta-analysis of 65 trials. Stat. Med. **21**, 2641–2652 (2002)

Bennett, D.A., Latham, N.K., Stretton, C., Anderson, C.S.: Capture–recapture is a potentially useful method for assessing publication bias. J. Clin. Epidemiol. **57**, 349–357 (2004)

Borenstein, M., Hedges, L.V., Higgins, J.P.T., Rothstein, H.R.: Introduction to Meta-Analysis. Wiley, Hobken (2009)

Brockwell, S.E., Gordon, I.R.: A comparison of statistical methods for meta-analysis. Stat. Med. **20**, 825–840 (2001)

Chang, M.: Meta-analysis with mixture of matched and unmatched paris. A paper manuscript in preparation (2011)

Curtin, F., Altman, D.G., Elbourne, D.: Meta-analysis combining parallel and cross-over clinical trials. I: Continuous outcomes. Stat. Med. **21**, 2131–2144 (2002)

Deeks, J.J.: Issues in the selection of a summary statistic for meta-analysis of clinical trials with binary outcomes. Stat. Med. **21**, 1575–1600 (2002)

DerSimonian, R., Laird, N.: Meta-Analysis in clinical trials. Control. Clin. Trials **7**, 177–188 (1986)

Engels, E.A., Schmid, C.H., Terrin, N., Olkin, I., Lau, J.: Heterogeneity and statistical significance in meta-analysis: An empirical study of 125 meta-analyses. Stat. Med. **19**, 1707–1728 (2000)

Feller, R.A.: An Introduction to Probability Theory and Its Applications, vol. 2, 2nd edn. Wiley, New York (1957)

Fiocco, M. Putter, H., van Houwelingen, J.C.: Meta-analysis of pairs of survival curves under heterogeneity: A Poisson correlated gamma-frailty approach. Stat. Med. **28**, 3782–3797 (2009)

Fleiss, J.L.: Statistical Methods for Rates and Proportions, 2nd edn. Wiley-Interscience, New York (1993)

Gelfand, L.A., Strunk, D.R., Tu, X.M., Noble, R.E.S., DeRubeis, R.J.: Bias resulting from the use of 'assay sensitivity' as an inclusion criterion for meta-analysis. Stat. Med. **25**, 943–955 (2006)

Higgins, J.P.T., Whitehead, A., Turner, R.M., Omar, R.Z., Thompson, S.G.: Meta-analysis of continuous outcome data from individual patients. Stat. Med. **20**, 2219–2241 (2001)

Jackson, D.: The implication of publication bias for meta-analysis' other parameter. Stat. Med. **25**, 2911–2921 (2006)

Jüni, P., Witschi, A., Bloch, R., Egger, M.: The hazards of scoring the quality of clinical trials for meta-analysis. J. Am. Med. Assoc. **282**, 1054–1060 (1999)

Khan, K.S., Bachmann, L.M., ter Riet, G.: Systematic reviews with individual patient data meta-analysis to evaluate diagnostic tests. Eur. J. Obstet. Gynecol. Reprod. Biol. **108**, 121–125 (2003)

Kokoska, S., Zwillinger, D.: Standard Probability and Statistical Tables and Formula. Chapman & Hall/CRC, Boca Raton (2000)

Kuhnert, R., Böhning, D.: A comparison of three different models for estimating relative risk in meta-analysis of clinical trials under unobserved heterogeneity. Stat. Med. **26**, 2277–2296 (2007)

Lan K.K.G, Hu, M., Cappelleri, J.C.: Applying the law of the iterated logarithm to cumulative meta-analysis of a continuous endpoint. Stat. Sin. **13**, 1135–1145 (2003)

Liberati, A., Altman, D.G., Tetzlaff, J., Mulrow, C., Gøtzsche, P.C., Ioannidis, J.P., et al.: The PRISMA statement for reporting systematic reviews and meta-analyses of studies that evaluate health care interventions: Explanation and elaboration. PLoS Med. **6**(7), e1000100 (2009). doi:10.1371/journal.pmed.1000100

Light, R.J., Pillemer, D.B.: Summing Up: The Science of Reviewing Research. Harvard University Press, Boston (1984)

Mantel, N., Haenszel, W.: Statistical aspects of the analysis of data from retrospective studies of disease. J. Nat. Cancer Inst. **22**, 719–748 (1959)

Moher, D., Cook, D.J., Eastwood, S., Olkin, I., Rennie, D., Stroup, D., for the QUORUM group: Improving the quality of reporting of meta-analysis of randomised controlled trials: The QUORUM statement. Lancet **354**, 1896–1900 (1999)

Moodie, P.F., Nelson, N.A., Koch, G.G.: A non-parametric procedure for evaluating treatment effect in the meta-analysis of survival data. Stat. Med. **23**, 1075–1093 (2004)

Motoda, H., Ohara, K.: Apriori. In: Wu, X., Kumar, V. (eds.) The Top Ten Algorithms in Data Mining. CRC/Chapman & Hall, Boca Raton (2009)

Normand, S.L.T.: Tutorial in biostatistics, meta-analysis: Formulating, evaluating, combining, and reporting. Stat. Med. **18**, 321–359 (1999)

Pagliaro, L., D'Amico, G., Sörensen, T.I., Lebrec, D., Burroughs, A.K., Morabito, A., Tiné, F., Politi, F., Traina, M.: Prevention of rst bleeding in cirrhosis – a meta-analysis of randomized trials of nonsurgical treatment. Ann. Intern. Med. **117**, 59–70 (1992)

Parmar, M.K.B., Torri, V., Stewart, L.: Extracting summary statistics to perform meta-analysis of the published literature for survival endpoints. Stat. Med. **17**, 2815–2834 (1998)

Pogue, J.M., Yusuf, S.: Cumulating evidence from randomized trials: Utilizing sequential monitoring boundaries for cumulative meta-analysis. Control. Clin. Trials **18**, 580–593 (1997)

Poli, R., Langdon, W.R., McPhee, N.F.: (2008). A field guide to genetic programming, Creative Commons Attribution. England & Wales License, UK.

Riley, R.D., Dodd, S.R., Craig, J.V., Thompson, J.R., Williamson, P.R.: Meta-analysis of diagnostic test studies using individual patient data and aggregate data. Stat. Med. **27**, 6111–6136 (2008a)

Riley, R.D., Lambert, P.C., Staessen, J.A., Wang, J., Gueyffier, F., Thijs, L., Boutitie, F.: Meta-analysis of continuous outcomes combining individual patient data and aggregate data. Stat. Med. **27**, 1870–1893 (2008b)

Robins, J., Breslow, N., Greenland, S.: Estimators of the Mantel-Haenszel variance consistent in both sparse data and large-strata limiting models. Biometrics **42**, 311–323 (1986)

Sadooghi-Alvandi, S.M., Nematollahi. A.R., Habibi, R.: On the distribution of the sum of independent uniform random variables. Stat. Pap. **50**, 171–175 (2009)

Smith, T.C., Spiegelhalter, D.J., Thomas, A.: Bayesian approaches to random-effects meta-analysis: A comparative study. Stat. Med. **14**, 2685–2699 (1995)

Sutton, A.J., Abrams, K.R., Jones, D.R., Sheldon, T.A., Song, F.: Methods for Meta-Analysis in Medical Research. Wiley, Ontario (2000)

Sutton, A.J., Abrams, K.R., Jones, D.R.: Generalized synthesis of evidence and the threat of dissemination bias: The example of electronic fetal heart rate monitoring (EFM). J. Clin. Epidemiol. **55**, 1013–1024 (2002)

Sutton, A.J., Cooper, N.J., Jones, D.R., Lambert, P.C., Thompson, J.R., Abrams, K.R.: Evidence-based sample size calculations based upon updated meta-analysis. Stat. Med. **26**, 2479–2500 (2007)

Sutton, A.J., Higgins, J.P.T.: Recent developments in meta-analysis. Stat. Med. **27**, 625–650 (2008)

Sutton, A.J., Kenrick, D., Coupland, C.A.C.: Meta-analysis of individual- and aggregate-level data. Stat. Med. **27**, 651–669 (2008)

Thompson, S.G., Pocock, S.J.: Can meta-analyses be trusted? Lancet **338**, 1127–1130 (1991)

Tobias, A., Saez, M., Kogevinas, M.: Meta-analysis of results and individual patient data in epidemiological studies. J. Mod. Appl. Stat. Methods, **3**, 176–185 (2004)

Tritchler, D.: Modeling study quality in meta-analysis. Stat. Med. **18**, 2135–2145 (1999)

Tudor, S.C., Williamson, P.R., Marson, A.G.: Investigating heterogeneity in an individual patient data meta-analysis of time to event outcomes. Stat. Med. **24**, 1307–319 (2005)

Turner, R.M., Omar, R.Z., Yang, M., Goldstein, H., Thompson, S.G.: A multilevel model framework for meta-analysis of clinical trials with binary outcomes. Stat. Med. **19**, 3417–3432 (2000)

Whitehead, A.: A prospectively planned cumulative meta-analysis applied to a series of concurrent clinical trials. Stat. Med. **16**, 2901–2913 (1997)

Whitehead, A.: Meta-Analysis of Controlled Clinical Trials. Wiley, Chichester (2002)

Chapter 8
Data Mining and Signal Detection

8.1 Common Data Mining Methods

8.1.1 Supervised, Unsupervised, and Reinforcement Learning

Data mining, a the confluence of multiple intertwined disciplines such as statistics, machine learning, pattern recognition, database systems, information retrieval, the World Wide Web, visualization, and many application domains, has made great progress in the past decade. Statistics plays a vital role in successful machine learning or data mining in which we are constantly dealing with streamed data, which are usually of vast volume, changing dynamically, possibly infinite, and containing multidimensional features. The contents and methods to be discussed in this chapter often appear under bioinformatics, data mining, signal detection, or pharmacovigilance.

Learning algorithms in data mining fall into three categories (supervised, unsupervised, and reinforcement learning) based on the type of feedback that the learner can get. In supervised learning, the learner will give a response $\hat{y}$ based on input x and will be able to compare his response $\hat{y}$ to the target (correct) response y. In other words, the "student" presents an answer $\hat{y}_i$ for each x_i in the training sample, and the supervisor provides either the correct answer and/or an error associated with the student's answer. If (X, Y) are random variables represented by some joint probability density $P(X, Y)$, then supervised learning can be formally characterized as a density estimation problem where one is concerned with determining properties of the conditional density $P(Y|X)$. Usually the properties of interest are the "location" parameters μ that minimize the expected error at each x (Hastie et al. 2001),

$$\mu(x) = \arg\min_{\theta} E_{Y|X} L(Y, \theta),$$

where $L(Y, \theta)$ is the loss function.

In unsupervised learning, the learner receives no feedback from the supervisor at all. Instead, the learner's task is to re-represent the inputs in a more efficient way,

M. Chang, *Modern Issues and Methods in Biostatistics*, Statistics for Biology and Health, DOI 10.1007/978-1-4419-9842-2_8, © Springer Science+Business Media, LLC 2011

as clusters or a reduced set of dimensions. Unsupervised learning is based on the similarities and differences among the input patterns. In this case, one has a set of n observations $(x_1, \ldots, x_n)$ of a random p-vector X having joint density $P(X)$. The goal is to directly infer the properties of this probability density without the help of a supervisor or teacher providing a correct answer or degree of error for each observation (Hastie et al. 2001).

Reinforcement learning is an active area in artificial intelligence study or machine learning that concerns how a learner should take actions in an environment so as to maximize some notion of long-term reward. Reinforcement learning algorithms attempt to find a policy (or a set of action rules) that maps states of the world to the actions the learner should take in those states. In economics and game theory, reinforcement learning is considered a rational interpretation of how equilibrium may arise. A Markov decision process is considered a reinforcement learning model.

Unlike supervised learning, in reinforcement learning, the correct input-output pairs are never presented. Furthermore, there is a focus on on-line performance, which involves finding a balance between exploration (of uncharted territory) and exploitation (of current knowledge).

8.1.2 Link Analysis

In many situations, finding causality relationships is the goal. When there are a larger number of variables, the task is not trivial. However, association is a necessary condition for a causal relationship. Finding the set of events that correlate with many others is often the focus and a subject for further research. Link analysis provides a way to find the event set with high density. Finding sale items that are highly related (or frequently purchased together) can be very helpful for stocking shelves, cross-marketing in sales promotions, catalog design, and consumer segmentation based on buying patterns. A commonly used algorithm for such density problems is the so-called Apriori (Motoda and Ohara, 2009, in Wu and Kumar 2009, p. 61).

Link analysis explores the associations between large numbers of objects of different types. Link analysis can be used to examine the adverse effects of medications during postmarketing surveillance (Fig. 8.1), determining whether a particular adverse event can be linked to just one medication or a combination of medications. Link analysis can examine specific patient characteristics to determine whether they might correlate with both the adverse event and the medication (Cerrito 2003). Link analysis has also been used in page ranking of webpages.

8.1.2.1 PageRank Algorithm

The name "PageRank" is a trademark of Google, and the PageRank process has been patented (U.S. Patent 6,285,999). However, the patent is assigned to Stanford

Fig. 8.1 Link analysis in
drug AE (adverse event)
relationship

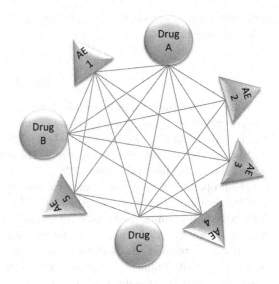

University and not to Google. Google has exclusive licensing rights on the patent from Stanford University. The university received 1.8 million shares of Google stock in exchange for use of the patent according to wikipedia.org.

The PageRank algorithm (Brin and Page 1998) first forms the so-called adjacency matrix A, whose element is 1 if page links to page and 0 otherwise. Then a probability transition matrix W is constructed by renormalizing each row of A to sum to 1. Imagine a random web surfer who randomly clicks a hyperlink on the page with a probability of $(1 - p_\varepsilon)$ to jump to another page or enter randomly a url to a new page with a probability of p_ε. The process continues until the web surfer stops. This process defines a Markov chain on the webpages with transition matrix $p_\varepsilon U + (1 - p_\varepsilon) W$, where U is the transition matrix of uniform transition probabilities ($U_{ij} = 1/n$ for all i, j). The vector of PageRank scores s is then defined to be the stationary distribution of this Markov chain. Equivalently, s is the principal right eigenvector of the transition matrix $(\varepsilon U + (1 - \varepsilon) W)'$. Here again the apostrophe represents the transpose of the matrix (Golub and Van Loan 1996; Langville and Meyer 2005)

$$(\varepsilon U + (1 - \varepsilon) M)' s = s. \tag{8.1}$$

8.1.2.2 HITS Algorithm

Another popular algorithm is the Kleinberg HITS algorithm (Kleinberg 1999), which is also an eigenvector-based method; it essentially computes principal eigenvectors of particular matrices related to the adjacency graph to determine "authority," a. The HITS algorithm posits that an article has high "authority" weight if it is linked by many pages with high "hub" weight and that a page has high hub weight if it links to many authoritative pages. The HITS algorithm iterates the following equations:

$$\begin{cases} a^{(t+1)} = (A'A)a^{(t)}, \\ h^{(t+1)} = (AA')h^{(t)}. \end{cases} \tag{8.2}$$

When the iterations are initialized with the vector of ones $(1, \ldots, 1)'$, this is the power method of obtaining the principal eigenvector of a matrix (Golub and Van Loan 1996). From (8.2) we know that $a^* = a^{(\infty)}$ and $h^* = h^{(\infty)}$ are the principal eigenvectors of $A'A$ and AA', respectively. The authoritativeness of page i is then taken to be a^* and likewise for hubs h^*.

The properties of (AA') determine the stability of the ranks generated by the HITS algorithm under small perturbations. The HITS, the PageRank, and other link-analysis algorithms can be used for identifying "authoritative" or "influential" articles, given hyperlink or citation information. The questions are: will such algorithms be reliable and will they give consistent answers? Ng et al. (2001) analyzed such algorithms when they can be expected to give stable ranks under small perturbations to the linkage patterns.

8.1.3 Nearest-Neighbors Method

Probably the simplest of all machine learning algorithms is the k nearest neighbors (kNN) method, in which an object is classified by a majority vote of its neighbors, with the object being assigned to the class most common among its k nearest neighbors. The kNN is a type of instance-based learning, or lazy learning, where the function is only approximated locally and all computation is deferred until classification. Despite its simplicity, kNN has been used in many classification problems such as handwritten digits, satellite imaging scenes, and electrocardiograms (EKGs or ECGs).

The kNN can be used for regression by simply assigning the property value for the object to be the average of the values of its k nearest neighbors.

$$\hat{y} = Ave\left(y_i | x_i \in N_k\left(x\right)\right), \tag{8.3}$$

where $N_k\left(x\right)$ is the set of k points nearest to x. We may weigh neighbors differently according to the distances. e.g.; to choose weight to be the reciprocal of the distance to the neighbor.

The neighbors are taken from a set of objects for which the correct classification (or, in the case of regression, the value of the property) is known. This can be thought of as the training set for the algorithm, though no explicit training step is required. The kNN can be effective when the decision boundary is very irregular (Hastie et al. 2001, 2009).

8.1.4 Kernel Method

The kernel method is a natural extension of the kNN method. The localization is achieved via two steps: (1) fitting a local model (e.g., a polynomial model) and (2) using a weighting function or kernel $K_\lambda (x_0, x_i)$, which assigns a weight to x_i based on its distance from x_0. The index parameter λ in the kernel K_λ is used to determine the width of the neighborhood. These memory-based methods in principle require little or no training. In general, larger λ implies lower variance but higher bias.

For a local linear regression, if the squared error is used, the kernel method becomes the following minimization problem at each target point x_0:

$$\min_{a(x_0), \beta(x_0)} \sum_{i=1}^{N} K_\lambda (x_0, x_i) \left[y_i - \alpha (x_0) - \beta (x_0) x_i \right]^2. \tag{8.4}$$

The estimate is then $\hat{y} = \hat{f}(x_0) = \hat{\alpha}(x_0) + \hat{\beta}(x_0)x_0$.
The kernel function can be an Epanechnikov quadratic kernel,

$$\begin{cases} K_\lambda (x_0, x) = D \left(\dfrac{||x - x_0||}{\lambda} \right), \\ D(t) = \dfrac{3}{4} \left(1 - t^2\right) I \left(|t| \leq 1\right). \end{cases} \tag{8.5}$$

Kernel density estimation (or the Parzen window method) is an unsupervised learning method. If a random sample $x_1, \ldots, x_n$ is independently drawn from a probability density $f_X (x)$, we can estimate $f_X (x)$ using

$$\hat{f}_X (x; \lambda) = \frac{1}{n} \sum_{i=1}^{n} \frac{1}{\lambda_i} K \left(\frac{x - x_i}{\lambda_i} \right), \tag{8.6}$$

where $K(\cdot)$ is some kernel and λ_i is a smoothing parameter called the bandwidth. A commonly used kernel is the standard Gaussian function with a constant bandwidth $\lambda_i = \lambda$. Thus the variance is controlled indirectly through the parameter λ.

Binary kernel discrimination has thus far mostly been used for distinguishing between active and inactive compounds in the context of virtual screening (Wilton et al. 2006; Harper et al. 2001).

8.1.5 Support Vector Machine

Linear discriminant analysis is based on the construction of the hyperplane that minimizes the misclassification error. Similarly, a support vector machine (SVM) is used to construct a hypersurface (multiple hyperplanes) that minimizes the misclassification or regression error.

The classifier is defined as

$$G\left(x\right) - \text{sgn}\left(x_i^T \beta + \beta_0\right).$$ (8.7)

The parameters β and β_0 that determine the hypersurface are obtained by solving the following optimization:

$$\min \|\beta\|,$$ (8.8)

$$\text{subject to} \begin{cases} y_i\left(x_i^T \beta + \beta_0\right) \geq 1 - \xi_i \ \forall i, \\ \xi_i \geq 0. \end{cases}$$ (8.9)

The interpretation of β is that $\|\beta\|$ is the distance or margin that separates the two classes. When the slack variable $\xi_i = \xi$ (constant), (8.8) defines a hyperplane. The computational details of (8.8) can be found elsewhere (e.g., Hastie et al. 2001, 2009).

8.1.6 Tree Methods

Tree methods are simple and popular methods in data mining and machine learning. The goal is to predict an outcome variable y based on input variables $x = (x_1, \ldots, x_n)$. There are so-called classification and regression trees (CARTs). In a regression tree, y is treated as continuous variable, and in a classification tree, it is treated as a discrete variable.

In the tree method, each input variable $x_i (i = 1, \ldots, p)$ is divided into categories in terms of value (e.g., age divided into age groups) sequentially (Fig. 8.2). A binary tree is a simple one in which x_i is divided into two categories. At the end of the tree are the leaves, denoted by R_j $(i = 1, 2, \ldots, m)$. R_j represents a classification of x. A value c_j is attached to each leaf. The prediction with the tree method is

$$\hat{y} = \sum_{i=1}^{m} c_i I\left(x \in R_i\right),$$ (8.10)

where c_i is a constant and $I(x \in R_i)$ is an indicator function, which is equal to 1 if $x \in R_i$ and 0 otherwise. Here are two questions that the tree methods try to answer: (1) For a given tree structure, how should the constant c_i be determined so that the error can be minimized? (2) How should the tree be constructed so that the error can be minimized?

Suppose we have observations $(x_{1j}, \ldots, x_{pj}, y_j)$, where $j = 1, \ldots n$. We take a subset $(x_{1j}, \ldots, x_{pj}, y_j)$, where $j = 1, \ldots n_t; n_t < n$. To determine the constant c_i, we minimize the error or impurity measure,

$$Err = \frac{1}{n_t} \sum_{j=1}^{n_t} (y_j - \hat{y}_j)^2,$$ (8.11)

Fig. 8.2 Tree structure

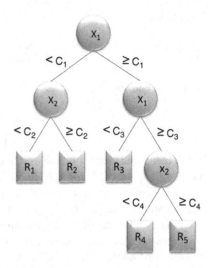

which leads to

$$c_i = ave\left(y_j | x_j \in R_i\right). \qquad (8.12)$$

Here we have assumed there are no missing data.

Knowing how to determine c_i in the minimization, we now can determine the tree structure to further minimize the error. The process is recursive. We split one x_i each time into categories from $i = 1$ to p and calculate the error Err_i from (8.11). Then we find the index i with minimum error,

$$i_{(1)} = \arg\min_i \left(Err_i\right). \qquad (8.13)$$

After we find the first index $i_{(1)}$, we further split the second variable and the second-best index $i_{(2)}$ and search among the rest of the $p - 1$ variables using the same criterion of minimizing the error given by (8.13). However, this time there are two variables that are split in the search process. This recursive process continues until all variables x_i have been split.

In a classification tree, if the classification problem has K categories (i.e., $y_1, \ldots, y_K$), the proportion of the kth class observations in a node can be written as

$$\hat{p}_{jk} = \frac{1}{n_t} \sum_{x_i \in R_j} I\left(y_i = k\right), \qquad (8.14)$$

where $I(A) = 1$ if $A = True$ and 0 otherwise.

The common impurity measures are misclassification error,

$$\frac{1}{n_t} \sum_{x_i \in R_j} I\left(y_i \neq k\right) = 1 - \hat{p}_{jk}; \qquad (8.15)$$

Gini index,

$$\sum_{k=1}^{K} \hat{p}_{jk} \left(1 - \hat{p}_{jk}\right) ; \tag{8.16}$$

and gross entropy or deviance,

$$\sum_{k=1}^{K} \hat{p}_{jk} \ln \hat{p}_{jk}. \tag{8.17}$$

Note that the number of leaves in the binary tree is much less than the number of unique categories (2^p) formulated by the n input variables.

There are, for example, several obvious questions in the tree methods: How many classes should the tree have? How do we determine the tree depth? How do we split the data for training and validation? A large training set will usually make the model better. The question is: Do you want a better model without knowing how good it is (if all the data available are used for training only) or a worse model with information on the quality of the model?

A single big tree is not stable because a single error in classification can propagate to the leaves. Therefore, different methods have been proposed as remedies, such as bagging, boosting, and random forests. The boosted trees can be used for regression-type and classification-type problems.

8.1.6.1 Bagging

Bagging (bootstrap aggregating) is a variance reduction method that averages predictions from multiple tree models. The tree models are generated by multiple sampling from training sets with replacement,

$$\hat{y}_{bag} = \frac{1}{N_b} \sum_{i=1}^{N_b} \hat{y}_i. \tag{8.18}$$

Bagging is also known as bootstrap aggregating.

8.1.6.2 Boosting

A week classifier $G_i(x)$, with value either -1 or 1, is one whose misclassification error rate is only slightly better than random guessing. A boost sequentially applies the weak classification algorithm to repeatedly reweigh the data, thereby producing a sequence of weak classifiers $G_i(x), i = 1, 2, \ldots, n_t$. The predictions from all of them are then combined through a weighted majority vote to produce the final prediction,

$$G(x) = \text{sgn} \left(\sum_{i=1}^{n_t} \alpha_i G_i(x) \right), \tag{8.19}$$

where $\alpha_1, \alpha_2, \ldots, \alpha_{n_t}$ are computed by the boosting algorithm in such a way that more accurate classifiers in the sequence will get larger weights.

The data modifications at each boosting step consist of applying weights $w_1, \ldots, w_{n_t}$ to each of the training observations (x_i, y_i), $i = 1, 2, \ldots, n_t$, such that the weight shifts more to misclassified observations. Initially all of the weights are set to $w_i = 1/n_t$, so that the first step simply trains the classifier on the data in the usual manner. At step i, those observations that were misclassified by the classifier $G_{i-1}(x)$ induced at the previous step have their weights increased, whereas the weights are decreased for those that were classified correctly. Thus, as iterations proceed, observations that are difficult to correctly classify receive ever-increasing influence. Each successive classifier is thereby forced to concentrate on those training observations that are missed by previous ones in the sequence (Hastie et al. 2001).

8.1.6.3 Random Forests

A random forest is an ensemble classifier that consists of many decision trees and outputs the class that is the mode of the class's output by individual trees. The method was introduced by Ho (1998) and Breiman (2001). The method combines Breiman's "bagging" idea and the random selection of features. There are many versions of random forest algorithms. Here is the basic one.

Each tree is constructed using the following algorithm:

1. Choose p for the number of variables in the classifier and n_t for the number of training cases.
2. Choose $m \ll p$ input variables for determining the decision at a node of the tree.
3. Choose a training set for this tree by choosing n times with replacement from all available training cases.
4. For each node of the tree, randomly choose m variables, from which the decision at that node is made. Calculate the best split based on these m variables in the training set.

8.1.7 Artificial Neural Network

An artificial neural network (ANN), or simply neural network (NN), is an artificial intelligence method for system modeling. An ANN mimics the mechanism of a human neural network using adaptive weights between the layers in the network to model very complicated systems. It can be used in supervised learning (classification) and predictions, and can be locally linear (having a relationship between two adjacent layers), but collectively it shows global nonlinear behavior.

An ANN is configured for a specific application, such as pattern recognition or data classification, through a learning process. Learning in biological systems

Fig. 8.3 A multilayer
feedforward ANN

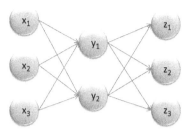

Input Layer   Hidden Layer   Output Layer

involves adjustments to the synaptic connections that exist between the neurons;
the same is true for ANNs. An ANN features adaptive learning (an ability to learn
how to do tasks based on the data given for training or initial experience) and self-
organization (creating its own organization or representation of the information it
receives at the learning phase).

What we know about how the brain trains itself to process information is very
limited. In the human brain, a typical neuron collects signals from others through
a host of fine structures called dendrites. The neuron sends out spikes of electrical
activity through a long, thin strand known as an axon, which splits into thousands
of branches. At the end of each branch, a structure called a synapse converts the
activity from the axon into electrical effects that inhibit or excite activity from the
axon into electrical effects that inhibit or excite activity in the connected neurons.
When a neuron receives an excitatory input that is sufficiently large compared with
its inhibitory input, it sends a spike of electrical activity down its axon. Learning
occurs by changing the effectiveness of the synapses so that the influence of one
neuron on another changes (Chang 2010).

The multiple-layer ANN model in Fig. 8.3 is an example of a perceptron with a
hidden layer where data are not measurable or observable.

The local models (link functions) for the hidden layer and the output layer are

$$y_k = G_a \left(\Sigma_i a_{ik} x_i \right), \tag{8.20}$$

and

$$z_m = G_b \left(\Sigma_j b_{jm} y_j \right), \tag{8.21}$$

respectively. The squared error loss is expressed as

$$E = \frac{1}{2} \sum_m \left(\hat{z}_m - z_m \right)^2, \tag{8.22}$$

where $\hat{z}_m$ and z_m are the observed and model outputs at the mth node, respectively.

Therefore we have

$$
\begin{cases}
\dfrac{\partial E}{\partial b_{ik}} = -G_b'\, (\hat{z}_k - z_k)\, y_i, \\[3mm]
\dfrac{\partial E}{\partial a_{ik}} = -G_b'\, G_a'\, x_i \sum_m \left[(\hat{z}_m - z_m)\, b_{km}\right].
\end{cases}
\tag{8.23}
$$

Given these derivatives, a gradient descent update at the $(r + 1)$th iteration can be formed,

$$
\begin{cases}
b_{ik}^{(r+1)} = b_{ik}^{(r)} + \beta^{(r)} G_b'\, (\hat{z}_k - z_k)\, y_i, \\[3mm]
a_{ik}^{(r+1)} = a_{ik}^{(r)} + \alpha^{(r)} G_b'\, G_a'\, x_i \sum_m \left[(\hat{z}_m - z_m)\, b_{km}\right],
\end{cases}
\tag{8.24}
$$

where $\alpha^{(r)}$ is the learning rate at the rth iteration.

Equations 8.23 and 8.24 formulate a back-propagation training algorithm for updating coefficients a_{ik} and b_{ik}. The computer pseudocode is available elsewhere (Chang 2010).

The performance of an ANN depends on the weights and the link function. A commonly used link function is the additive logit function, given by

$$
G(x) = \frac{1}{1 + \exp(-f(x))}; \quad G'(x) = G(x)\,(1 - G(x))\,\frac{df(x)}{dx},
\tag{8.25}
$$

where $f(\cdot)$ is a real function.

8.1.8 Unsupervised to Supervised Learning

We are going to discuss a very interesting method that converts the unsupervised problem into a supervised problem.

The density estimation problem can be stated as finding a subset s_j of data (or support S_j), $j = 1, \ldots, p$, such that

$$
P\left[\cap_{j=1}^{p} \left(X_j \in s_j\right)\right]
\tag{8.26}
$$

is high.

To solve this unsupervised density problem, we can convert it to the supervised problem (Hastie et al. 2001).

Let $x_1, x_2, \ldots, x_n$ be the i.i.d. random sample from an unknown p.d.f. $g(x)$. Let $x_{n+1}, x_{n+2}, \ldots, x_{n+n_0}$ be the i.i.d. random sample from a reference (e.g., uniform) p.d.f., $g_0(x)$. Assign weight $w = n_0/(n_0 + n)$ to each observation from $g(x)$ and $w_0 = n/(n_0 + n)$ to each observation from $g_0(x)$. Then the resulting pooled data with $n + n_0$ observations can be viewed as a sample drawn from the mixture density $(g(x) + g_0(x))/2$. Let $Y = 1$ to each sample point from $g(x)$ and $Y = 0$ to each sample point from $g_0(x)$. Then

$$\mu(x) = E(Y|x) = \frac{g(x)}{g(x) + g_0(x)} \tag{8.27}$$

can be estimated by supervised learning using the combined sample

$$(y_1, x_1), (y_2, x_2), \ldots (y_{n+n_0}, x_{n+n_0}), \tag{8.28}$$

as the training dataset. The resulting estimate $\hat{\mu}(x)$ can be inverted to provide an estimate for $g(x)$:

$$\hat{g}(x) = g_0(x) \frac{\hat{\mu}(x)}{1 - \hat{\mu}(x)}. \tag{8.29}$$

Similarly, for logistic regression, since the log odds ratio is given by

$$f(x) = \ln \frac{g(x)}{g_0(x)}, \tag{8.30}$$

$g(x)$ can be estimated by

$$\hat{g}(x) = g_0(x) e^{\hat{f}(x)}. \tag{8.31}$$

8.1.9 K-Means Algorithm

The k-means algorithm is one of the simplest and most popular clustering methods. Let data be $X = \{x_i; i = 1, \ldots, n\}$ and cluster $C = \{c_j; j = 1, \ldots, k\}$. For a given k, the goal of clustering is to find C such that

$$\min_{c_j; j} \left(\sum_{i=1}^{n} ||x_i - c_j|| \right). \tag{8.32}$$

The k-means algorithm is described as follows:

1. Randomly choose k data points from X as the initial cluster C.
2. Reassign all $x_i \in X$ to the closest cluster mean c_j.
3. Update all $c_j \in C$ with the means of their corresponding clusters.
4. Repeat steps 2 and 3 until the cluster assignments don't change.

The convergence of the algorithm is guaranteed in a finite number of iterations. However, when the distance $\sum_{i=1}^{n} ||x_i - c_j||$ is a nonconvex function, the convergence can lead to a local optimum. The algorithm is also sensitive to outliers and could lead to some empty clusters. Here we have assumed that k is fixed. The clustering problem with variable k is very challenging computationwise.

8.1.10 Genetic Programming

Genetic programming (GP), inspired by biological evolution, is an evolutionary computation (EC) technique that automatically solves problems without requiring the user to know or specify the form or structure of the solution in advance. At the most abstract level GP is a systematic, domain-independent method for getting computers to solve problems automatically starting from a high-level statement of what needs to be done (Poli et al. 2008). The idea of GP is to evolve a population of computer programs such that, generation by generation, GP stochastically transforms populations of programs into new populations of programs that will effectively solve the problem under consideration. Like evolution in nature, It has been very successful at developing novel and unexpected ways of solving problems (Chang 2010). GP is considered a reinforced learning approach.

8.1.11 Cellular Automata Method

Cellular automata (CAs) are a class of simple computer simulation methods used to model both temporal and spatiotemporal processes. They normally consist of large numbers of identical cells that form a lattice or drift (like a chessboard) with defined interaction rules.

Cellular automata were invented in the late 1940s by von Neumann and Ulam (von Neumann 1966) and have been used to model a wide range of artificial intelligence, image processing, virtual music creation, and physical science applications (Wolfram 2002). Cellular automata also have a long history in biological modeling. Indeed, one of the first and most interesting CA simulations in biology was Conway's Game of Life (Berlekamp et al. 1982). CAs are simple but can do virtually everything that any computer can do. For example, there is a finite initial state such that any paragraph of English prose, when properly coded as a sequence of gliders, will result in a "spell-checked" paragraph of English prose (again coded as a sequence of gliders).

The rule of CAs can be defined in many ways. Here is a simple example.

Example 8.1. An occupant of a cell with less than two neighbors will, sadly, die of loneliness; with two or three neighbors she will continue into the next generation; and with four or more neighbors she will die of overexcitement.

The objects (cells, proteins, or reagents) in a CA simulation usually do not move: they only appear, change properties, or disappear. Object properties, attributes, or information are the only things that "move" in CA simulations. Variations on the CA model, known as dynamic cellular automata (DCAs), actually enable objects to exhibit motions (Wishart et al. 2005). We can apply random-walk or other stochastic processes to DCA. Depending on the implementation of the DCA algorithm, molecules can move one or more cells in a single time step. DCA models permit considerably more flexibility in simulating biological processes (Materi and Wishart 2007).

There are CA applications in the pharmaceutical industry, such as drug release in bio-erodible microspheres (Zygourakis and Markenscoff 1996), lipophilic drug diffusion (Kier et al. 1997; Wishart et al. 2005), drug-carrying micelle formation (Kier et al. 1996), the progression of HIV/AIDS and HIV treatment strategies (Peer et al. 2004), and simulation of different drug therapies or combination therapies. The CA model has the capacity to model the extreme timescales (days to decades) efficiently and to simulate the spatial heterogeneity of viral infections.

8.1.12 Agent-Based Models

In an agent-based model (ABM) of a biological system, agents represent biological entities (molecule or drug, gene, cell, metabolites, proteins, tissue, organ, body, humanecosystem, etc.). The term "agent" is used to indicate a "conscious" computer program entity with potential learning capabilities that is characterized by some degree of autonomy and synchrony with regard to its interactions with other agents and its environment. An agent must be distinguishable from its environment by some kind of spatial, temporal, or functional attribute.

The first step in devising an agent-based model is to identify the entities to be modeled. There are many possible levels of entities, from molecule, to cell, to humanecosystem, that can be chosen for modeling and simulation. An appropriate selection of the entity level is important to the success of the simulation.

A quite interesting observation on agent-based simulation is that by using simple agents who interact locally with simple rules of behavior and actions limited to merely responding befittingly to environmental cues without necessarily striving for an overall goal, we have as a result a synergy that leads to a higher-level whole with much more intricate behavior than that of each component agent. Agents, though, as discrete, diverse, and heterogeneous entities, besides having their own goals and behavior, share the ability to adapt and modify their behavior to their environment, placing their autonomy characteristic at a more sophisticated level (Politopoulos 2007). This is again the general phenomenon called "micro-motivated and macro-consequence."

In the medical field, ABMs have been used for real-time signaling induced in osteocytic networks by mechanical stimuli (Ausk et al. 2005), studying social behavior of cells and understanding important clinical problems (Walker et al. 2006), investigating the patterns in tumor systems and the dynamics of cell motility and aggregation, studying the theory and approaches for stem cell organization in the adult human body (d'Inverno and Prophet 2005), modeling the effect of exogenous calcium on keratinocyte and HaCat cell proliferation and differentiation (Walker et al. 2006), simulating bacterial chemotaxis (Emonet et al. 2005), modeling the calcium-dependent cell migration events in wound healing (Walker et al. 2006), developing optimal breast cancer vaccination protocols (Lollini et al. 2006), and predicting clinical trial outcomes of different anticytokine treatments for sepsis

(An 2004). In An's study, an ABM model of the innate immune response was constructed using extensive literature data and information about all the relevant cell types, cell functions, and cell mediators (cytokines).

8.2 Signal Detection and Analysis

8.2.1 Pharmacovigilance

There is no unified definition of the term "signal" in pharmacovigilance. One commonly cited definition is from the WHO (World Health Organization), which defines a safety signal as reported information on a possible causal relationship between an adverse event and a drug, the relationship being unknown or incompletely documented previously. Another popular definition, given by the PhRMA working group (Almenoff et al. 2005), is that a signal is a relationship between a drug and event that is strong enough, using a predefined threshold or criteria set by an analyst, to warrant further evaluation.

When a safety signal is identified, further investigation is generally warranted to determine whether an actual connection exists. Data contained in spontaneous adverse event reports are collected from patients, health care providers, lawyers, health authorities, the medical literature, and other sources. This information is entered by pharmaceutical companies into their safety databases so that, first, serious events meeting certain reporting criteria can be reported to regulators in an expedited manner, and, second, so that the adverse event data can be analyzed cumulatively for potential safety signals. Where a spontaneously reported serious adverse event meets expedited reporting criteria, it must be reported to regulatory agencies within 15 days, depending on the nature of the event. All spontaneous reports received by the FDA are entered into the Adverse Event Reporting System (AERS), a database designed to support the FDA's postapproval safety monitoring. The AERS contains data for all approved medicines and therapeutic biologic products, with a goal of providing a vehicle for signal detection by the agency (www.pfizer.com/medicinesafety, August 2008). The most recent FDA Sentinel Initiative, the Observational Medical Outcomes Partnership (OMOP), has the goal of developing a nationwide electronic safety monitoring system to strengthen the FDA's ability to monitor postmarket performance of a product. The system will enable the FDA to partner with existing data owners (e.g., insurance companies with large claims databases, owners of electronic health records). The data sources remain with the original owners behind existing firewalls. Owners would run queries per clients' requests and convey summary results of their queries to the network according to strict privacy and security safeguards. This initiative was a response to the U.S. Congress's request. In 2007, Congress (FDA Amendments Act) asked the FDA to develop postmarket safety surveillance and analysis (25 million patients by 2010; 100 million by 2012) guidance and do it in collaboration with others.

The postapproval spontaneous safety reporting systems maintained by pharmaceutical companies and regulatory agencies contain substantially larger volumes of data than preapproval databases, which are mainly based on clinical study data. Although useful, spontaneous reports have some limitations, such as no "denominators" for calculating the AE rate. Patients can take more than one medication. In such instances, one bad medicine can make others look good.

According to Pfizer (www.pfizer.com/medicinesafety, August 2008), safety signals that warrant further investigation include, but are not limited to:

- new adverse events, not currently documented in the product label, especially if serious and in rare untreated populations;
- an apparent increase in the severity of an adverse event that is already included in the product label;
- occurrence of serious adverse events known to be extremely rare in the general population;
- previously unrecognized interactions with other medicines, dietary supplements, foods, or medical devices;
- identification of a previously unrecognized at-risk population, such as populations with specific genetic or racial predisposition or coexisting medical conditions;
- confusion about a product's name, labeling, packaging, or use;
- concerns arising from the way a product is used (e.g., adverse events seen at doses higher than normally prescribed, or in populations not recommended, in the label);
- concerns arising from a failure to achieve a risk management goal.

8.2.2   Traditional Hypothesis Test

Hypothesis-testing for drug safety can be confusing. For example, the ICH E9 Guideline (EMEA 1998) states that for safety data "statistical adjustments for multiplicity to quantify the type-I error are appropriate, but the type-II error is usually of more concern," whereas the CPMP Points to Consider on Multiplicity (CPMP 2002), on the other hand, states that "an adjustment for multiplicity is counterproductive for considerations of safety."

The confusion can come from the way the hypothesis test is formulated in a clinical trial. Suppose we are investigating the safety issue in a two-arm parallel trial using hypothesis testing. We may use hypothesis

$$H_o : R_T - R_C \leq \delta \text{ versus } R_T - R_C > \delta \tag{8.33a}$$

or

$$H_o : R_T - R_C > \delta \text{ versus } R_T - R_C \leq \delta, \tag{8.33b}$$

where δ is usually a positive value and R_T and R_C are adverse event rates in the test and control groups, respectively. In clinical trials, due to low event rates in tier 1 AE (see Chap. 10), the power for (8.33a) is usually low and it is often unable to detect safety problems. However, if (8.33b) is used, an insufficient sample size will lead to potential false safety warnings (i.e., acceptance of $H_o : R_T - R_C > \delta$) and a conclusion that the AE rate is higher in the treatment group than in the control.

8.2.3 Sequential Probability Ratio Test

A commonly used method for pharmacovigilance is the sequential likelihood ratio test or the sequential probability ratio test (SPRT).

Wald's SPRT tests a null hypothesis $H_o : f = f_0$ versus a simple alternative hypothesis $H_a : f = f_1$, based on independent observations $x_1, \ldots, x_i, \ldots$ that have a common density function f. As the ith observation arrives, the log-likelihood ratio statistic Λ_i is calculated as

$$\Lambda_i = \ln \frac{L(x|H_a)}{L(x|H_o)} = \ln \frac{\prod_{j=1}^i f_1(x_i)}{\prod_{j=1}^i f_0(x_i)}. \tag{8.34}$$

The stopping rule is as follows:

1. If $\Lambda_i \le A$, stop monitoring and accept H_o.
2. If $A < \Lambda_i < B$, continue monitoring.
3. If $\Lambda_i \ge B$, stop monitoring and accept H_a.

Here A and B are constants and $0 < A < B$.

A and B are chosen to maintain the prespecified type-I and type-II error rates. Exact values of A and B are difficult to calculate analytically, but Wald showed an approximation to the thresholds, $A \approx \ln\left(\frac{\beta}{1-\alpha}\right)$, $B \approx \ln\left(\frac{1-\beta}{\alpha}\right)$, where α and β are the type-I and type-II error rates, respectively. This approximation is based on the assumption of negligible excess of the likelihood ratio over the threshold when the test ends, which is often true in practice.

Suppose the random variable C_t, the number of adverse events up until and including time t, follows a Poisson distribution with its mean being μ_t and $r\mu_t$ for some $r > 1$ under the null and the alternative hypotheses, respectively, where μ_t is a known function reflecting the baseline risk of adverse events adjusted for the time a person exposed and some confounders like age or sex. The relative risk (RR) of the drug equals 1 under the null hypothesis (H_o) and equals $r > 1$ under the alternative hypothesis (H_a). The test statistic Λ_t for the sequential probability ratio test becomes

$$\Lambda_t \equiv \ln \frac{P(C_t = c_t | H_a)}{P(C_t = c_t | H_o)} = \ln \frac{\exp(-r\mu_t)(r\mu_t)^{c_t}/c_t!}{\exp(-\mu_t)(\mu_t)^{c_t}/c_t!} = (1 - r)\mu_t + c_t \ln r, \tag{8.35}$$

where c_t is a realization of C_t.

8.2.3.1 Maximum SPRT

Because the performance of Wald's SPRT depends heavily on the prespecified value r for the alternative hypothesis (Abt 1998), an inappropriate specification of r for the alternative hypothesis may fail to detect the excess risk or delay the detection. To overcome the difficulty of correctly specifying a single-point alternative hypothesis, Kulldorff (2006) generalized Wald's SPRT by proposing the maximum SPRT (MaxSPRT) for a null hypothesis $H_o : f = f_0$ versus a composite alternative hypothesis $H_a : f = f_1$ using the likelihood ratio:

$$\Lambda_i = \ln \frac{\sup\limits_{\theta \in \Theta_o \cup \Theta_a} L(x_1, \ldots, x_i | \theta)}{\sup\limits_{\theta \in \Theta_o} L(x_1, \ldots, x_i | \theta)} = \ln \frac{\prod_{j=1}^{i} f_1\left(X_i | \hat{\theta}\right)}{\prod_{j=1}^{i} f_0\left(X_i | \hat{\theta}_0\right)}, \qquad (8.36)$$

where $\hat{\theta} = \arg\sup\limits_{\theta \in \Theta_o \cup \Theta_a} L(x_1, \ldots, x_i | \theta)$ and $\hat{\theta}_0 = \arg\sup\limits_{\theta \in \Theta_o} L(x_1, \ldots, x_i | \theta)$.

Under the Poisson distribution, the test statistic for the MaxSPRT is given by

$$\Lambda_t = \ln \left(\frac{\max\limits_{r>1} P(C_t = c_t | RR = r)}{P(C_t = c_t | RR = 1)} \right)$$

$$= \ln \max\limits_{r>1} \frac{\exp(-r\mu_t)(r\mu_t)^{c_t}/c_t!}{\exp(-\mu_t)(\mu_t)^{c_t}/c_t!}. \qquad (8.37)$$

Because the MLE of r is c_t/μ_t, we can write the log-likelihood ratio for the MaxSPRT as

$$\Lambda_t = \mu_t - c_t + c_t \ln \frac{c_t}{\mu_t}, \qquad (8.38)$$

where the indicator function $I(\cdot)$ was defined previously. The critical values for the stopping rules are provided by Li and Kulldorff (2010).

8.2.3.2 Conditional MaxSPRT

It is known that for a homogeneous Poisson process with rate $\lambda > 0$, P_k, the cumulative person time from the beginning of the surveillance until the kth event, is a sum of k i.i.d. random variables from the exponential distribution with rate λ_v and thus follows an Erlang distribution, which is a special case of the gamma distribution with shape k and scale $1/\lambda_v$. According to Li and Kulldorff (2010), V, the total person time in the historical data, is in general greater than the cumulative person time for the observed events c, as it is extremely rare that the historical data ends right after the last observed event. However, for simplicity, we assume they do. Thus, as a sum of the i.i.d. random variables c from the exponential distribution with rate λ_h, V is also gamma-distributed with shape c and scale $1/\lambda_h$. Right after the kth adverse event in the surveillance population, the joint likelihood of the historical data and the current data L_k is

$$L_k = \lambda_h^c \exp\left(-\lambda_h V\right) \lambda_v^k \exp\left(-\lambda_v P_k\right), \tag{8.39}$$

and the test statistic is defined as

$$\Lambda_k = \ln \frac{\max_{\lambda_v \geq \lambda_h} P\left(L_k | \lambda_h, \lambda_v\right)}{\max_{\lambda_0} P\left(L_k | \lambda_h = \lambda_v = \lambda_0\right)} = \ln \frac{\max_{\lambda_v \geq \lambda_h} e^{-\lambda_h V - \lambda_v P_k} \lambda_h^c \lambda_v^k}{\max_{\lambda_v = \lambda_h = \lambda_0} e^{-\lambda_0(V + P_k)} \lambda_0^c \lambda_0^k}$$

$$= I\left(\frac{k}{c} > \frac{P_k}{V}\right) \left[c \ln \frac{c\left(1 + P_k/V\right)}{c + k} + k \ln \frac{k\left(1 + P_k/V\right)}{\left(P_k/V\right)\left(c + k\right)}\right]. \tag{8.40}$$

Conditioning on the number of adverse events, the only random part in Λ_k is the ratio of the person-times P_k/V. Furthermore, under the null hypothesis, the distribution of the ratio P_k/V does not depend on the value of λ_0 simply because $P_k/V = \lambda_0 P_k/\lambda_0 V$ and the distributions of $\lambda_0 P_k$ and $\lambda_0 V$ depend on c and k only. Therefore, under H_0, the distribution of Λ_k and the joint distribution of $(\Lambda_1, \Lambda_2, \ldots, \Lambda_k)$ for any $k \geq 1$ depend on c and k only. The critical values for decision-making are provided by the authors (Li and Kulldorff 2010).

8.2.4 Disproportional Analysis

Pharmacovigilance spontaneous reporting systems are primarily devoted to early detection of the adverse reactions of marketed drugs. They maintain large spontaneous reporting databases (SRDs) for which several automatic signaling methods have been developed (Ahmed et al. 2010). The commonly used public safety databases include FDA Spontaneous Report System (SRS) (postmarketing surveillance of all drugs since 1969), FDA Adverse Event Reporting System (AERS), FDA/CDC Vaccine Adverse Events (VAERS), World Health Organization Collects Similar Data across Countries, and others.

The methods for disproportional analysis of drug safety are often considered as data mining approaches since they are applied to these larger databases. The most commonly used methods are the proportional reporting ratio (PRR), the reporting odds ratio (ROR), the Bayesian confidence propagation neural network (BCPNN) and the multi-gamma Poisson shrinker (MGPS or GPS). Currently, none of these methods is defined as a reference method. The BCPNN method is used for the WHO safety database, the MGPS method for the AERS, and the ROR and PRR methods for the European Medicines Agency EudraVigilance database (Ahmed et al. 2010).

Table 8.1 Drug-event pairs

	Target event	Other events	All events
Target drug	a	b	n_{td}
Other drugs	c	d	n_{od}
All drugs	n_{te}	n_{oe}	n

8.2.4.1 Nonparametric Method

A basic disproportional analysis method is a nonparametric one based on a two-way table for any particular drug and event, as shown in Table 8.1, where the count numbers of drug-event pairs are generated by the reports in a spontaneous reporting database. This is not the same as the number of reports because each report could generate multiple drug-event pairs.

The degree of reporting association is measured by the statistic

$$\lambda = \frac{a}{E(a)}, \tag{8.41}$$

where the reporting ratio, $E(a)$, denotes the expected number of reports mentioning the target drug and target event. A value of λ larger than 1 indicates a drug-event reporting association. If the value of λ is large, the drug will be "flagged for follow-up."

Different definitions of $E(a)$ lead to different estimators of λ, e.g.,

reporting ratio: $E(a) = \frac{n_{td}n_{te}}{n}$,
proportional reporting ratio: $E(a) = \frac{n_{td}c}{n_{od}}$,
odds ratio: $E(a) = \frac{bc}{d}$.

8.2.4.2 GPS Method

The parameter λ can also come from the model. Two commonly used methods are the empirical Bayes method (DuMouchel 1999), employed by the FDA, and the fully Bayesian method (Bate et al. 1998), used by the World Health Organization (WHO). In the empirical Bayes approach models, parameters for the posterior distributions are determined by the MLE. The empirical Bayes (FDA) and Bayes (WHO) approaches flag a drug-event pair for follow-up if the lower 5% quantile of λ (the posterior distribution of λ) exceeds a critical value of λ_0. The choice of values for λ_0 is somewhat arbitrary and there is no consensus in the pharmacovigilance community as to the appropriate critical value to use (Gould 2007).

Both empirical Bayes and Bayes methods utilize a mixture of gamma distributions accounting for multiplicity (see Sect. 10.1.5). The method can be described as follows.

Assume m_{ij}, the number of spontaneous reports mentioning the drug-event pair associated with the ith drug and the jth event, is a realization from a Poisson distribution with parameter $\mu_{ij} = \lambda_{ij}E_{ij}$ and p.d.f.

$$f\left(m_{ij}; \mu_{ij}\right) = \frac{\mu_{ij}^{m_{ij}} e^{-\mu_{ij}}}{n_i!}, \tag{8.42}$$

where E_{ij}, assumed known, denotes the number of reports that would be expected to mention the ith drug-jth event pair.

The mixture model has p.d.f.

$$g_{mix}\left(\lambda_{ij}; \omega\right) = \omega g\left(\lambda_{ij}; a_0, b_0\right) + (1-\omega)g\left(\lambda_{ij}; a_1, b_1\right), \tag{8.43}$$

where $0 \le \omega \le 1$ is the weight; $g\left(\lambda_{ij}; a_0, b_0\right)$ and $g\left(\lambda_{ij}; a_1, b_1\right)$. Here $g\left(\cdot; \cdot; \cdot\right)$ is the gamma distribution given by

$$g\left(\lambda; a, b\right) = b\left(b\lambda\right)^{a-1} \exp\left(-b\lambda\right)/\Gamma\left(a\right). \tag{8.44}$$

Integrating (8.43) out with respect to λ_{ij} and using (8.42), we obtain

$$f\left(m_{ij}\right) = \omega f_0\left(m_{ij}\right) + (1-\omega) f_1\left(m_{ij}\right), \tag{8.45}$$

where

$$f_k\left(m_{ij}\right) = \frac{1}{m_{ij} B\left(a_k, m_{ij}\right)} \left(\frac{b_k}{b_k + E_{ij}}\right)^{a_k} \left(\frac{E_{ij}}{b_k + E_{ij}}\right)^{m_{ij}}, \quad k = 0, 1. \tag{8.46}$$

Estimates of ω, a_0, b_0, a_1, and b_1 are obtained by maximizing the likelihood,

$$\max_{\omega, a_0, b_0, a_1, b_1} \prod_{i,j} f\left(m_{ij}\right). \tag{8.47}$$

The empirical Bayes approach given by the following posterior density of λ_{ij} is still a mixture of the gamma density:

$$f\left(m_{ij}\right) = \omega_{ij}^* g\left(\lambda_{ij}; a_0 + m_{ij}, b_0 + E_{ij}\right) + \left(1 - \omega_{ij}^*\right) g\left(\lambda_{ij}; a_1 + m_{ij}, b_1 + E_{ij}\right), \tag{8.48}$$

where

$$\omega_{ij}^* = \left[1 + \frac{1-\omega}{\omega} \frac{f_1\left(n_i\right)}{f_0\left(n_i\right)}\right]^{-1}. \tag{8.49}$$

The initial strategy of DuMouchel was to rank the cells according to the posterior expectation of $\log_2(\lambda_{ij})$; later he ranked them according to the 5% quantile $Q_{0.05}$ of the posterior distribution of λ_{ij}, and a threshold of 2 for this quantile was recommended by Szarfman et al. (2002) on the basis of several retrospective studies. The GPS software is available online at ftp://ftp.research.att.com/dist/gps/.

Gould (2007) discussed the posterior based on the Bayes approach. The result turns out to be the same formulation as (8.49) but with a different weight ω^*.

8.2.4.3 FPR and FNR

Ahmed et al. (2010) proposed the Bayesian false positive rate and false negative rate, respectively denoted by FDR and FNR. The quantity $d_{ij} \in \{0, 1\}$ represents the decision to generate a signal ($d_{ij} = 1$) or not ($d_{ij} = 0$). Define by v_{ij} the posterior probability for the alternative hypothesis to be true,

$$FDR = \frac{\sum_{ij} (1 - v_{ij}) d_{ij}}{\sum_{ij} d_{ij}} \text{ and } FNR = \frac{\sum_{ij} (1 - d_{ij}) v_{ij}}{n_{cell} - \sum_{ij} d_{ij}},$$

where n_{cell} is the number of cells and v_{ij} is the posterior probability for the alternative hypothesis to be true, which can be calculated based on GPS or BNPNN.

8.2.5 Group Sequential Method

In Chap. 7, we discussed the cumulative meta-analysis using (7.62), which is derived from the Law of the Iterated Logarithm. This method can be used directly for sequential safety monitoring. Here we discuss a group sequential method based on a combination of stagewise p-values. From Chap. 4, we know that when $p_i \sim U(0, 1)$, the sum of stagewise p-values $T_k = \sum_{i=1}^{k} p_i$ has p.d.f. (Sadooghi-Alvandi and Nematollahi 2009)

$$f_k(x) = \begin{cases} \frac{1}{(k-1)!} \sum_{i=0}^{k} (-1)^i \binom{k}{i} (x-i)^{k-1} I(x-i) & \text{for } 0 \le x \le k, \\ 0, & \text{otherwise,} \end{cases} \quad (8.50)$$

where the indicator function $I(x - i)$ is defined as 1 if $x - i > 0$ and 0 otherwise. As $k \to \infty$, T_k approaches the normal distribution $N(k/2, k/12)$.

Therefore, for the statistic, the average of stagewise p-values (with large k) is

$$T_k = \frac{1}{k} \sum_{i=1}^{k} p_i \sim N\left(0.5, \frac{1}{12k}\right) \text{ under } H_o. \quad (8.51)$$

Using the error spending function $\alpha^*(k) = \frac{1}{2} k^c$ for the stopping rules, the constant c can be easily determined for large k.

Note that this method is valid as long as p_i $(i = 1, \ldots, k)$ is stochastically larger than uniform p_i. Therefore, it is valid even when the variability of the interstudy τ is large.

8.2.6 Data Mining Approach

In postmarketing pharmacovigilance, a primary task is to assign an adverse event to its treatment cause or treatments in the case of interaction or to classify subjects into treatments based on their adverse events. To this end, Southworth and O'Connell (2009) quantify the ability of all the adverse events to classify subjects by treatment. In this setting, the response variable is the treatment classification and the explanatory variables are the adverse events experienced by each subject. The authors a variety of tree ensemble methods, including bagging (Breiman 1996), boosting (Friedman 2001), random forests (Breiman 2001), and boosted randomized trees, to the model formulation. These methods fit a sequence of trees through bootstrapping and give all adverse events a chance to classify subjects into treatment groups. In contrast, a single tree produced by a greedy algorithm may get stuck in a local optimum as mentioned earlier. Southworth and O'Connell use observations left out of the bootstrap sample for each tree (out-of-bag patients/observations) to estimate the prediction accuracy of the model and relative importance of the adverse events in classifying the treatment. They use both the permutation and split improvement measures of variable importance in the analysis. In the random forests, the number of variables considered at each split is set to be $\log_2(n_{ae}) + 1$, where n_{ae} is the number of adverse event terms in the analysis. The bagging method allows all interactions between adverse events available within individual trees in the forest. Examples are provided by the authors (Southworth and O'Connell 2009).

8.3 Challenges

The challenges of data mining in the biological and medical fields come from multiple sources. Large-scale databases from genetic mapping, microarray studies, functional genomics, protein-protein and protein-ligand interactions, structural biology, and open source journal articles are growing at rapid rates. The challenge in systems biology is to connect all the dots from the diverse molecular, cellular, organism, and environmental data sources to deduce how subsystems and whole organisms work using dimension reduction technologies. We need to decipher the language of life – the language of the genome, protein folding, and biology pathways.

Establishment of the structure activity relationship (SAR) in drug development is a challenging task. Over ten million nonredundant chemical structures cover the actual chemical space, out of which only about 1,000 are currently approved as drugs. The complexity of the 3D structures of proteins and ligands, and their relative locations that determine the interactions, raise numerous computational challenges in collecting, indexing, searching, and mining these vast data sources. Mining the diverse data sources from private and public sectors is a crucial component in piecing together the bigger picture.

Proteomics, the large-scale study of proteins, particularly their structures and functions, becomes very attractive to biological scientists and bioinformaticians. The proteome is the complete set of proteins in the cell under a set of conditions. It is a dynamic and complex system that is characterized in terms of structure, protein expression level, localization (subcellular location), post-translational modifications, and protein interactions.

Functional annotation of the proteome comprehensively categorizes the information to help address questions such as: Why is a given protein produced (biological process)? What kind of molecule is it (molecular function)? Where is it found (cellular localization)? However, during this massive discovery process using data mining, reducing the false discovery rate (FDR) becomes critically important. FDR is usually high because of multiple-testing procedures as discussed in Chap. 1. The same occurs in signal detection due to the large number of repeated analyses.

Another important aspect in data mining is the dimensionality reduction. Computational limitation requires a large reduction in parameter space. However, a large reduction may not be possible because evolution has made man a very robust creature with large redundancy so that when one part fails other parts will take over the same functional role.

Regarding the accessibility of data, there are privacy issues. Data from internal data warehouses in different companies usually are not shared. Data from different health institutes cannot be easily shared either. These medical data can be multimedia, which will raise another layer of challenges.

Text mining (e.g., in medical records) is an important aspect in modern life sciences. Text mining involves the preprocessing of document collections (text categorization, information extraction, term and sentence extraction), the storage of the intermediate representations, the techniques to analyze these intermediate representations, and visualization of the results. There are several challenges in such text mining, including entity extraction and autonomous text analysis. Most text analysis systems rely on accurate extraction of entities and relations from the documents. However, the accuracy of the entity extraction systems in some of the domains reaches only 70–80% and creates a noise level that prohibits the adoption of text mining systems by a wider audience. Therefore, it is desirable to have a domain-independent language with high accuracy. Text analysis systems today are pretty much user-guided, and they enable users to view various aspects of the corpus. There is still a lot to be done before we have a text analysis system that is totally autonomous and will analyze huge corpora and come up with truly interesting findings that are not captured by any single document in the corpus and were not known before.

Similar to the classic Turing test, the AI agents in text mining systems will be able to pass standard reading comprehension tests such as the SAT, GRE, and GMAT, and will understand medical records (free text field). The systems can utilize the Web when answering the test questions. We should emphasize interactive text mining rather than the classic static text mining approach. These interactive data mining systems will be able to work with physicians or other endusers. These AI data mining agents can learn from each other. We expect these AI agents will eventually not only understand existing knowledge but also to discover and create new knowledge.

In pharmacovigilance signal detection or data mining, there are many challenges. We try to determine the adverse event rate, but without a denominator or the number of patients who took the drug. It is not reliable to use sales or prescription data for determining the denominator. For this reason, we have constructed internal denominators from an independence model. However, this approach also faces challenges; i.e., data reliability because of substantial under-reporting to the FDA, uncertainty about the cause of a reported reaction, and different reporting rates of adverse events by drug.

8.4 Exercises

8.1. Construct a link-analysis model for a practical problem in a biological or medical field, and perform the analysis.

8.2. Assume $y = x + \exp(2\sin(x)) + \varepsilon$, where the random error ε has the standard normal distribution. Perform a comparative analysis between the nearest-neighbors method, kernel method, and support vector machine.

8.3. Prove the constants c_i given by (8.12) will minimize the error given by (8.11).

8.4. Following the idea of Southworth and O'Connell (2009), perform data mining to identify the treatment code for blinded data from a clinical trial.

8.5. In Sect. 8.1.8, for general weights ω_0 and ω, what is the corresponding expression $\mu(x)$ in (8.27)? Study the effect of ω_0 and ω on the variance of $\hat{\mu}(x)$.

Further Readings and References

Abt, K.: Poisson sequential sampling modified towards maximal safety in adverse event monitoring. Biomed J. **40**, 21–41 (1998)

Ahmed, C., Dalmasso, F., Haramburu, F., Thiessard, F., Broët, P., Tubert-Bitter, P.: False discovery rate estimation for frequentist pharmacovigilance signal detection methods. Biometrics **66**, 301–309 (2010)

Ahmed, I., Haramburu, F., Fourrier-Réglat, A., Thiessard, F., Kreft-Jais, C., Miremont-Salamé, G. et al.: Bayesian pharmacovigilance signal detection methods revisited in a multiple comparison setting. Stat. Med. **28**, 1774–1792 (2009)

Almenoff, J., Tonning, J.M., Gould, A.L., et al.: Perspectives on the use of data mining in pharmacovigilance. Drug Saf. **28**(11), 981–1007 (2005)

An, G.: In-silico experiments of existing and hypothetical cytokine-directed clinical trials using agent based modeling. Crit. Care Med. **32**(10), 2050–2060 (2004)

Ausk, B.J, Gross, T.S., Srinivasan, S.: An agent based model for real-time signaling induced in osteocytic networks by mechanical stimuli. J. Biomech. **39**, 2638–2646 (2005)

Balakin, K.V. (ed.): Pharmaceutical Data Mining: Approaches and Applications for Drug Discovery. Wiley, Hoboken (2010)

Bate, A., Lindquist, M., Edwards, I.R., Olsson, S., Orre, R., Lansner, A., De Freitas, R.M.A Bayesian neural network method for adverse drug reaction signal generation. Eur. J. Clin. Pharmacol. **54**, 315–321 (1998)

Berlekamp, E.R., Conway, J.H., Guy, R.K.: Winning Ways for Your Mathematical Plays. Academic Press, London (1982)

Breiman, L.: Bagging predictors. Mach. Learn. **24**, 123–140 (1996)

Breiman, L.: Random forests. Mach. Learn. **45**, 5–32 (2001)

Brin, S., Page, L.: The anatomy of a large-scale hypertextual (Web) search engine, in the seventh international World Wide Web conference. Comput. Netw. ISDN Syst. **30**, 1–767 (1998)

Carroll, K.: Analysis of progression-free survival in oncology trials: Some common statistical issues. Pharm. Stat. **6**, 99–113 (2007)

Cerrito, P.B.: Data mining and biopharmaceutical research. In: Chow, S.C. (ed.) Encyclopedia of Biopharmaceutical Statistics. Marcel Dekker, Boca Raton (2003)

Chang, M.: Monte Carlo Simulation for the Pharmaceutical Industry. CRC, Boca Raton (2010)

Committee for Proprietary Medicinal Products (CPMP): Points to Consider on Switching between Superiority and Non-inferiority. London (2000)

Committee for Proprietary Medicinal Products (CPMP): Points to Consider on Multiplicity Issues in Clinical Trials. London (2002)

Crowe, B.J., Xia, H.A., Berlin, J.A., Watson, D.J., Shi, H., et al.: Recommendations for safety planning, data collection, evaluation and reporting during drug, biologic and vaccine development: A report of the safety planning, evaluation, and reporting team. Clin. Trials **6**, 430–440 (2009)

d'Inverno, M., Prophet, J.: Multidisciplinary investigation into adult stem cell behaviour. In: Priami, C., Merelli, E., Gonzalez, P., Omicini, A. (eds.) Transactions on Computational Systems Biology III. Lecture Notes in Computer Science, vol. 3737, pp. 49–64. Springer, Berlin (2005)

DuMouchel, W.: Bayesian data mining in large frequency tables, with an application to the FDA spontaneous reporting system (Discussion pp. 190–202). Am. Stat. **53**, 177–190 (1999)

EMEA: ICH Topic E9: Statistical principles for clinical trials. http://www.ema.europa.eu/pdfs/human/ich/036396en.pdf (1998). Accessed 10 Oct 2010

Emonet, T., Macal, C.M., North, M.J., Wickersham, C.E., Cluzel, P.: AgentCell: A digital single-cell assay for bacterial chemotaxis. Bioinformatics **21**, 2714–2721 (2005)

Friedman, J.H.: Greedy function approximation: A gradient boosting machine. Ann. Stat. **29**(5), 1189–1232 (2001)

Golub, G.H., Van Loan, C.F.: Matrix Computations. Johns Hopkins University Press, Baltimore (1996)

Gould, A.L.: Accounting for multiplicity in the evaluation of signals obtained by data mining from spontaneous report adverse event databases. Biom. J. **49**, 151–165 (2007)

Hand, D., Mannila, H., Smyth, P.: Principles of Data Mining. MIT Press, Cambridge (2001)

Harper, G., Bradshaw, J., Gittins, J.C., Green, D.V.S., Leach, A.R.: Prediction of biological activity for high-throughput screening using binary kernel discrimination. J. Chem. Info. Comput. Sci. **41**, 1295–1300 (2001)

Hastie, T., Tibshirani, R., Friedman, J.: The Elements of Statistical Learning. Springer, London (2001, 2nd edn., 2009)

Ho, T.: The random subspace method for constructing decision forests. IEEE Trans. Pattern Anal. Mach. Intell. **20**(8), 832–844 (1998)

June, A., Joseph, T.M., Gouid, L.A., Ana, S. Manfred, H., Rita, O.H., et al.: Perspectives on the use of data mining in pharmacovigilance. Drug Saf. **28**(11), 981–1007 (2005)

Kier, L.B., Cheng, C.K., Testa, B., Carrupt, P.A.: A cellular automata model of micelle formation. Pharm. Res. **13**, 1419–1422 (1996)

Kier, L.B., Cheng, C.K., Testa, B., Carrupt, P.A.: A cellular automata model of diffusion in aqueous systems. J. Pharm. Sci. **86**, 774–778 (1997)

Kleinberg, J.: Authoritative sources in a hyperlinked environment. J. ACM **46**(5), 577–603 (1999)

Kulldorff, M.: A maximized sequential probability ratio test for drug and vaccine adverse event surveillance. Presented at the Vaccine Safety Datalink Annual Meeting, Berkeley, 11 May 2006

Langville, A.N., Meyer, C.D.: Deeper inside PageRank. Internet Math. **1**(3), 335–380 (2005)

Li, L.: A conditional sequential sampling procedure for drug safety surveillance. Stat. Med. **28**, 3124–3138 (2009)

Li, L., Kulldorff, M.: A conditional maximized sequential probability ratio test for pharmacovigilance. Stat. Med. **29**, 284–295 (2010)

Lollini, P.L., Motta, S., Pappalardo, F.: Discovery of cancer vaccination protocols with a genetic algorithm driving an agent-based simulator. BMC Bioinfom. **7**, 352–352 (2006)

Materi, W., Wishart, D.S.: Computational systems biology in drug discovery and development: Methods and applications. Drug Discov. Today **12**(7/8) (2007)

Mehrotra, D.V., Heyse, J.F.: Multiplicity considerations in clinical safety analysis. Stat. Meth. Med. Res. **13**, 227–238 (2004)

Ng, A.Y., Zheng, A.X., Jordan, M.I.: Link analysis, eigenvectors and stability. In: Proceedings of the Seventeenth International Joint Conference on Artificial Intelligence, pp. 903–910. Morgan Kaufmann Publishers, San Francisco (2001)

Peer, M.A., Shah, N.A., Khan, K.A.: Cellular automata and its advances to drug therapy for HIV infection. Indian J. Exp. Biol. **42**, 131–137 (2004)

Poli, R., Langdon, W.R., McPhee, N.F.: A field guide to genetic programming, Creative Commons Attribution. England & Wales License, UK (2008)

Politopoulos, I.: Review and Analysis of Agent-Based Models in Biology. University of Liverpool, Liverpool (2007)

Posch, M., Zehetmayer, S., Bauer, P.: Hunting for significance with the false discovery rate. J. Am. Stat. Assoc. **104**, 832–840 (2009).

Sadooghi-Alvandi, S.M., Nematollahi, A.R.: On the distribution of sum of independent uniform random variables. Stat. Pap. **50**, 171–175 (2009)

Spiegelhalter, D.J., Best, N.G., Carlin, B.P., van der Linde, A.: Bayesian measures of model complexity and fit (with discussion). J. R. Stat. Soc. B Ser. **64**, 583–640 (2002)

Southworth, H., O'Connell, M.: Data mining and statistically guided clinical review of adverse event data in clinical trials. J. Biopharm. Stat. **19**, 803–817 (2009)

Szarfman, A., Machado, S., O'Neill, R.: Use of screening algorithms and computer systems to efficiently signal higher-than-expected combinations of drugs and events in the US FDA's spontaneous reports database. Drug Saf. **25**(6), 381–392 (2002)

von Neumann, J.: Elementary cellular automata. In: Burks, A. (ed.) The Theory of Self-Reproducing Automata. University of Illinois Press, Urbana-Champaign (1966)

Walker, D.C., Hill, G., Wood, S.M., Smallwood, R.H., Southgate, J.: Agent-based computational modeling of wounded epithelial cell monolayers. IEEE Trans. Nanobiosci. **3**, 153–163 (2006)

Wilton, D.J., Harrison, R.F., Willett, P.: Virtual screening using binary kernel discrimination: analysis of pesticide data. J. Chem. Info. Model. **46**, 471–477 (2006)

Wishart, D.S., Yang, R., Arndt, D., Tang, P., Cruz, J.: Dynamic cellular automata: an alternative approach to cellular simulation. In Silico Biol. **5**, 139–161 (2005).

Wolfram, S.: A new kind of science. Wolfram Media. http://www.wolframscience.com (2002). Accessed 15 Oct 2010

Wu, X., Kumar, V.: The Top Ten Algorithms in Data Mining. Chapman and Hall/CRC, Boca Raton (2009)

Zygourakis, K., Markenscoff, P.A.: Computer-aided design of bioerodible devices with optimal release characteristics: A cellular automata approach. Biomaterials **17**, 125–135 (1996)

Chapter 9
Monte Carlo Simulation

9.1 Random Number Generation

Monte Carlo simulation is the technique to mimic a dynamic system or process using a computer program. Computer simulations, as an efficient and effective research tool, have been used virtually everywhere, including in biostatistics, engineering, finance, and other areas. To perform simulations, we often need to draw random samples from a certain probability distribution. Typically, the simplest and most important random sampling procedure is sampling from the uniform distribution over $(0, 1)$, denoted by $U(0, 1)$. The computer-generated "random" number is not truly random because the sequence of numbers is determined by the so-called seed, an initial number. Random variates from other distributions can often be obtained by applying a transformation to uniform variates. There are usually several algorithms available to generate random numbers from a particular distribution. The algorithms differ in speed, accuracy, and the computer memory required. Many software packages have implemented various algorithms to generate random numbers with different probability distributions. Here we introduce a few commonly used algorithms.

9.1.1 Inverse c.d.f Method

The inverse c.d.f. (cumulative distribution function) method, if available, is a direct method of generating a sample with a given distribution.

Theorem 9.1. *Let* $\{F(z),\ a \leq z \leq b\}$ *denote a distribution with inverse distribution*

$$F^{-1}(u) = \inf\{z \in [a, b] : F(z) \geq u, 0 \leq u \leq 1\}. \tag{9.1}$$

Let U *denote a random variable from the uniform distribution* $U(0, 1)$. *Then* $Z = F^{-1}(U)$ *has the c.d.f.* F.

M. Chang, *Modern Issues and Methods in Biostatistics*, Statistics for Biology and Health, 233
DOI 10.1007/978-1-4419-9842-2_9, © Springer Science+Business Media, LLC 2011

Algorithm 9.1 Inverse c.d.f. Method

Objective: generate Z from $\{F(z), a \leq z \leq b\}$ using the inverse c.d.f. method.
Generate U from $U(0, 1)$
$Z := F^{-1}(U)$
Return Z
§

The proof is straightforward because $\Pr(Z \leq z) = \Pr\left(F^{-1}(U) \leq z\right) = \Pr[U \leq F(z)] = F(z)$. The algorithm for implementing the inverse c.d.f. method is simple (Algorithm 9.1).

The inverse c.d.f. relationship exists between any two continuous (nonsingular) random variables. If X is a continuous random variable with c.d.f. F and Y is a continuous random variable with c.d.f. G, then $X = F^{-1}(G(Y))$ over the ranges of positive support. To use this relationship is actually to match percentile points of one distribution, F, with those of another distribution, G.

Although the inverse method is simple, the closed form of F^{-1} is not always available. When F does not exist in a closed form, the inverse c.d.f. method can be applied by solving equation $F(x) - u = 0$ numerically.

The inverse c.d.f. method also applies to discrete distributions. Suppose the discrete random variable X has mass points of $m_1 < m_2 < m_3 < \ldots$ with associated probabilities of $p_1, p_2, p_3, \ldots$, and the distribution function

$$F(x) = \sum_{m_i \leq x} p_i. \tag{9.2}$$

To use the inverse c.d.f. method, we generate a realization u of the uniform random variable U, then deliver the realization of the target distribution as x, where x satisfies the relationship

$$F(x - \Delta x) < u \leq F(x), \tag{9.3}$$

where $\Delta x > 0$ is a small increment of x determining the precision of the histogram.

9.1.2 Acceptance-Rejection Methods

The acceptance-rejection method is an elegant method for random number generation. For generating realizations of a random variable X with p.d.f. $f(x)$, the acceptance-rejection method generates random numbers by using realizations of another random variable, Y, with a simpler distribution, g. The method is based on the following theorem (Fishman 1996, p. 171).

Theorem 9.2. (Von Neuman 1951) Let $\{f(z), a \leq z \leq b\}$ denote a p.d.f. with factorization

$$f(z) = cg(z)h(z), \tag{9.4}$$

where $h(z) \geq 0$, $\int_a^b h(z) \, dz = 1$, $c = \sup_z [f(z)/h(z)]$, and $0 \leq g(z) \leq 1$.

Algorithm 9.2 Acceptance-Rejection Method

Objective: Generate a random number from distribution g.
rejection :=**True**
While rejection:
    Generate y from p.d.f. g
    Generate u from $U(0, 1)$
    If $u < f(y)/cg(y)$, **Then** rejection := **False**
Endwhile
Return y
§

Let Z denote a random variable with p.d.f. $\{h(z)\}$ and let U be the standard uniform distribution $U(0, 1)$. If $U \leq g(Z)$, then Z has the p.d.f. $\{f(z)\}$.

The algorithm with acceptance-rejection method is presented in Algorithm 9.2.

9.1.3 Markov Chain Monte Carlo

A Markov chain $\{X_n\}$ with a countable state space S and transition probability matrix $P \equiv [p_{ij}]$ is said to be irreducible if for any two states i and j the probability of the Markov chain visiting j starting from i is positive, i.e., for some $n \geq 1$, $p_{ij}^{(n)} \equiv P(X_n = j | X_0 = i) > 0$.

Theorem 9.3. *(Law of Large Numbers for Markov chains) Let $\{X_n\}_{n \geq 0}$ be an irreducible Markov chain with countable states, a transition probability matrix P, and a stationary probability distribution $\pi \equiv (\pi_i : i \in S)$. Then, for any bounded function $h: S \to \mathbb{R}$ and for any initial distribution of X_0*

$$\frac{1}{n} \sum_{i=0}^{n-1} h(X_i) \to \sum_j h(j) \pi_j \tag{9.5}$$

in probability as $n \to \infty$.

A similar Law of Large Numbers holds when the state space S is not countable.

Monte Carlo simulations based on this theorem are called MCMC. For example, to calculate $\sum_j h(j) \pi_j$, we can use an irreducible Markov chain $\{X_i\}$ with state space S and stationary distribution π. Let the stochastic process run sufficiently long. Then the integral of h with respect to π reduces to:

$$\sum_j h(j) \pi_j = \frac{1}{n} \sum_{i=0}^{n-1} h(X_i). \tag{9.6}$$

A discrete-time Markov chain is the basis for several schemes for generating random numbers, either continuous or discrete, multivariate or univariate. The differences in the various methods using Markov processes come from differences in the transition kernel. To generate variate from an arbitrary distribution $\pi = (\pi_i > 0, i \in \mathcal{L})$ on a finite state space $\mathcal{L} = \{0, 1, \ldots, v - 1\}$, we use the Metropolis-Hastings method (Chang 2010).

9.2   Clinical Trial Simulation

9.2.1   Adaptive Trial Simulation

Clinical trial simulation (CTS) is a powerful tool for supporting strategic decision-making in clinical trials. CTS is very intuitive, easy to implement with minimal cost, and can be done in a short time. The utilities of CTS include (1) sensitivity analysis and risk assessment, (2) estimation of the probability of success (power), (3) design evaluation and optimization, (4) cost, time, and risk reduction, (5) clinical development program evaluation and prioritization, (6) prediction of long-term benefits using short-term outcomes, (7) validation of trial design and statistical methods, and (8) streamlining communication among different parties. Within regulatory bodies, CTS has been frequently used for assessing the robustness of results, validating statistical methodology, and predicting long-term benefits of accelerated approvals.

In classical designs, CTS not only can be used to simulate the power of a hypothesis test for a complex trial, but also allows us to calculate the probability of success. CTS plays an important role in adaptive design for the following reasons: First, statistical theory for adaptive designs is often complicated under some relatively strong assumptions, and CTS is useful in modeling very complicated situations not only to control the type-I error but also to calculate the power and generate many other important operating characteristics such as the expected sample size, conditional power, and unbiased estimates. Second, CTS can be used to evaluate the robustness of the adaptive design against protocol deviations. Moreover, CTS can be used as a tool to monitor trials, predict outcomes, identify potential problems, and provide early remedies.

As discussed in Chap. 4, there are four major components of adaptive designs in the frequentist paradigm: (1) type-I error rate or α-control, determination of stopping boundaries, (2) calculation of power or sample size and probability of success, (3) in trial monitoring: calculation of the conditional power or futility index, and (4) in analysis after the completion of the trial, calculation of adjusted p-values, unbiased point estimates, and confidence intervals.

9.2.1.1 Sample Size Reestimation

A sample size reestimation (SSR) design refers to an adaptive design that allows for sample size reestimation based on the review of interim analysis results.

For a two-stage SSR of a two-group trial, the sample size per group for the second stage can be calculated based on the target conditional power cP (Chap. 4),

$$
\begin{cases}
n_2 = \frac{2\hat{\sigma}^2}{\hat{\delta}^2}\left(z_{1-\alpha_2+p_1} - z_{1-cP}\right)^2, & \text{for MSP,} \\[2mm]
n_2 = \frac{2\hat{\sigma}^2}{\hat{\delta}^2}\left(z_{1-\alpha_2/p_1} - z_{1-cP}\right)^2, & \text{for MPP,} \\[2mm]
n_2 = \frac{2\hat{\sigma}^2}{\hat{\delta}^2}\left(\frac{z_{1-\alpha_2}}{w_2} - \frac{w_1}{w_2}z_{1-p_1} - z_{1-cP}\right)^2, & \text{for MINP,}
\end{cases}
\tag{9.7}
$$

where, for the purpose of calculation, $\hat{\delta}$ and $\hat{\sigma}$ are taken to be the observed treatment effect and standard deviation at stage 1.

An algorithm for a two-stage design with SSR based on MSP (see Chap. 4) is presented in Algorithm 9.3.

Algorithm 9.3 Two-Stage Sample Size Reestimation with MSP

Objective: Return power and PE for two-stage adaptive design.
Input treatment difference δ and common σ, stopping boundaries $\alpha_1, \alpha_2, \beta_1$, n_1, n_2, target conditional power for SSR, the maximum sample size $n_{\max}$, clinical meaningful and commercial viable $\delta_{\min}$, target conditional power cP, and the number of simulation runs $nRuns$.
power := 0
PE := 0
For $iRun$:= 1 **To** $nRuns$
    $T := 0$
    Generate u from $N(0,1)$
    $z_1 = \delta\sqrt{n_1/2}/\sigma + u$
    $p_1 = 1 - \Phi(z_1)$
    If $p_1 > \beta_1$ **Then Exitfor**
    If $p_1 \leq \alpha_1$ **Then** power := power+1/$nRuns$
    If $p_1 \leq \alpha_1$ **And** $\hat{\delta}_1 \geq \delta_{\min}$ **Then** PE := PE+1/$nRuns$
    If $\alpha_1 < p_1 \leq \beta_1$ **Then**
        $n_2 := \frac{2\sigma^2}{\delta_1^2}\left(z_{1-\alpha_2+p_1} - z_{1-cP}\right)^2$
        Generate u from $N(0,1)$
        $z_2 = \delta\sqrt{n_2/2}/\sigma + u$
        $p_2 = 1 - \Phi(z_2)$
        $T := p_1 + p_2$
        If $T \leq \alpha_2$ **Then** power := power+1/$nRuns$
        $\hat{\delta} = (\hat{\delta}_1 n_1 + \hat{\delta}_1 n_2)/(n_1 + n_2)$
        If $T \leq \alpha_2$ **And** $\hat{\delta} \geq \delta_{\min}$ **Then** PE := PE+1/$nRuns$
    Endif
Endfor
Return {power, PE}
§

9.2.2 Dynamic Drug Supply

The conventional way for drug supply in a clinical trial separates the supply chains for each stratum or treatment group. In this approach, an initial drug shipment would be made for each stratum. Resupply shipments would then follow, based on fixed trigger levels for each stratum. However, keeping the supply chains separate requires a high initial outlay and can result in a lot of waste if a site does not enroll as anticipated. This conventional drug supply can be particularly problematic for adaptive trials.

Hamilton and Ho (2004) described a dynamic drug supply method as follows: To randomize a patient, a site would call the IVRS and enter some basic patient identifiers such as ID number and date of birth, along with the stratum to which the patient belonged. The system would then access the randomization and treatment kit lists and read back to site personnel the blinded kit number assigned to that patient. A fax confirming patient information and the assigned kit number would then be automatically generated by the system and sent to the site.

Their logistic steps for the dynamic supply are:

1. At site initiation, ship enough drug to cover the first y patients enrolling into the study, regardless of strata.
2. After each patient is randomized, recalculate the patient coverage based on the randomization list and current levels of drug supply at the site.
3. If the patient coverage falls below a lower resupply threshold x, ship enough drug to replenish supply to an upper resupply threshold y. That is, ship enough drug so that the next y patients can be enrolled into the study, regardless of strata.

The implementation aspect of the dynamic supply can be further elaborated as follows: In the original study, the dynamic drug supply scheme was implemented utilizing a telephone-based interactive voice response system. The system was designed in such a way that when a site completed regulatory and contractual requirements, sponsor personnel could go to a secure administrative Web page and activate that site. Upon activation, the system would examine the randomization list for that site and calculate the amount of drug needed to cover the first y patients, regardless of strata. Notifications via email and fax would then be sent to the central drug repository indicating which drug kits to ship and the shipment number to appear on the waybill. When the site received the drug shipment, they were instructed to register the shipment number with the IVRS, making those drug kits available to be used to randomize patients at the site.

The steps to randomize a patient via IVRS are similar to the conversional approach. After each patient was successfully randomized, the IVRS would recalculate patient coverage at the site. If patient coverage dropped below x patients, another calculation was made by the IVRS to determine which kit types were necessary to bring the coverage back up to cover the next y patients. An automatic notification would then be sent to the central drug repository, indicating which drug kits to be shipped to the site.

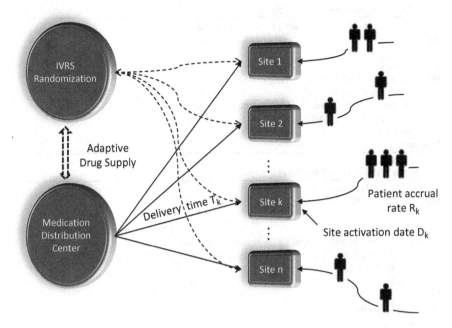

Fig. 9.1 Sketch of adaptive medication supply system

9.2.2.1 Adaptive Drug Supply

In adaptive drug supply (Chang 2010) (Fig. 9.1), recommendations are to use the prerandomization based on all possible scenarios and associated probabilities for the next n patients at each site. The size of n can typically be 2–10, but depends on the time and cost required for the drug shipment and available medication packaging (e.g., placebo, 1, 2, 3, ..., units). With all these random variables, we can do the dynamic shipment to ensure a probability (p) of covering the drug supply. The "trigger/resupply" or "floor/ceiling" system of inventory control with joint replenishment can be used with IVRS at centers and depots.

Algorithms 9.4a and b provide a way to simulate adaptive drug supply, where m_i is the number of patients recruited during the time interval for the drug shipment from the warehouse to the ith clinic site, which is equal to the time required for the drug shipment to the ith site multiplied by the patient accrual rate at the ith site. p is the target probability of having sufficient drug at the site. The drug amount D_c will provide a probability (p) of covering the drug supply needed for the site; D_c is also used as the trigger level for resupply in the algorithm.

Algorithm 9.4a Adaptive Drug Supply

Objective: Return the amount of drug required for a trial.
Input p and $\{m_i\}$ for sites.
mDrug $:= \sum_i n_{i0}$
$\{d_i\} := \{n_{i0}\}$
When each patient is enrolled at site i
    $D_c := \text{DrugCoverage}(p)$
    Calculate the drug inventory d_i at the site
    If $d_i < D_c$ **Then** mDrug$:=$ mDrug $+ D_c$
    Return mDrug
Endwhen

Algorithm 9.4b Function DrugCoverage (p)

Objective: Function used in Algorithm 9.4a.
For $i := 1$ **To** 10000
    $D_i := 0$
    For $j := 1$ **To** m_i
        Randomize patient j based on randomization rule.
        Determine the drug package x required for patient j.
        $D_i := D_i + x$
    Endfor
Endfor
Sort D_i in ascending order
Return $D_{10000 \cdot pro}$

9.2.3 Bootstrapping Methods

Bootstrapping is a resampling method that estimates the distribution of an estimator by sampling with replacement from the original sample. Bootstrapping is useful when the analytical form of distribution is not available or unknown. Bootstrapping is often used for deriving robust estimates of standard errors and confidence intervals of a population parameter like a mean, median, proportion, odds ratio, correlation coefficient, or regression coefficient.

Suppose $x_1, x_2, \ldots, x_n$ is i.i.d. from probability distribution F. The empirical distribution function $\hat{F}$ is defined to be the discrete distribution that put $1/n$ on each value x_i $(i = 1, \ldots, n)$,

$$\hat{\Pr}\{A\} = \frac{\#\{x_i \in A\}}{n}. \tag{9.8}$$

9.2.3.1 The Plug-in Principle

The plug-in principle is a simple method of estimating parameters from samples. The plug-in estimate of a parameter $\theta = t(F)$ is defined as (Efron and Tibshirani 1994; Chernick 2007)

$$\hat{\theta} = t\left(\hat{F}\right). \tag{9.9}$$

Algorithm 9.5 Bootstrapping Distribution of Estimator

Objective: Return bootstrapping distribution of estimator $\theta\,(x_1, \ldots, x_n)$.
Input observations $\{x_1, \ldots, x_n\}$ and $n\,Runs$.
For $i := 1$ **To** $n\,Runs$
    For $j := 1$ **To** n
        Draw k from the equal distribution $U_c\,(n)$
        $y_j^{(i)} := x_k$
    Endfor
    $\hat{\theta}_i := \theta\left(y_1^{(i)}, y_2^{(i)} \ldots, y_m^{(i)}\right)$
Endfor
Sort $\left\{\hat{\theta}_1, \hat{\theta}_2, \ldots, \hat{\theta}_{n\,Runs}\right\}$
Return $\left\{\hat{\theta}_1, \hat{\theta}_2, \ldots, \hat{\theta}_{n\,Runs}\right\}$
§

In other words, we estimate the function $\theta = t\,(F)$ of the probability distribution F using the same function of the empirical distribution $\hat{F}$, $\hat{\theta} = t\left(\hat{F}\right)$.

Algorithm 9.5 is an algorithm for the plug-in principle.

Having obtained the sorted $\left\{\hat{\theta}_1, \hat{\theta}_2, \ldots, \hat{\theta}_{n\,Runs}\right\}$, its median, quantiles, mean, standard error, and confidence interval can be easily calculated.

9.2.3.2 Resampling Methods in Clinical Trials

Confidence intervals (CI) and hypothesis tests are common statistical analyses in clinical trials. The following is a clinical trial example with two parallel groups of sample size n per group. Assume the total number of responses observed is m and the observed proportions in groups 1 and 2 are $\hat{p}_1$ and $\hat{p}_2$, respectively. In Algorithm 9.6, the goal is to calculate the confidence interval for the difference between the response rates p_1 and p_2. The main step in the bootstrap approach is to sort the bootstrap values for $T_k = p_2 - p_1$ $(k = 1, 2, \ldots)$. With these sorted values T_k, the confidence interval and the p-value are ready to obtain. Because the CI and p-value can be calculated based on the assumption of the null hypothesis condition, meaning there is no treatment effect, the response data can be pooled and the treatment code can be scrambled. In Algorithm 9.6, the pooled data represented by $\{x_1, x_2, \ldots, x_{2n}\}$, for each simulation run, the treatment code is randomly assigned for each observation x_i and the response rates, p_1 and p_2, are calculated for the two groups, from which the test statistic $T_k := p_2 - p_1$ is calculated. These T_ks are then sorted to calculate the confidence interval for the rate difference. The histogram of T_k is the empirical distribution of the test statistic T_k under the null hypothesis; by comparing this distribution with the observed value $\hat{T} = \hat{p}_2 - \hat{p}_1$, the p-value can be calculated.

Algorithm 9.6 Bootstrapping CI for Rate Difference

Objective: Return a bootstrap $100(1 - \alpha)\%$ CI for $\hat{p}_2 - \hat{p}_1$.
Input n, m, $\hat{p}_1$, $\hat{p}_2$, and binary responses $\{x_1, x_2, \ldots, x_{2n}\}$.
For $k := 1$ **To** nRuns
$\quad$ $p_1 := 0$
$\quad$ $p_2 := 0$
$\quad$ **For** $i := 1$ **To** $2n$
$\quad\quad$ Generate a random sample u from $U_c(n)$
$\quad\quad$ **If** $u = 1$ **Then** $p_1 := p_1 + x_i/n$
$\quad\quad$ **If** $u = 2$ **Then** $p_2 := p_2 + x_i/n$
$\quad$ **Endfor**
$\quad$ $T_k := p_2 - p_1$
Endfor
Sort $\{T_1, T_2, \ldots, T_{nRuns}\}$ in ascending order
$CI := \left\{ T_{\lfloor \alpha \cdot nRuns \rfloor}, T_{\lceil (1-\alpha) \cdot nRuns \rceil} \right\}$
Return CI and $\{T_1, T_2, \ldots, T_{nRuns}\}$
§

9.3   Molecular Design and Simulation

9.3.1   The Landscape of Molecular Design

As mentioned earlier, Pharmaceutical R & D expense has increased dramatically over the past 15 years, while the number of NDAs approved has been relatively flat. Innovative and cost-effective drug discovery approaches become inevitable for any pharmaceutical company to stay competive. Molecular design and modeling is a promising new field, in which computer simulations and a chemical compound database are used to screen, model, and design NMEs in order to reduce the discovery cost and accelerate the discovery process. The reasons why this in-silico method can help in this aspect are because (1) the number of compounds that can be examined by a human mind is limited compared with the capacity throughput of virtual, computer-based storage, modeling, and virtual screening systems, and (2) compound supply is also limited. Many different companies use blind screening for the same compound libraries even after many of the compounds have been proven structurally unfavorable, which often turns out to be a waste of time and resources. Computer-based design of activity enriched screening libraries can be of great value here, and (3) the traditional biochemical screening assays can be very expensive, especially for cell-based systems or when elaborate protein purification schemes are required. Costs have been estimated to fall somewhere between \$0.02 and \$10 per well. When considering a screening library containing one million compounds with multiple measurements, the sum adds up (Schneider and Baringhaus 2008).

There are approximately 8,000 drug targets, of which 5,000 could be "hit" by small druglike molecules. Only about 3,000 targets out of the 5,000 are pharmacological interest, and only 200–500 targets are addressed by marketed drugs – there are many more targets to be explored in the future. It is estimated that out of the 20,000–25,000 human genes supposed to code for about 3,000 druggable targets, only a subset of the pharmacological space (about 800 proteins) has currently been investigated by the pharmaceutical industry (Paolini et al. 2006). Over ten million nonredundant chemical structures cover the actual chemical space, out of which only about 1,000 are currently approved as drugs. Chemogenomics is the new interdisciplinary field that attempts to fully match target and ligand space, and ultimately identify all ligands of all targets. The 8,000 drug targets can be further categorized into seven different classes: proteases (19%), kinases (12%), other enzymes (17%), G-protein coupled receptors (GPCRs, 16%), ion channel (13%), nuclear receptor (4%), and other targets (19%).

The steps in the standard drug lead approach include (1) identifying the target (e.g., enzyme, receptor, ion channel, transporter), (2) determining the DNA and/or protein sequence, (3) elucidating the structures and functions of proteins, (4) proving the therapeutic concept in animals ("knock-outs"), (5) developing an assay for HTS, (6) mass screening, and (7) selecting lead structures.

A goal of Monte Carlo molecular design is to identify novel substances that exhibit desired properties. An example would be a particular biological activity profile including a selective binding to a single target or desired activity modulation of multiple targets simultaneously. This design certainly must include proper physicochemical and ADMET (absorption, distribution, metabolism, excretion, and toxicity) properties of the novel compounds (Schneider and Baringhaus 2008).

9.3.2 The Drug-Likeness Concept

The term "druglike" describes various empirically found structural characteristics of molecular agents that are associated with pharmacological activities. It is not strictly defined but provides a general concept of what makes a drug a drug. Drug-likeness may be considered as the overall likelihood that a molecular agent can be turned into a drug. Therefore, it is a measure of complex physicochemical and structural features of the compound that can be used to guide the rational design of lead structures that can be further optimized to become a drug.

The well-known QSAR (quantitative structure-activity relationship) Lipinski's rule-of-five is often used in rational drug design to reduce the risk of costly late-stage preclinical and clinical failures. The guidelines predict that poor passive absorption or permeation of an orally administered compound is more likely if the compound meets at least two of the following criteria (Lipinski et al. 1997):

1. molecular weight greater than 500 Da;
2. high lipophilicity (expressed as clogP > 5);
3. more than five hydrogen-bond donors, expressed as the sum of OHs and NHs;
4. more than ten hydrogen-bond acceptors, expressed as the sum of Os and Ns;
5. containing more than five rotatable bonds to limit its conformational freedom.

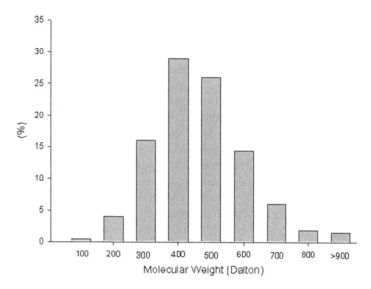

Fig. 9.2 Weight distribution of druglike molecules

These guidelines were developed based on an empirical pharmaceutical database. For example, Fig. 9.2 is the distribution of molecular weights of 4,500 selected druglike molecules containing marketed drugs and drug candidates. We can see that most druglike molecules weight between 300 and 600 Da.

9.3.2.1 Tanimoto Similarity Index

The rationale behind a similarity search is the so-called similar property principle: structurally similar molecules are likely to have similar chemical or physiological properties. A variety of methods are used in these searches, including 2D and 3D shape similarity, graph theory, vector space models based on 2D fingerprints, and machine learning methods.

Similarity searching can be achieved by comparing representations of molecules with respect to the substructure elements they contain. A popular similarity index is the Tanimoto (Jaccard) index defined by

$$T_{AB} = \frac{n_{AB}}{n_A + n_B - n_{AB}}, \tag{9.10}$$

where n_A is the number of bits set to 1 (indicating a certain substructure) in molecule A, n_B is the number of bits set to 1 in molecule B, and n_{AB} is the number of set bits common to both A and B. The possible value of T_{AB} ranges between 0 (maximal dissimilarity) and 1 (identical bitstrings). However, $T_{AB} = 1$ implies A and B have identical fingerprint but does not necessarily mean that the two molecules A and B are identical.

Ligands A and B can be viewed as fingerprint vectors, and the quantity

$$D_{AB} = 1 - T_{AB} \qquad (9.11)$$

is called the distance in vector space. For the distance, the following triangular inequality holds (Lipkus 1999):

$$|D_{AB} - D_{AC}| \le D_{BC} \le D_{AC} + D_{AB}. \qquad (9.12)$$

From (9.12) we can obtain the following bound on the Tanimoto similarity index:

$$T_{BC} \le 1 - |T_{AB} - T_{AC}|. \qquad (9.13)$$

This bound (9.13) has been improved by Baldi and Hirschberg (2009).

9.3.2.2 Bayesian Network for Similarity Search

In a similarity search, a Bayesian network (BN) is a simple and popular way of doing probabilistic inference that formalizes the way to synchronize the evidence using the Bayes rule:

$$P(H|E) = P(E|H)P(H)/P(E).$$

A Bayesian network is a directed acyclic graph and has the following properties:

- Nodes of the BN represent random variables and the parents of a node are those judged to be direct causes of it.
- The roots of the network are the nodes without parents.
- The arcs represent causal relationships between these variables, and the strengths of these casual influences are expressed by conditional probabilities.
- Let $X = \{x_1, \ldots, x_n\}$ be a set of parents of y (child node), where $x_i \cap x_j = \phi$ (empty) for $i \ne j$ and x_i is a direct cause of y. The influence of X on y can be quantified with the conditional probability $P(y|X)$.

9.3.3 *Molecular Docking*

A ligand (drug candidate) has to bind the protein closely enough in order to have a drug effect. This requires the ligand to have the right shape and orientation to fit the "pocket" of the protein target. Molecular docking is a computer-based technology to find the binding orientation of a ligand (small molecule) to the protein target in order to predict the affinity and activity of the small molecule. Hence docking plays an important role in the rational design of drugs. The docking methods can be geometry or energy-based. Here we only discuss the energy minimization approach.

9.3.3.1 Energy Minimization Approach

The design of ligands that interact with a target receptor always yields a low energy ligand-receptor complex. The free energy (Gibbs energy) change ΔG for a receptor-ligand interaction was defined by Gibbs in 1873 as

$$\Delta G = \Delta H - T \Delta S, \tag{9.14}$$

where ΔH and $T \Delta S$ are enthalpic and entropic terms, respectively, contributing to the change in the free energy of binding ΔG.

This ligand conformation is not necessarily the global minimum-energy conformation. However, typical bioactive ligand conformations are close to global minimum conformations in water, which might differ substantially from conformations in a vacuum.

Free-energy differences between two states are almost independent of high-energy contributions. This allows an approximation of each state by its mean partition function, taking into account only relevant low-energy conformations weighted by their Boltzmann probability. The energy differences between the two states can be quantified from Monte Carlo or molecular dynamics (MD) simulations (Schneider and Baringhaus 2008).

9.3.3.2 Monte Carlo Simulated Annealing

In solid physics, annealing is known as a thermal process for obtaining the lowest-energy states of a solid. The processes are governed by molecular dynamics in which the system starts at a high-temperature state with its particles being relatively free to move around. The temperature then slowly deceases and the particles are forced to line up to achieve the local energy minimization. In this process, the system is cooled down slowly; otherwise, if it cools too fast, the particles will not have enough time to line up (Liu 2001). In Monte Carlo simulated annealing, during each constant temperature cycle, random perturbations are made to the ligand's current orientation and conformation. The new state is accepted if its energy is lower than the energy of the preceding state. Otherwise, the configuration is accepted probabilistically based upon a Boltzmann equation (Höltje et al. 2008). The probability of acceptance is given by

$$P_a = \exp \left(-\frac{\Delta E}{k_B T} \right), \tag{9.15}$$

where ΔE is the difference in energy from the previous step, T is the absolute temperature in Kelvin, and k_B is the Boltzmann constant.

From (9.15), we can see that the higher the temperature of the cycle, the higher the probability that the new state is accepted. When the energy change ΔE is negative, P_a will be larger than 1. Therefore, regardless of the direction of the energy change in Monte Carlo simulated annealing, the acceptance probability for a state can be written as

Algorithm 9.7 Simulated Annealing

Objective: Docking with simulated annealing
Set up initial ligand's coordinates.
Input temperature sequence $\{T_i\}$, k_B, and a small $\varepsilon > 0$.
For $i := 1$ **To** K
    Make random perturbations to the ligand's current orientation and
    conformation.
    Calculate the incremental energy ΔE
    Generate random number u from $U(0,1)$
    If $u < P_a = \min\left(1, e^{-\frac{\Delta E}{k_B T_i}}\right)$ **Then** accept new state
      If $\Delta E < \varepsilon$ **Then Exitfor**
Endfor
Return current state of the ligand
§

$$P_a = \min\left(1, e^{-\frac{\Delta E}{k_B T}}\right). \tag{9.16}$$

Keep in mind that the final state in Monte Carlo simulated annealing usually depends on the initial placement of the ligand because the algorithm does not explore the solution space exhaustively. The algorithm for the simulated annealing is presented in Algorithm 9.7.

9.3.3.3 Scoring Functions

A scoring function is a measure of interaction between a ligand and a receptor; it is a measure of the drug-likeness of a ligand. The scoring function can be the free energy of binding given by the Gibbs-Helmholtz equation (9.14), where ΔG relates to the binding constant K_i through the equation

$$\Delta G = -RT \ln K_i, \tag{9.17}$$

where R is the gas constant.

The binding free-energy difference between a ligand and a reference molecule can be accurately calculated using energy perturbation Miyamoto and Kollman (1993). However, such a time-consuming approach is not practical for virtual screening to compute energies for thousands of protein-ligand complexes. A fast method is desirable. A scoring function, monotonic in ΔG, can be calculated quickly and the resulting conformation rankings based on a score function will be the same as those by the ΔG.

Höltje and colleagues (2008) categorize scoring functions into three groups: empirical scoring functions, force-field-based functions, and knowledge-based potential of mean force. Scoring functions can be used in two ways (1) during the docking process, they serve as fitness functions in the optimal placement of the ligand; and (2) when the docking is completed, they are used to rank each ligand of the database for which a docking solution has been found.

9.4 Biological Pathway Simulation

9.4.1 Biology Pathways

A *biological pathway* is a molecular interaction network in biological processes. The pathways can be classified into the fundamental categories: metabolic, regulatory, and signal transduction. There are about 10,000 pathways, nearly 160 pathways involving 800 reactions.

A *metabolic pathway* is a series of chemical reactions occurring within a cell, catalyzed by enzymes, resulting in either the formulation of a metabolic product to be used or stored by the cell, or the inhibition of another metabolic pathway. Pathways are important to the maintenance of homeostasis within an organism.

A *gene regulatory pathway* or *genetic regulatory pathway* is a collection of DNA segments in a cell that interact with each other and with other substances in the cell, thereby governing the rates at which genes in the network are transcribed into mRNA. In general, each mRNA molecule goes on to make a specific protein or its particular structural properties. The protein can be an enzyme for breakdown of a food source or toxin. By binding to the promoter region at the start of other genes, some proteins can turn the genes on, initiating or inhibiting the production of another protein.

A *signal transduction pathway* is a series of processes involving a group of molecules in a cell that work together to control one or more cell functions, such as cell division or cell death. Molecular signals are transmitted between cells by the secretion of hormones and other chemical factors, which are then picked up by different cells. After the first molecule in a pathway receives a signal, it activates another molecule, and then another, until the last molecule in the signal chain is activated. Abnormal activation of signaling pathways can lead to a disease such as cancer. Drugs are being developed to block these disease pathways.

Systems biology is a newly emerging, multidisciplinary field that studies the mechanisms underlying complex biological processes by treating these processes as integrated systems of many interacting components (Materi and Wishart 2007). Quantitative studies in systems biology require the utilization of computer modeling and simulation, which has given rise to a new discipline called computational systems biology (CSB).

The modeling and simulation can be carried out on different temporal and spatial scales, ranging from nanometers to meters and milliseconds to days. Conventionally, "fine grain" models simulate the events that concern short times (ms) or small (nm) dimensions, and coarse "grain models" simulate the events that concern longer times (s) or larger (mm or cm) dimensions.

9.4.2 Petri Nets

A Petri net (PN) is a mathematical network model for simulating a dynamic system such as an electronic process, traffic system, or biological pathway. Petri nets were proposed by Carl Adam Petri in 1962 in his PhD thesis in computer science. PN has gained an increasing attention in the biological sciences and drug development in the past 10 years. PN research papers dominate the field in simulations of life sciences and PNs have been adopted more and more by the pharmaceutical industry.

The basic elements in PNs include *places* (or stelle) to symbolize the states or conditions of the system, *transitions* to symbolize the actions in the system, *tokens* to symbolize the resources responsible for the changes of the system, *directed arcs* to indicate the directions of token (resource) travel, and *weights* for the directed arcs representing the minimum required tokens for firing (executing action). Graphically, a place is often denoted by a circle; a transition is denoted by a rectangle; tokens are allocated in places; places and transitions are connected by directed lines (arcs); and weights are values next to the corresponding arcs. When the number of tokens in a *place* meets the minimum requirement for firing (execution), some of the tokens are moving from one place to another – the firing rules. Figure 9.3 is a PN representation of the chemical reaction of water.

The mathematical definition of a PN can be described as follows.

Definition 9.1. A Petri net is a 5-tuple $PN = (P, T, F, W, M_0)$ where

- $P = \{p_1, \ldots p_K\}$ is the set of K *places*,
- $T = \{t_1, \ldots t_N\}$ is the set of N transitions, with $P \cap T = \emptyset$ and $P \cup T \neq \emptyset$,
- $F = I \subseteq (P \times T) \cup O \subseteq (T \times P)$ is the flow relation defining the set of directed arcs,
- $W : F \to (\mathbb{N} \setminus \{0\})$ ($\mathbb{N} = \{0, 1 \ldots\}$) is the arc weight function, and
- $M_0 = \{m_{01}, \ldots, m_{0K}\} \in \mathbb{N}^K$ is the initial marking, i.e., an integer number of tokens associated to each place initially.

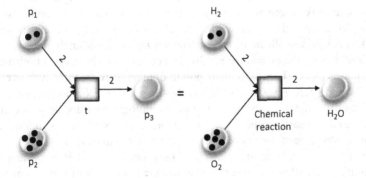

Fig. 9.3 PN representing chemical reaction of water

Note that the preset I corresponds to all the directed arcs from places to transitions, whereas postset O corresponds to all the directed arcs from transitions to places. $M(p)$ often denotes the number of tokens in place p in marking M.

The state of a Petri system is characterized by the distribution of tokens in the places. The dynamics of PN is characterized by the firing mechanism. A place may contain zero or several tokens, which may be interpreted as resources. There may be several input and output arcs between a place and a transition. The number of these arcs is represented as the weight of a single arc. A transition is enabled if each of its input places contains at least as many tokens as the corresponding input arc weight indicates. When an enabled transition is fired, its input arc weights are subtracted from the input place markings and its output arc weights are added to the output place markings. Formally, we have the following definition.

Petri nets can be of different types: (1) place/transition PNs (colored or non-colored) or (2) time-dependent PNs (discrete PN, continuous PN, hybrid PN for mixtures of continuous and discrete systems, and stochastic PN).

9.4.2.1 Why Petri Nets

Biological networks or pathways are extremely complicated, and their mechanisms are difficult to understand using the traditional 2D representation. Using a Petri net, we can have a coherent presentation of the very diverse forms of information and solve the problem by means of computer simulation. Petri nets offer a general framework for analyzing the dynamic properties of large systems, either from a qualitative or a quantitative point of view. The mathematical properties of standard Petri nets are well studied and can be used for model validation. PNs can be used on an abstract level with specification of limited resources possible and allow for combining all these different abstract levels within one model. PNs allow for integration of qualitative and quantitative analyses. Petri nets have an executable graphical representation, supporting the intuitive understanding of the system modeled and the communication between experimentally and theoretically working scientists. There are movable objects, the animation of which visualizes possible flows through the network. Model animation helps us experience the network behavior and allows us to test whether the model actually does behave in the desired manner (Koch and Heiner 2008). Petri nets can be used as both analysis and prediction tools. There exist many public-domain software tools such as editors, animators, and analyzers. One of the nice features with a PN is its scalability to fit the constantly updated knowledge of systems biology. Any update to the current knowledge can be easily implemented in the previous PN by simply modifying the relevant substructure of the PN without recreating a completely new PN.

There are biological interpretations for most properties of a PN. For example, the reachability of a marking from some other marking in the PN model of a metabolic pathway determines the possibility of forming a specified set of product metabolites from another set of reactant metabolites, using some sequence of reactions that is dictated by the PN's firing sequence(s).

9.4.2.2 Petri Net Dynamics

PN dynamics include *reachability, liveness,* and *boundedness.* They all relate to the initial marking. A reachability study concerns whether a marking under consideration can be reached from the initial marking; liveness study addresses whether any transition will eventually be fired for the given initial marking; and a boundedness study investigates whether the number of tokens at each place is bounded for any initial marking of the Petri net.

There are three commonly used abstract levels in the simulation, (1) molecular level (biochemical network), (2) gene cross-regulation level (genetic network), and (3) tissue level (intercellular network), in which the biological cells are believed to operate with a steady state of the internal metabolites. Note that the same compound can be presented using multiple places in the same network if they play different biological roles.

9.4.3 Biological Pathway Simulations

9.4.3.1 Petri Net for Metabolic Pathways

A metabolic pathway is a series of enzymatic reactions consuming certain metabolites and producing others. These metabolites usually participate in more than one metabolic pathway, forming a complex network of reactions.

The S-transformation of biochemical reactions can be modeled using PNs in which (1) places can be metabolites, reactants, products, genes, cells, and enzymes, (2) transitions can be reactions, catalysis, activation, and inhibition, and (3) weighted arcs can be stoichiometries (Chang 2010).

9.4.3.2 Stochastic PN for Regulatory Pathways

Regulation of gene expression (or gene regulation) includes the processes (amount and timing) turning the information in genes into gene products (RNA or protein). The majority of known mechanisms regulate protein coding genes. Any step of the gene's expression may be modulated, from DNA-RNA transcription to the post-translational modification of a protein. The stages where gene expression is regulated are chromatin domains, transcription, post-transcriptional modification, RNA transport, translation, mRNA degradation, and post-translational modification. Gene regulation is essential for viruses, prokaryotes, and eukaryotes, as it increases the versatility and adaptability of an organism by allowing the cell to express protein when needed. The first discovered (by Jacques Monod) example of a gene regulation system was the lac operon, in which proteins involved in lactose metabolism are expressed by E. coli only in the presence of lactose and absence of glucose (Chang 2010).

9.4.3.3 Hybrid PN for Regulatory Pathways

In many cases, molecular concentration is considered continuous rather than discrete. How do we deal with actual molecule numbers? If we represent each molecule by one token, it is not feasible for simulations; if one token stands for, for example, 1 mol of a substance, it might not be accurate enough. The solution is to allow continuous values for certain places, which leads to the so-called hybrid Petri nets (HPNs) (Chang 2010).

An HPN can have continuous and discrete tokens in places. Discrete places have tokens, whereas continuous places contain real variables. Discrete transitions fire after a certain delay. Continuous transitions fire continuously at a given rate.

Chen and Hofestädt (2003) conducted a case study on the urea cycle disorder, a genetic disease caused by a deficiency of one enzyme in the urea cycle that is responsible for removing ammonia from the bloodstream. In urea cycle disorders, the nitrogen, a waste product of the metabolite, is not removed from the body. Ammonia then reaches the brain through the blood, where it causes irreversible brain damage, coma, and/or death.

The metabolic behavior is modeled using continuous places and transitions, whereas gene regulations are modeled by discrete net elements. The regulation both on genomic and metabolic levels can be simulated. A generalization of hybrid Petri nets (hybrid function Petri nets) was developed by Matsuno et al. (2003). The typical examples they studied included a metabolic pathway (the glycolysis) and a signaling pathway (the Fas legand induced apoptosis). The effectiveness of PN-based biopathway modeling was demonstrated in the circadian rhythm in *Drosophila* and the apoptosis induced by the Fas ligand. The simulations of these models were performed with the software tool Genomic Object Net.

9.5 PK and PD Modeling and Simulation

9.5.1 Pharmacokinetic Simulation

For a drug to interact with a target, it is necessary for the drug to present sufficient concentration in the fluid medium surrounding the cells with receptors. Pharmacokinetics is the study of the kinetics of absorption, distribution, metabolism, and excretion (ADME) of a drug. It analyzes the way the human body works with a drug after it has been administered, and the transportation of the drug to the specific site for drug-receptor interactions.

In what follows, we will discuss the ADME mechanisms to guide our PK modeling and simulation. There are two schools of modeling and simulation approaches. One is to model the complex ADME directly, treating the whole body as one entity – the macro-approach. The mixed-effect population PK model is an example of this type of statistical modeling. There are nearly 100 commercial software products

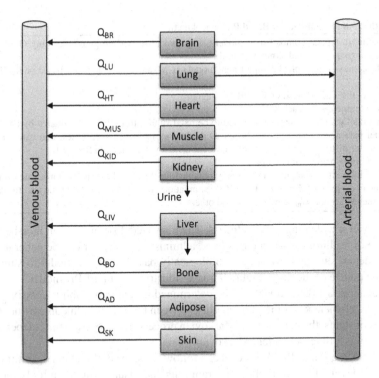

Fig. 9.4 Physiology-based pharmacokinetic model

available (see, e.g., www.boomer.org/pkin/soft.html for such a list) for this type of modeling and most PK specialists are familiar with the approach and software. I am not going to discuss this approach. Alternatively, we can use low-level modeling, which either models the four components of ADME separately or models the mechanisms at the organ level as for the physiologically based pharmacokinetic (PBPK) model (Fig. 9.4) and then integrate the low-level components into a higher-level model. The integration is accomplished through simulation.

The law governing the drug concentration $C(t)$ over time t is the diffusion equation:

$$\frac{dC(t)}{dt} = kC(t). \tag{9.18}$$

It is interesting that the model is mathematically equivalent to the survival model (6.1). Therefore, the same method can deal with two complete problems in two completely different disciplines.

PBPK model structures are based on the actual physiological and biochemical structure of the species being described, allowing the physiological and biochemical parameters in the model to be changed from those for the test species to those appropriate for humans to perform animal to human extrapolations and predict drug

Algorithm 9.8 Physiologically Based Pharmacokinetics

1. Construct a typical compartment model using object-oriented programming (any OOP computer language or visual simulation tool).
2. Make copies of the typical compartment model (TCM) and that customized based on the PBPK model
3. Connect the TCMs based on the PBPK diagram.
4. Input parameters for each TCM:
   The model parameters can be assumed to be fixed values, from data, or validated by data. The model parameters can also be chosen as random variables. In such cases, one can generate parameter distributions for each compartment using the technique in Sect. 9.1.
5. Determining output parameters:
   Many different PK outputs can be easily obtained for the model for each compartment (organ) or the body as a single entity. The PBPK simulation model can also output the traditional PK parameters such as C_{max}, AUC, $t_{1/2}$, and others.

effects over a wide range of conditions. The improved dose metric can then be used in place of traditional dose metrics (e.g., administered dose) or can be generated as a time-dependent input for a more biologically based response model to simulate the time course of the drug. Figure 9.4 is an illustration of a PBPK model.

In general, a PBPK model can be determined by the permeability matrix $[k_{ij}]$, where the element k_{ij} is the permeability between the ith and jth compartments. If k_{ij} are constants, the network is a Markovian process; if $k_{ij} \geq 0$ are time-dependent, the model is a time-dependent Markovian chain.

Implementation of PBPK models can follow the steps outlined in Algorithm 9.8. If you know any object-oriented programming and visual simulation tools such as ExtentSim, building a PBPK model is a straightforward job programming-wise. However, determining the parameters and validating the model are still challenging.

9.5.1.1 Markov Chain with Constant Permeability

It is possible to include fixed and known covariates in the time-independent permeability k_{ij} from state (compartment) i to state (compartment) j. The total permeability for state m is defined as $k_m = \Sigma_{i \neq j} k_{ij}$. In this model, the transition probabilities can be evaluated by means of exponential functions:

$$dP_{kl}(t)/dt = \Sigma_m P_{km}(t) G_{ml}, \qquad (9.19)$$

where $G_{ml} = -k_{ml}$ $(m \neq l)$ and $G_{mm} = k_m$.

In general, we can show that

$$P_{kl}(v, t) = P_{kl}(0, t - v). \qquad (9.20)$$

The solution can be described by means of the matrix exponential function, where the matrix of transition probabilities satisfies (Hougaard 2001)

$$P(v, t) = \exp\{G(t - v)\} = \sum_{r=0}^{\infty} \frac{G^r (t - v)^r}{r!}. \qquad (9.21)$$

The eigenvalues of G are usually distinct, and the solutions for the transition probabilities are the sums of exponential functions, where the rate constants are the eigenvalues of G. Sometimes it might be most convenient to evaluate them explicitly knowing that the transition probabilities are of the form

$$P_{kl}(v,t) = \sum_r \alpha_{klr} \exp\{-\beta_r(t-v)\}, \tag{9.22}$$

where $-\beta_r$, $r = 1,\ldots,S$ are the eigenvalues of G. The solution is only valid when the eigenvalues are distinct. The eigenvalues are found as the solutions to the general matrix determinant equation

$$|G + \beta I| = 0, \tag{9.23}$$

where I is the identity matrix. The eigenvectors are required to satisfy a set of boundary conditions and a set of balance equations,

$$P_{kk}(t,t) = 1, \text{ and } P_{kl}(t,t) = 0 \text{ for } k \neq l, \tag{9.24}$$

which can be expressed as, respectively,

$$\sum_r \alpha_{kkr} = 1, \text{ and } \sum_r \alpha_{klr} = 0 \text{ for } k \neq l. \tag{9.25}$$

The balance equations specify that the solutions have to satisfy Eq. 9.23. This can generally be written as

$$-\alpha_{klr}\beta_r = \sum_m \alpha_{kmr}k_{ml}, \tag{9.26}$$

for each r.

9.5.2 Pharmacodynamic Simulation

9.5.2.1 Objectives of Pharmacodynamics

Pharmacodynamics is the study of the relationship between the drug concentration at the site of action and the pharmacological response (biochemical and physiological effects). According to the occupancy theory, originated by Clark (1933), the drug effect is a function of the following processes: binding of drug to the receptor, drug-induced activation (or inhibition) of the receptor, and propagation of this initial receptor activation (or inhibition) into the observed pharmacological effect, where the intensity of the pharmacological effect is proportional to the number of receptor

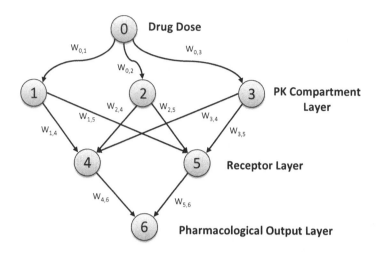

Fig. 9.5 Artificial neural network for PD

sites occupied by drug. The interaction of a drug molecule with a receptor causes a chain of reactions (events) that could lead to a desirable pharmacological effect or undesirable side effect. Therefore, the relationship between pharmacokinetic and pharmacodynamic properties is a focus of pharmacodynamics. In PK, we study the relationship between dose regimen and plasma drug concentration (PK); in PD, we study the time course of the concentration in relation to the pharmacological (positive or negative) responses using modeling and simulation. The goal is to use pharmacokinetics to develop dosing regimens that will result in plasma concentrations in the therapeutic window and yield the desired therapeutic or pharmacological response.

In general, a typical PK-PD curve for an ideal drug can be divided into three stages: (1) low dose level, where no biological effect will be seen; (2) moderate dose level, where pharmacological or clinical effects are expected to be seen, but some infrequent adverse events will also be observed; and (3) pharmacological response has no significant changes but toxicity increases dramatically. We should choose a dose regimen to avoid situations (1) and (3) and target situation (2).

The commonly used models are logistic and E_{max} models (Chang 2010). Here we consider the artificial neural network (ANN). There are many possible ANNs for pharmacodynamic analyses. Figure 9.5 presents an ANN with four layers: input, PK compartment, receptor, and pharmacological output layers.

The layer structure such as the one in ANNs is very common in our lives. The nodes in each layer perform similar roles but differ in magnitude or efficiency (weights differ). Once some nodes fail, other nodes in the same layer will take more "responsibilities" or weights to accomplish the mission. There are plenty of examples where several units in a system have the same functionality but differ in efficiency or time (it seems that redundant equals robust). For example, many people can accomplish the same task, but their speed and quality of outcomes differ. There are many cells that carry out similar functions or several biological pathways that could cause the same disease. For this reason, we can consider them the nodes in the same layer in an ANN and use a linear combination for the outcome.

Keep in mind that, in the regression method, less significant parameters are removed from the final model to avoid overfitting. In an ANN, no parameters are removed from the model, but the weights are adjusted gradually based on observed (training) data using algorithms such as the back-propagation method discussed in Chap. 8.

9.6 Implementation Challenges

The precision of simulation results will depend on the model assumptions, machine memory, and quality of the random number generation. Let's illustrate the precision of simulation using a trivial example for which the exact answer is known. Suppose we want to know the probability of $x < 0.000001$, where random variable x has a uniform distribution in $[0, 1]$. We draw a sample x_i ($i = 1$ to $10,000,000$) and inspect the number of observations within $[0, 0.000001)$. Ideally, we should find 10 such observations. However, we can't always expect 10; otherwise, x is not random at all. If it is one off from 10 (i.e., 11 or 9), it will be 11% off in precision. In addition, pseudorandom numbers are not completely random: x may not be truly uniform over an arbitrary small interval of $[0,1]$, and x will repeat the whole sequence after a certain point. The largest size of nonrepeated sequence is called the period of a random number sequence.

The second problem is computer power. The currently available power from a single computer or a small-scale parallel computing network is good enough for clinical trial simulations but not sufficient for complex biological simulation and molecular modeling. The large number of pathways (10,000) and reactions involved (800 identified) demand more computing power. The same is true for molecular modeling: 3D molecular docking itself requires a large amount of CPU time, and, on top of that, finding the structure-activity relationship adds another layer of complexity. The emerging IT platform cloud-computing technology, could be a better solution. Cloud computing is an IT platform that aims at global information and computer resource exchanges. It is predicted that computing will 1 day be the fifth utility (after water, electricity, gas, and telephony). This computing utility, like all four other existing utilities, will provide computing services that are considered essential to meet the everyday needs of individuals and communities.

Sensitivity analyses, often used in simulation, can be used to answer "What if" questions and serve as a supporting tool in optimization. These sensitivity analyses provide insights about how the model behaves and thus can be used as a model validation tool. The analyses allow us to make earlier preparations if the actual course deviates from our initial predictions. However, to determine a small set of "what if" scenarios that are just enough to cover what is likely to happen is not always easy. Many other challenges in simulation are the same as those in modeling using pharmaceutical decision and game theory (Chap. 2), and will not be repeated here.

Keep in mind that computer simulations require the ability to rapidly integrate knowledge and experiences from different disciplines into the decision-making process and hence require a shift to a more collaborative working environment among disciplines.

9.7 Exercises

9.1. The log-normal distribution $LN\left(\mu, \sigma^2\right)$ p.d.f. is given by

$$f\left(x\right) = \frac{1}{\sqrt{2\pi}\sigma x} \exp\left(-\frac{(\ln x - \mu)^2}{2\sigma^2}\right).$$

Devise a computer algorithm for generating samples from this distribution.

9.2. Use Monte Carlo to evaluate the value of π from the formula $\pi = \frac{4}{\sqrt{2}}$ $\int_0^1 \frac{1+x^2}{1+x^4}dx$.

9.3. Use Monte Carlo to evaluate the constant $e = \frac{\pi}{2} / \int_0^\infty \frac{\cos x}{1+x^2}dx$.

9.4. Implement Algorithm 9.3 using a computer language, and design an adaptive trial (see Chap. 4).

9.5. Implement Algorithm 9.4 and run simulations.

9.6. Implement Algorithm 9.6 and run simulations.

9.7. Carry out a comparative study on software products available for molecular design and docking.

9.8. Conduct research and give the mathematical definitions and biological interpretations of the following terms in a Petri net: reachability, coverability, liveness, boundedness, P-invariance, and T-invariance. Hint: See Chang (2010).

9.9. Develop a computer algorithm using the pseudocode for the PBPK model presented in Fig. 9.4.

9.10. Develop a back-propagation algorithm for the ANN defined in Fig. 9.5.

Further Readings and References

Baldi, P., Hirschberg, D.S.: An intersection inequality sharper than the Tanimoto triangle inequality for efficiently searching large databases. J. Chem. Inf. Model. **49**(8), 1866–1870 (2009)

Chang, M.: Clinical trial simulations in early development phases. In: Chow, S.C. (ed.) Encyclopedia of Biopharmaceutical Statistics. Taylor and Francis, New York (2007)

Chang, M.: Monte Carlo Simulation for the Pharmaceutical Industry. Chapman and Hall/CRC, Boca Raton (2010)

Chen, M., Hofestädt, R.: Quantitative Petri net model of gene regulated metabolic networks in the cell. In Silico Biol. **3**(3), 347–365 (2003)

Chernick, M.: Bootstrap Methods: A Guide for Practitioners and Researchers, 2nd edn. Wiley-Interscience, New York (2007)

Clark, A.: Applied Pharmacology, 5th edn. Churchill, London (1933)

Efron, B., Tibshirani, R.: An Introduction to the Bootstrap. Chapman and Hall/CRC, Boca Raton (1994)

Fishman, G.: Monte Carlo, Concepts, Algorithms and Applications. Springer, New York (1996)

Hamilton, S., Ho, K.F.: Efficient drug supply algorithms for stratified clinical trials by focusing on patient coverage-not just site supplies-this dynamic approach significantly reduces drug waste. Appl. Clin. Trials Feb 1 (2004)

Höltje, H., Sippl, W., et al.: Molecular Modeling: Basic Principles and Applications, 3rd edn. Wiley-VCH, Frankfurt (2008)

Hougaard, P.: Analysis of Multivariate Survival Data. Springer-Verlag, New York (2001)

Koch, I., Heiner, M.: Petri net. In: Junker, B.H. (eds.) Analysis of Biological Networks. Wiley, Hoboken (2008)

Lipinski, C.A., Lombardo, F., Dominy, B.W., Feeney, P.J.: Experimental and computational approaches to estimate solubility and permeability in drug discovery and development settings. Adv. Drug Deliv. Rev. **23**, 3–25 (1997)

Lipkus, A.: A proof of the triangle inequality for the Tanimoto distance. J. Math. Chem. **26**, 263–265 (1999)

Liu, J.S.: Monte Carlo Strategies in Scientific Computing. Springer, New York (2001)

Materi, W., Wishart, D.S.: Computational systems biology in drug discovery and development: Methods and applications. Drug Discov. Today **12**(7/8), 295–303 (2007)

Matsuno, H., et al.: Biopathways representation and simulation on hybrid functional Petri net. In Silico Biol. **3**, 389–404 (2003)

Miyamoto, S., Kollman, P.A.: Absolute and relative binding free energy calculations of the interaction of biotin and its analogs with streptavidin using molecular dynamics/free energy perturbation approaches. Proteins **16**, 226–245 (1993)

Paolini, G.V., Shapland, R.H.B., van Hoorn, W.P., Mason, J.S., Hopkins, A.L.: Global mapping of pharmacological space. Nat. Biotechnol. **24**, 805–815 (2006)

Schneider, G., Baringhaus, K.H.: Molecular Design: Concepts and Applications. Wiley-VCH Verlag, Frankfurt (2008)

Szarfman, A., Machado, S.G., O'Neill, R.T.: Use of screening algorithms and computer systems to efficiently signal higher-than-expected combinations of drugs and events in the US FDA's spontaneous reports database. Drug Saf. **25**(6), 381–392 (2002)

Taylor, H.M., Karlin, S.: An Introduction to Stochastic Modeling, 3rd edn. Academic, San Diego (1998)

Von Neuman, J.: Various technigues used in connection with random digits. National Bureau of Standards Applied Math Series **3**, 36–38 (1951)

Chapter 10
Bayesian Methods and Applications

10.1 Bayesian Paradigm

This introductory section will provide some key elements in the Bayesian paradigm and a quick review of basic Bayesian methods. It is intended mainly for those who are new to Bayesianism or Bayesian applications in biostatistics.

10.1.1 Bayesian Inference

There are different statistical paradigms or theoretical frameworks that reflect different philosophies or beliefs. These differences have provoked quite a few controversies. However, within each paradigm or axiom system, consistency and completeness are expected. Our discussions in this chapter will focus on the Bayesian paradigm.

Definition 10.1. A Bayesian statistical model is made of a parametric statistical model, $f(x|\theta)$, and a prior distribution of the parameters, $\pi(\theta)$.

The Bayes Theorem places causes (observations) and effects (parameters) on the same conceptual level since both have probability distributions. It is considered a major step from the notion of an unknown parameter to the notion of a random parameter (Robert 1997). However, it is important to distinguish x and θ: x is usually observable, but θ is usually latent.

Denote the prior distribution by $\pi(\theta)$ and the sample distribution by $f(x|\theta)$. The following are four basic elements of the Bayesian approach:

1. the joint distribution of (θ, x), given by

$$\varphi(\theta, x) = f(x|\theta) \pi(\theta), \qquad (10.1)$$

M. Chang, *Modern Issues and Methods in Biostatistics*, Statistics for Biology and Health, 261
DOI 10.1007/978-1-4419-9842-2_10, © Springer Science+Business Media, LLC 2011

2. the marginal distribution of x, given by

$$m(x) = \int \varphi(\theta, x) \, d\theta = \int f(x|\theta) \, \pi(\theta) \, d\theta, \tag{10.2}$$

3. the posterior distribution of θ, given by the Bayes formula

$$\pi(\theta|x) = \frac{f(x|\theta) \, \pi(\theta)}{m(x)}; \text{ and} \tag{10.3}$$

4. the predictive probability distribution, given by

$$P(y|x) = \int P(x|y, \theta) \, \pi(\theta|x) \, d\theta. \tag{10.4}$$

Example 10.1. Beta Posterior Distribution: Assume that $X \sim Bin(n, p)$ and $p \sim Beta(\alpha, \beta)$. The sample distribution is given by

$$f(x|p) = \binom{n}{x} p^x (1-p)^{n-x}, \quad x = 0, 1, \ldots, n. \tag{10.5}$$

The prior about the parameter p is given by

$$\pi(p) = \frac{1}{B(\alpha, \beta)} p^{\alpha-1} (1-p)^{\beta-1}, \quad 0 \leq p \leq 1, \tag{10.6}$$

for the beta function $B(\alpha, \beta) = \frac{\Gamma(\alpha)\Gamma(\beta)}{\Gamma(\alpha+\beta)}$.

The joint distribution then is given by

$$\varphi(p, x) = \frac{\binom{n}{x}}{B(\alpha, \beta)} p^{\alpha+x-1} (1-p)^{n-x+\beta-1}, \tag{10.7}$$

and the marginal distribution is

$$m(x) = \frac{\binom{n}{x}}{B(\alpha, \beta)} B(\alpha + x, n - x + \beta). \tag{10.8}$$

Therefore the posterior distribution is given by

$$\pi(p|x) = \frac{p^{\alpha+x-1} (1-p)^{n-x+\beta-1}}{B(\alpha + x, \beta + n - x)} = Beta(\alpha + x, \beta + n - x). \tag{10.9}$$

Example 10.2. Normal Posterior Distribution: Assume that X has a normal distribution: $X \sim N(\theta, \sigma^2/n)$ and $\theta \sim N(\mu, \sigma^2/n_0)$. The posterior distribution can be written as

$$\pi(\theta|X) \propto f(X|\theta) \, \pi(\theta) \tag{10.10}$$

or

$$\pi(\theta|X) = Ce^{-\frac{(X-\theta)^2 n}{2\sigma^2}} e^{-\frac{(\theta-\mu)^2 n_0}{2\sigma^2}}, \tag{10.11}$$

where C is a constant. We immediately recognize that (10.11) is the normal distribution of $N(\frac{n_0\mu + nX}{n_0 + n}, \frac{\sigma^2}{n_0 + n})$.

We now wish to make predictions concerning future values of X, taking into account our uncertainty about its mean θ. We may write $X = (X - \theta) + \theta$, so that we can consider X the sum of two independent quantities: $(X - \theta) \sim N(0, \sigma^2/n)$ and $\theta \sim N(\mu, \sigma^2/n_0)$. The predictive probability distribution is given by

$$X \sim N\left(\mu, \sigma^2\left(\frac{1}{n} + \frac{1}{n_0}\right)\right). \tag{10.12}$$

If we have already observed the mean of the first n_1 observations $\bar{x}_{n_1}$, the predictive distribution is given by

$$X|x_{n_1} \sim N\left(\frac{n_0\mu + n_1\bar{x}_{n_1}}{n_0 + n_1}, \sigma^2\left(\frac{1}{n_0 + n_1} + \frac{1}{n}\right)\right). \tag{10.13}$$

10.1.1.1 Conjugate Family

We have noticed that, in Examples 10.1 and 10.2, the posterior distributions are the same as the priors. In general, a family F of probability distributions on Θ is said to be conjugate if, for every $\pi \in F$, the posterior distribution $\pi(\theta|x)$ also belongs to F. Commonly used conjugate families are presented in Table 10.1.

10.1.1.2 Point Estimate

The Bayesian point estimate is the posterior expectation of the parameter, given by

$$E(\theta) = \int \pi(\theta|x)\theta d\theta. \tag{10.14}$$

Parallel to the frequentist confidence interval, the Bayesian credible interval (BCI) describes the variability of the parameter θ.

Table 10.1 Commonly used conjugate families

Model $f(x|\theta)$	Prior $\pi(\theta)$	Posterior $\pi(\theta|x)$
Normal $N(\theta, \sigma^2)$	$N(\mu, \tau^2)$	$N\left(\frac{\sigma^2\mu + \tau^2 x}{\sigma^2 + \tau^2}, \frac{\sigma^2\tau^2}{\sigma^2 + \tau^2},\right)$
Poisson $P(\theta)$	$G(\alpha, \beta)$	$G(\alpha + x, \beta + 1)$
Gamma $G(v, \theta)$	$G(\alpha, \beta)$	$G(\alpha + v, \beta + x)$
Binomial $Bin(n, \theta)$	$Beta(\alpha, \beta)$	$Beta(\alpha + x, \beta + n - x)$
Neg. Bin $NB(m, \theta)$	$Beta(\alpha, \beta)$	$Beta(\alpha + m, \beta + x)$

Definition 10.2. For $0 < \alpha < 1$, a $100(1-\alpha)\%$ credible set for θ is a subset $C \in \Theta$ such that

$$P\{C|X = x\} = 1 - \alpha. \tag{10.15}$$

The BCI usually is not unique. The commonly used equal-tailed credible interval does not necessarily have the smallest size. The smallest-sized credible interval is defined by the highest posterior density (HPD).

Definition 10.3. Suppose the posterior density for θ is unimodal. Then the HPD interval for θ is the interval

$$C = \{\theta : \pi(\theta|X = x) \geq k\}, \tag{10.16}$$

where k is chosen such that

$$P(C|X = x) = 1 - \alpha. \tag{10.17}$$

10.1.1.3   Hypothesis Testing

For the hypothesis test,

$$H_o : \theta \in \Theta_0 \text{ versus } H_a : \theta \in \Theta_a, \tag{10.18}$$

we would use the posterior odds ratio (POR) $\frac{P(\Theta_0|x)}{P(\Theta_a|x)}$; a small value of POR is strong "evidence" against the null hypothesis H_o.

We can separate the POR into the prior component and current evidence from the current data

$$\frac{P(\Theta_0|x)}{P(\Theta_a|x)} = \frac{P(\theta \in \Theta_0)}{P(\theta \in \Theta_a)} BF, \tag{10.19}$$

where the Bayes factor (BF) is defined as

$$BF = \frac{\int_{\Theta_0} f(x|\theta) \pi_0(\theta) \, d\theta}{\int_{\Theta_a} f(x|\theta) \pi_a(\theta) \, d\theta}. \tag{10.20}$$

The BF is independent of the prior and equal to the POR when $P(\theta \in \Theta_0) = P(\theta \in \Theta_a)$. The BF may be more useful in practice than the POR because the prior is subjective and varies from individual to individual, and it is difficult to convince everyone to use a particular individual prior. In general, we reject H_o if the $BF \leq k_0$, where k_0 is a small value, e.g., 0.1. A small value of the BF implies strong evidence in favor of H_a or against H_o.

10.1.1.4 Bayesian *p*-value

Suppose we want to test the null hypothesis that $H_o : \theta \leq 0$ against an alternative hypothesis that $H_a : \theta > 0$.

The frequentist *p*-value is the probability of having the observed treatment difference or larger under the condition $\theta = 0$; i.e., Pr(more extreme data$|\theta = 0$). The Bayesian *p*-value, calculated from the posterior distribution, is the probability of $\theta \leq 0$ (no treatment effect) given the observed data, i.e., Pr($\theta \leq 0|$data).

Bayesian significance is claimed when the Bayesian *p*-value is less than or equal to the so-called Bayesian significance level α, a predetermined constant that does not have to be the same as the frequentist significance level. Spiegelhalter et al. (2004) provided examples in clinical trials using the concept of the Bayesian *p*-value.

10.1.1.5 Asymptotic Property

Using Taylor's expansion near $\tilde{\theta}_n$, we have

$$\ln \pi (\theta|X_n) = \ln \pi \left(\tilde{\theta}_n|X_n\right) + \left(\theta - \tilde{\theta}_n\right) \frac{\partial}{\partial \theta} \ln (\theta|X_n) |_{\tilde{\theta}_n}$$
$$-\frac{1}{2} \left(\theta - \tilde{\theta}_n\right)' \tilde{I}_n \left(\theta - \tilde{\theta}_n\right) + o \left(||\theta - \tilde{\theta}_n||^3\right), \quad (10.21)$$

where the generalized observed Fisher information matrix is given by

$$\tilde{I}_n \left(\theta - \tilde{\theta}_n\right) = -\frac{\partial^2}{\partial \theta_i \partial \theta_j} \ln (\theta|X_n) |_{\theta = \tilde{\theta}_n}. \quad (10.22)$$

Here we have assumed that $\ln (\theta|X_n)$ is sufficiently differentiable and has finite derivatives at $\tilde{\theta}_n$ with respect to θ.

Theorem 10.1. *If* $\ln (\theta|X_n)$ *is sufficiently differentiable and has finite derivatives at* θ_0 *with respect to* θ, *then for any prior* $\pi_0(\theta)$,

$$P \left(\lim_{\substack{n \to \infty \\ \tilde{\theta}_n \to \theta_0}} \int \pi_n (t|X_1, \ldots, X_n) - \frac{\sqrt{\tilde{I}(\theta_0)}}{\sqrt{2\pi}} \exp \left(-\frac{1}{2} t^2 \tilde{I}(\theta_0)\right) dt = 0 \right) = 1,$$
$$(10.23)$$

where $\pi_n(t|X_1, \ldots, X_n)$ *is the posterior density of* $t = \sqrt{n}(\theta - \tilde{\theta}_n)$ *given* $X_1, \ldots, X_n$.

10.1.2 Model Selection

Suppose i.i.d. samples x are drawn from a density $f(x|\theta)$ with an unknown parameter θ. Then we face a model selection problem:

$$\begin{cases} M_0 : X \sim f(x|\theta) \text{ where } \theta \in \Theta_0, \\ M_1 : X \sim f(x|\theta) \text{ where } \theta \in \Theta_1. \end{cases} \tag{10.24}$$

Let $\pi_i(\theta)$ be the prior density conditional on M_i being the true model. We can use the Bayes factor BF_{01} for model selection:

$$BF_{01} = \frac{\int_{\Theta_0} f(x|\theta)\,\pi_0(\theta)\,d\theta}{\int_{\Theta_1} f(x|\theta)\,\pi_1(\theta)\,d\theta}. \tag{10.25}$$

We know that the Bayes factor is the ratio of the posterior odds ratio of the hypotheses to the corresponding prior odds ratio. Thus, if the prior probability $P(M_0) = P(\Theta_0)$ and $P(M_1) = P(\Theta_1) = 1 - P(\Theta_0)$, then

$$P(M_0|x) = \left\{ 1 + \frac{1 - P(\Theta_0)}{P(\Theta_0)} \frac{1}{BF_{01}(x)} \right\}^{-1}. \tag{10.26}$$

Therefore, if conditional prior densities π_0 and π_1 can be specified, we should simply use the Bayes factor BF_{01} for model selection. If $P(\Theta_0)$ is also specified, the posterior odds ratio of M_0 to M_1 can be used.

However, the computation of the BF may not always be easy. In such cases, we can use the Bayesian information criterion (BIC). Using the Taylor series expansion, we have the approximation (Ghosh et al. 2006)

$$2\ln(BF_{01}) = 2\ln\left(\frac{f\left(x|\hat{\theta}_0\right)}{f\left(x|\hat{\theta}_1\right)} \right) - (\kappa_0 - \kappa_1)\ln n + O(1), \tag{10.27}$$

where κ_0 and κ_1 are the number of parameters in models M_0 and M_1, respectively, and n is the number of data points in x. Here the term $(p_0 - p_1)\ln n$ can be viewed as a penalty for using a more complex model. Alternatively, the Akaike information criterion (AIC),

$$\text{AIC} = 2\ln f\left(x|\hat{\theta}\right) - 2\kappa, \tag{10.28}$$

is often used, where κ is the number of parameters in the model. The AIC has a smaller penalty for more complex models than the BIC does.

10.1.3 Hierarchical Model

For modeling, it is often convenient and appropriate to use Bayesian statistical models hierarchically with several levels of conditional prior distributions.

Definition 10.4. A hierarchical Bayes model is a Bayesian statistical model, $(f(x|\theta), \pi(\theta))$, where the prior distribution $\pi(\theta)$ is decomposed into conditional distributions

$$\pi_1(\theta|\theta_1), \pi_2(\theta_1|\theta_2), \cdots, \pi_n(\theta_{n-1}|\theta_n) \qquad (10.29)$$

and a marginal distribution $\pi_{n+1}(\theta_n)$ such that

$$\pi(\theta) = \int_{\Theta_1 \times \cdots \times \Theta_n} \pi_1(\theta|\theta_1) \pi_2(\theta_1|\theta_2) \cdots \pi_n(\theta_{n-1}|\theta_n) \pi_{n+1}(\theta_n) \, d\theta_1 \cdots d\theta_n.$$

$$(10.30)$$

The parameters θ_i are called hyperparameters of level i.

Note that hierarchical structures do exist in frequentist models. See the following example.

Example 10.3. The following random-effect model can be viewed as a hierarchical model:

$$\boldsymbol{y}|\boldsymbol{\theta} \sim N(\boldsymbol{\theta}, \Sigma_1)$$
$$\boldsymbol{\theta}|\boldsymbol{\beta} \sim N(\boldsymbol{X\beta}, \Sigma_2). \qquad (10.31)$$

The mean of $\boldsymbol{y}$, $\boldsymbol{\theta}$, is decomposed into fixed effects, $\boldsymbol{X\beta}$, and random effects, and $\boldsymbol{Z\eta}$ is normal with mean 0 (the covariance Σ_2 can be singular).

10.1.3.1 Exchangeability

The parameters $(\theta_1, \ldots, \theta_n)$ are exchangeable in their joint distribution if the density $f(\theta_1, \ldots, \theta_n)$ is invariant with respect to permutations of the indexes $(1, \ldots, n)$.

The simplest form of exchangeable distribution has each of the parameters θ_j as an independent sample from a prior (or population) distribution governed by some unknown parameter vector ϕ; thus,

$$f(\theta|\phi) = \prod_{j=1}^{n} f(\theta_j|\phi). \qquad (10.32)$$

In general, ϕ is unknown, so our distribution for θ must average over our uncertainty in ϕ:

$$f(\theta) = \int \prod_{j=1}^{n} f(\theta_j|\phi) \pi(\phi) \, d\phi. \qquad (10.33)$$

10.1.3.2   Elimination of Nuisance Parameters

In a multivariate or hierarchical model, our interest may not be in the full parameter vector $\theta = (\theta_1, \ldots, \theta_n)$ but only certain components of θ. In the frequentist paradigm, there are three methods that can be used (Ghosh et al. 2006, p. 51): (1) constructing a conditional test, (2) using an invariance argument, and (3) using the profile likelihood defined as

$$L_p(\theta_1) = \sup_{\theta_2} f(x|\theta_1, \theta_{1+}) = f\left(x|\theta_1, \hat{\theta}_{1+}(\theta_1)\right), \qquad (10.34)$$

where θ_1 is the parameter of interest, $\theta_{1+} = (\theta_2, \theta_3, \ldots, \theta_n)$, and $\hat{\theta}_{1+}(\theta_1)$ is the MLE of θ_{1+} given the value of θ_1.

In the Bayesian paradigm, to eliminate the nuisance parameters we just integrate them out in the joint posterior. This "integrate out" approach can also be used on other quantities; e.g., analogous to profile likelihood,

$$L(\theta_1) = \int f(x|\theta_1, \theta_{1+}) \, \pi(\theta_{1+}|\theta_1) \, d\theta_{1+}. \qquad (10.35)$$

10.1.4   Bayesian Decision-Making

Statistical analyses and predictions are motivated by objectives. When we choose between models, we evaluate their consequences or impacts. The impact is characterized by a loss function in decision theory. The challenge is that different people have different perspectives on the loss and hence different loss functions. Loss functions are often vague and not explicitly defined, especially when we make decisions in our daily lives. Decision theory makes this loss explicit and deals with it with mathematical rigor.

In decision theory, statistical models involve three spaces: the observation space X, the parameter space Θ, and the action space A. Actions are guided by a decision rule $\delta(x)$. An action $\alpha \in A$ always has an associated consequence characterized by the loss function $L(\theta, a)$. In hypothesis-testing, the action space is $A = \{$accept, reject$\}$.

Because it is usually impossible to uniformly minimize the loss $L(\theta, a)$, in the frequentist paradigm, the decision rule δ is determined to minimize the following average loss:

$$\begin{aligned} R(\theta, \delta) &= E^{X|\theta}(L(\theta, \delta(x))) \\ &= \int_X L(\theta, \delta(x)) \, f(x|\theta) \, dx. \end{aligned} \qquad (10.36)$$

The rule $a = \delta(\mathbf{x})$ is often called an estimator in estimation problems. Commonly used loss functions are *squared error loss* (SEL), $L(\theta, a) = (\theta - a)^2$, *absolute loss*, $L(\theta, a) = |\theta - \alpha|$; and *0-1 loss*, $L(\theta, a) = I(|\alpha - \theta|)$, for example.

Definition 10.5. Bayesian expected loss is the expectation of the loss function with respect to the posterior measure,

$$\rho(\delta(\mathbf{x}), \pi) = E^{\theta|X} L(\delta(\mathbf{x}), \theta) = \int_{\Theta} L(\theta, \delta(\mathbf{x})) \, \pi(\theta|\mathbf{x}) \, d\theta. \qquad (10.37)$$

An action $a^* = \delta^*(\mathbf{x})$ that minimizes the posterior expected loss is called a Bayes action.

By averaging (10.36) over a range of θ for a given prior $\pi(\theta)$, we can obtain

$$r(\pi, \delta) = E^{\pi}(R(\theta, \delta))$$

$$= \int_{\Theta} \int_{X} L(\theta, \delta(\mathbf{x})) \, f(\mathbf{x}|\theta) \, \pi(\theta) \, d\mathbf{x} \, d\theta. \qquad (10.38)$$

The two notions in (10.37) and (10.38) are equivalent in the sense that they lead to the same decision.

Theorem 10.2. *An estimator minimizing the integrated risk $r(\pi, \delta)$ can be obtained by selecting, for every $x \in X$, the value $\delta(x)$ that minimizes the posterior expected loss, $\rho(a, \pi)$, because*

$$r(\pi, \delta) = \int_{X} \rho(a, \delta(\mathbf{x})|\mathbf{x}) \, m(\mathbf{x}) \, d\mathbf{x}. \qquad (10.39)$$

The Bayes estimators use uniform representations of loss functions.

10.1.5 Bayesian Approach to Multiplicity

In Chap. 1, we provided many multiplicity examples. Here are three more examples: (1) In analyses of gene expression microarrays, we are interested in the mean differential expression, μ_i, of genes $i = 1, \ldots, 10{,}000$, using hypothesis tests $H_0 : \mu_i = 0$ versus $H_1 : \mu_i \neq 0$. The multiplicity problem is that even if all $\mu_i = 0$, one would find that roughly 500 tests reject at, say, level $\alpha = 0.05$, so a correction for this effect is needed. (2) In pharmacovigilance for monitoring drug safety, we conduct a sequence of analyses on a cumulative adverse drug event database (Chap. 8). Without multiplicity control, all drugs will eventually be flagged unsafe. (3) In syndromic surveillance of the national defense and homeland security, many counties in the USA perform daily tests on the "excess" of some symptoms, wishing to have early detection of the outbreak of epidemics or bioterrorist attacks (Berger 2009).

We should be aware that Bayesian views on multiplicity are different from those of frequentists. Therefore, the Bayesian approach to multiplicity is different from the frequentist approaches. We also must not confuse the penalty on a more complex model (Occam's Razor principle) with the multiplicity penalty. When competing hypotheses are equal in other respects, the principle recommends selection of the hypothesis that introduces the fewest assumptions and postulates the fewest entities while still sufficiently answering the question.

Multiple tests in exchangeable settings are handled by a mixed model $y_i = w f_0 + (1 - w) f_1$, where f_0 and f_1 are distributions under signal and noise, respectively. The primary goal is to flag which y_is are signals and which are noise. We have seen an application of this approach to drug safety signal detections in Chap. 8.

The general empirical Bayes approach to such a problem can be outlined as follows:

1. Represent the hypothesis-testing problem, $H_i : \theta_i = 0$, as a model uncertainty problem: model M_i, with densities $f_i(x|\theta_i)$ for data x, given unknown parameters θ_i.
2. Specify prior distributions $\pi_i(\theta_i)$, and calculate the marginal likelihoods $m_i(x) = \int f_i(x|\theta_i) \pi_i d\theta_i$.
3. Specify the forms of prior probabilities, $P(M_i)$, of models to reflect the multiplicity issues.
4. Implement Bayesian model averaging based on

$$P(M_i|x) = \frac{P(M_i) m_i(x)}{\sum_j P(M_j) m_j(x)}. \tag{10.40}$$

The quantities of interest are $P(M_i|x)$, the probabilities of inclusion of θ_i (equivalent to $\theta_i \neq 0$) in the model and the distributions of the "signals" if the corresponding null is not true.

Example 10.4. Suppose data X arise from a normal linear regression model, with K possible regressors having associated unknown regression coefficients β_i, $i = 1, \ldots K$, and unknown variance σ^2. Consider selection from among the submodels $M_i, i = 1, \ldots, 2^K$, having only k_i regressors with coefficients $\boldsymbol{\beta}_i$ (a subset of $(\beta_1, \ldots, \beta_K)$) and resulting density $f_i(x|\boldsymbol{\beta}_i, \sigma^2)$. We consider Zellner-Siow priors $\pi_i(\beta_i, \sigma^2)$ for the prior density under M_i. The marginal likelihood of M_i is given by

$$m_i(x) = \int f_i(x|\beta_i, \sigma^2) \pi_i(\beta_i, \sigma^2) d\beta_i d\sigma^2. \tag{10.41}$$

Define Bernoulli variables $\gamma_i = 1$ if $\beta_i \neq 0$ and $\gamma_i = 0$ if $\beta_i = 0$. The standard modern practice in Bayesian variable-selection problems is to treat variable inclusions as exchangeable Bernoulli trials with common success probability $p(\gamma_i = 1)$

(called the inclusion probability), which implies that the prior probability of a model is given by

$$P(M_i) = p^{k_i} (1 - p)^{K-k_i}.$$ (10.42)

We discuss the empirical and full Bayes choice of the prior inclusion probability p.

1. Empirical Bayes exchangeable variable inclusion

Find the MLE $\hat{p}$ by maximizing the marginal likelihood of p (often called type-II maximum likelihood),

$$\hat{p} = \arg\max_{p\in[0,1]} \sum_j p^{k_j} (1 - p)^{K-k_j} m_j (x),$$ (10.43)

and use $P(M_i) = \hat{p}^{k_i}(1 - \hat{p})^{K-k_i}$ as the prior model probabilities. Thus, from (10.40), the posterior probability of M_i becomes

$$P (M_i|x) \propto \hat{p}^{k_i} (1 - \hat{p})^{K-k_i} m_i (x).$$ (10.44)

From (10.43), we can see that the empirical Bayes model does control for multiplicity in that $\hat{p}$ will be small if K is large due to many β_is that are zero. If $p_{i,\max} = \max_{\gamma_i=1, j\in(1,...,K)} P(M_j|x) > p_c$, β_i will be included. In other words, if model M_j includes $\beta_i \neq 0$ and a posterior $P(M_j|x) > p_c$, then β_i will be included. With that approach, the false positive (inclusion of $\beta_i = 0$ in any submodel M_j) rate can be controlled. Numerical examples can be found elsewhere (Scott and Berger 2010).

It is interesting to know (Scott and Berger 2010) that in the variable-selection problem, if the null model M_0 (including no β_i) has the (strictly) largest marginal likelihood among all models, then the type-II MLE of p is $\hat{p} = 0$. Similarly, if the full model M_F (including all β_is) has the (strictly) largest marginal likelihood, then the type-II MLE of p is $\hat{p} = 1$. As a consequence, the empirical Bayes approach here would assign final probability 1 to M_0 whenever it has the largest marginal likelihood and final probability 1 to M_F whenever it has the largest marginal likelihood. These are clearly very unsatisfactory answers. My suggestion for handling this problem is to add an artificial variable x_0 known to have the corresponding parameter $\beta_0 \neq 0$ and another variable x_{K+1} known to have the corresponding parameter $\beta_{K+1} = 0$. With these two artificial variables, we can ignore the posterior null model and full model because we know they are false. Of course, we can add more variables that have known β_i to improve model performance.

A good model should have higher probabilities to include any β_is that are not truly zero and lower probabilities to include any β_is that are truly 0. The separation of these two types of probabilities (the true and false inclusion probabilities) is determined by the curvature of $m_i(x)$, which is instructive in selecting the density $f_i(x|\theta_i)$ for model M_i.

2. Bayes exchangeable variable inclusion

Each variable, β_i, is independently in the model with unknown inclusion probability p. A commonly used prior is $p \sim Beta(p|a, b)$. Thus

$$P(M_i) = \int_0^1 p^{k_i}(1-p)^{K-k_i}\, Beta\,(p|a,b)\, dp = \frac{Beta\,(a+k_i, b+K-k_i)}{Beta\,(a,b)}.$$
(10.45)

For a uniform prior on p, $a = b = 1$, (10.45) reduces to

$$P(M_i) = \frac{k_i!\,(K-k_i)!}{(K+1)\,K!} = \frac{1}{K+1}\binom{K}{k_i}^{-1}.$$
(10.46)

Therefore the posterior model is

$$P(M_i|x) \propto \frac{1}{K+1}\binom{K}{k_i}^{-1} m_i(x).$$
(10.47)

Similar to the situation for the empirical Bayes model, it is clear that $P(M_i) \to 0$ as $K \to \infty$, and the separation of true and false inclusion probabilities is determined by the curvature of $m_i(x)$.

Scott and Berger (2010) show that the prior odds ratio (smaller/larger) is reduced as the number of variables K increases, and if one uses the posterior inclusion criterion $\geq p_c = 0.5$ to include β_i, the false positive (inclusion of noise variable) rate will be controlled – multiplicity control.

It should be pointed out that the equal prior probabilities $P(M_i) = 2^{-K}$ do not control for the multiplicity; it corresponds to a fixed prior inclusion probability $p = 1/2$ for each variable.

Note that the control of multiplicity by Bayesian variable inclusion usually reduces model complexity but is different from the usual Bayesian Occam's Razor effect that reduces model complexity. The latter operates through the effect of model priors $\pi_i(\beta_i, \sigma^2)$ on $m_i(x)$, penalizing models with more parameters, whereas multiplicity correction occurs through the choice of the $P(M_i)$.

The multiple associations that arise in fitting structured low-dimensional models in order to describe high-dimensional joint distributions (dimension reduction), such as Gaussian graphical models, can be found elsewhere (Carvalho and Scott 2009).

10.1.6 Bayesian Computation

A Markov chain is a sequence of random variables $\theta^{(1)}$, $\theta^{(2)}$,..., such that for any t the distribution of $\theta^{(t)}$ depends only on $\theta^{(t-1)}$. Markov chain Monte Carlo

(MCMC) is a general method based on drawing values of θ from approximate Markov chain distributions and then correcting those draws over time to better approximate the target posterior, $p(\theta|y)$. MCMC is an effective means of sampling from the posterior distribution of interest even when the form of that posterior has no known algebraic form.

The idea behind the simulation of a posterior distribution is that if we can easily simulate a sequence of θ_i $(i = 1, 2, \ldots)$ from an unnormalized conditional density $q(\theta|y)$, given observations y, we can construct an empirical distribution of θ using the normalization

$$\hat{\theta}_i = \frac{\theta_i}{\sum \theta_j}. \tag{10.48}$$

In other words, the histogram of $\hat{\theta}_i$ forms the desired empirical distribution. Using this empirical distribution, an inference (estimate, hypothesis test, CI) is a straightforward task. Once simulations have been obtained from the posterior distribution, $p(\theta|\tilde{y})$, sampling from the predictive distribution of future data, $\tilde{y}$, can be simple. For each draw of θ from the posterior distribution, we just draw one value $\tilde{y}$ from the predictive distribution, $p(\tilde{y}|\theta)$. The set of simulated $\tilde{y}$s from all the θs characterizes the posterior predictive distribution.

The key to Markov chain simulation is to create a Markov process whose stationary distribution is the target posterior distribution. If such an MC is found, then we can run the simulation long enough so that the distribution reaches approximately its stationary state. The number of simulation runs needed to reach the stationary state is called the "burning period."

There are two popular MCMC algorithms, Gibbs and Metropolis-Hastings (see, e.g., Chang 2010), described below.

10.1.6.1 Gibbs Algorithm

The Gibbs method is an iteration algorithm in which during each iteration cycle through the parameter $\theta_1, \theta_2, \ldots, \theta_n$, a typical $\hat{\theta}_i$ is drawn conditional on the value of all the others, $\theta_{-i} = \{\theta_1, \ldots, \theta_{i-1}, \theta_{i+1}, \ldots \theta_n\}$. Let's illustrate this with a simple bivariate normal distribution (Gelman et al. 2004).

Consider a single observation (y_1, y_2) from a bivariate normally distributed population with an unknown mean $\theta = (\theta_1, \theta_2)$ and a known covariance matrix $\left(\begin{smallmatrix} 1 & \rho \\ \rho & 1 \end{smallmatrix}\right)$. With a uniform prior distribution on θ, the posterior distribution is

$$\begin{pmatrix} \theta_1 \\ \theta_2 \end{pmatrix} | y \sim N \left(\begin{pmatrix} y_1 \\ y_2 \end{pmatrix}, \begin{pmatrix} 1 & \rho \\ \rho & 1 \end{pmatrix} \right). \tag{10.49}$$

At step t, draw a sample from each of the following marginal posterior distributions in turn:

$$
\begin{cases}
\text{draw } \hat{\theta}_1^{(t)} \text{ from } \theta_1|\theta_2, y \sim N\left(y_1 + \rho\left(\theta_2^{(t-1)} - y_2\right), 1 - \rho^2\right), \\
\text{draw } \hat{\theta}_2^{(t)} \text{ from } \theta_2|\theta_1, y \sim N\left(y_2 + \rho\left(\theta_1^{(t)} - y_1\right), 1 - \rho^2\right).
\end{cases}
\tag{10.50}
$$

The initial value $\theta^{(0)}$ can affect the convergence of the algorithm.

10.1.6.2 Metropolis Algorithms

The Metropolis algorithm is a general term for a family of Markov chain simulation methods for drawing samples from Bayesian posterior distributions. The method is an extension of the usual rejection-acceptance sampling method (Chap. 9). The algorithm proceeds as follows:

1. Draw a starting point $\theta^{(0)}$ at timestep $t = 0$, for which $p(\theta^{(0)}|y) > 0$, from a starting distribution $p_0(\theta)$.
2. Sample a proposal θ^* from a proposal distribution at timestep t, $J_t(\theta^*|\theta^{(t-1)})$, where J_t is symmetric; i.e., $J_t(\theta|\eta) = J_t(\eta|\theta)$.
3. Draw a sample u from the uniform distribution $U(0, 1)$.
4. If $u < \tilde{r}$, then $\theta^{(t)} = \theta^*$, otherwise, $\theta^{(t)} = \theta^{(t-1)}$, where $\tilde{r} = \frac{p(\theta^*|y)}{p(\theta^{(t-1)}|y)}$.
5. Increase the timestep t by 1 and go back to step 2.

The symmetry requirement for $J_i(\cdot|\cdot)$ can be removed if we define the quantity r as

$$
\tilde{r} = \frac{p\left(\theta^*|y\right) J_t\left(\theta^{(t-1)}|\theta^*\right)}{p\left(\theta^{(t-1)}|y\right) J_t\left(\theta^*|\theta^{(t-1)}\right)}.
\tag{10.51}
$$

The Metropolis algorithm with $\tilde{r}$ defined by (10.43) is called the Metropolis-Hastings algorithm.

To illustrate the algorithm, Gelman et al. (2004, p. 290) provided the following example. The target density is the bivariate unit normal, $p(\theta|y) = N(0|0, I)$, where I is the 2×2 identity matrix. The jumping distribution is also bivariate normal, centered at the current iteration, $J_t(\theta^*|\theta^{t-1}) = N(\theta^*|\theta^{t-1}, 0.2^2 I)$. At each step, the density ratio $r = N(\theta^*|0, I)/N(\theta^{t-1}|0, I)$ can be calculated. In general, the proposal distribution should be chosen such that (1) for any θ it is easy to sample from $J_t(\theta^*|\theta^{(t-1)})$; (2) the value r is larger (otherwise samples will be rejected too often, causing inefficiency) and is easy to compute; and (3) each step goes a reasonable distance in the parameter space.

10.1.6.3 Convergence

MCMC is convergent to the target posterior over time. To determine the time of convergence or the burning period, we can use multiple sequences with m overdispersed starting points. The convergence can be determined using the quantity

$$G = \frac{n-1}{n}W + \frac{1}{n}B, \tag{10.52}$$

where B and W are between- and within-sequence variances, i.e., the burning ends as soon as $G < \varepsilon$ (a small positive value).

10.2 Applications of Bayesian Methods

10.2.1 Clinical Trial Design

We are going to use an example to illustrate some differences between Bayesian and frequentist approaches in trial designs.

Example 10.5. Effect of Prior on Power: Consider a two-arm parallel design comparing a test treatment with a control. Suppose three historical trials show that the effect sizes are 0.1, 0.25, and 0.4. The three trials have approximately the same sample size and variance of the effect size.

For the two-arm trial, the power of the hypothesis test from the frequentist approach is a function of effect size ε,

$$\text{power}(\varepsilon) = \Phi\left(\frac{\sqrt{n}\varepsilon}{2} - z_{1-\alpha}\right), \tag{10.53}$$

where Φ is the c.d.f. of the standard normal distribution and $z_{1-\alpha} = \Phi^{-1}(1-\alpha)$.

With the Bayesian approach we consider the uncertainty of ε, with prior $\pi(\varepsilon) = 1/3$ for $\varepsilon = 0.1, 0.25$, and 0.4. The expected power can be calculated as

$$P_{\exp} = \int \Phi\left(\frac{\sqrt{n}\varepsilon}{2} - z_{1-\alpha}\right)\pi(\varepsilon)\,d\varepsilon. \tag{10.54}$$

Numerical integration is usually required for evaluation (10.46).

To illustrate the implication of (10.54), let's assume a one-sided $\alpha = 0.025$, $z_{1-\alpha} = 1.96$, and the prior

$$\pi(\varepsilon) = \begin{cases} 1/3, & \varepsilon = 0.1, 0.25, 0.4, \\ 0, & \text{otherwise.} \end{cases} \tag{10.55}$$

Conventionally, we use the average of the effect size, $\bar{\varepsilon} = 0.25$, to design the trial and calculate the sample size. For the two-arm balanced design with type-II error rate $\beta = 0.2$ or power $= 80\%$, the total sample from (10.45) is given by

$$n = \frac{4(z_{1-a} + z_{1-\beta})^2}{\varepsilon^2} = \frac{4(1.96 + 0.842)^2}{0.25^2} = 502. \tag{10.56}$$

With the Bayesian approach, the expected power from (10.54) with a sample size of 252 is the average of the three powers calculated using the three different effect sizes (0.1, 0.25, and 0.4), which turns out to be 66%, much lower than the 80% from the frequentist approach.

This is an example of a Bayesian-frequentist hybrid approach, i.e., the Bayesian approach is used for the trial design to increase the probability of success given the final statistical criterion, p-value $\leq \alpha = 0.025$.

10.2.2 Bayesian Adaptive Trial

How the response is related to the dose for a new investigational product is a question that is usually answered in a dose-finding or dose-response study. Dose-response trials may serve a number of objectives, among which the following two are particularly important: the investigation of the shape and location of the dose-response curve and the determination of a maximal dose beyond which additional benefit would be unlikely to occur. These objectives should be addressed using the data collected at a number of doses under investigation, including a placebo (zero dose) wherever appropriate. There are various sample size calculation methods available for dose-response trials with different endpoints (Chang and Chow 2006; Chang 2007b).

The continual reassessment method (CRM) is a model approach in which the parameters for the response model are continually updated based on the observed response data using a Bayesian approach. Actions taken (assigning the next patient an appropriate dose, modifying or dropping doses, and/or adjusting sample size) are based on the updated dose-response relationship. In principle, this method can be applied to many different problems, but here we use an oncology dose-escalation trial as an example.

10.2.2.1 Probability Model for Dose-Response

Let x be the dose or dose level, and $p(x)$ be the probability of response or response rate. The commonly used model for dose-response is the logistic model

$$p(x) = [1 + b \exp(-ax)]^{-1}, \tag{10.57}$$

where b can be a predetermined constant and a is a parameter to be updated based on observed data.

10.2.2.2 Prior Distribution of Parameter

The Bayesian approach requires the specification of the prior probability distribution of the unknown parameter a,

$$a \sim g_0(a), \tag{10.58}$$

where $g_0(a)$ is the prior probability. A beta distribution is often used.

When there is very limited knowledge about the prior, a noninformative prior can be used.

10.2.2.3 Likelihood Function

The next step is to construct the likelihood function. Given n observations with y_i ($i = 1, \ldots, n$) associated with dose x_{m_i}, the likelihood function can be written as

$$f_n(\mathbf{r}|a) = \prod_{i=1}^{n} [p(x_{m_i})]^{r_i} [1 - p(x_{m_i})]^{1-r_i}, \tag{10.59}$$

where

$$r_i = \begin{cases} 1, & \text{if a response is observed for } x_{m_i}, \\ 0, & \text{otherwise.} \end{cases} \tag{10.60}$$

10.2.2.4 Reassessment of Parameter: Posterior Distribution

The response model (10.57) is continually updated through the posterior distribution based on the cumulative response data observed from the trial thus far. In other words, the posterior probability of parameter a can be obtained as follows:

$$g_n(a|\mathbf{r}) = \frac{f_n(\mathbf{r}|a)g_0(a)}{\int f_n(\mathbf{r}|a)g_0(a)\, da}. \tag{10.61}$$

After obtaining $g_n(a|\mathbf{r})$, we can update the predictive probability using

$$p(x) = \int [1 + b \exp(-ax)]^{-1} g_n(a|\mathbf{r})\, da. \tag{10.62}$$

10.2.2.5 Assignment for the Next Patient

The updated dose-toxicity model is usually used to choose the dose level for the next patient. In other words, the next patient enrolled in the trial is assigned the currently estimated MTD (maximum tolerated dose) based on the dose-response model (10.57). In practice, this assignment is subject to safety constraints such as a limited dose jump. Assignment to a patient of the most updated MTD is intuitive. This way, the majority of the patients will be assigned to the dose levels near the MTD, which allows for a more precise estimation of the MTD.

10.2.2.6 Stopping Rule

There are many possible rules for stopping a trial. For example, when a fixed total number of subjects is reached, the trial will stop. However, this simple method often does not work well. An alternative is to fix the number of subjects at a dose level and whenever the number is reached at any dose level, the trial will stop. Simulations have shown that this is more efficient than fixing the total number of subjects (Chang 2008).

10.2.2.7 Extension of CRM

Extensive studies have been done along the lines of CRM and dose-finding studies: CRM for bivariate competing outcomes (Braun 2002), dose-finding based on toxicity-efficacy trade-offs (Thall and Cook 2004), dose-finding with two agents in phase-I oncology trials (Thall et al. 2003), a hybrid Bayesian adaptive design for dose-response trials (Chang and Chow 2005), a logistic regression for drug combination trials (Wang and Ivanova 2005), a dose-finding model using toxicity-efficacy odds-ratio contour (Yin et al. 2006), a quasi-likelihood approach to accommodating multiple toxicity grades (Yuan et al. 2007), the Bayesian model averaging approach, safety-efficacy modeling to time-to-event outcomes, copula regression for drug-combination trials (Yin and Yuan 2009a,b), and others.

For a combination of drugs, a single model may not fit the data well. In such cases, the average CRM can be used, in which multiple models are specified and the final average toxicity rate is the weighted average of the models,

$$\bar{p}(x) = \hat{\pi}_k(x) \Pr(M_k|D),$$

where D denotes the observed data and M_k is the kth model with toxicity rate $p_k(x; a_k)$ (e.g., a logistic model (10.57)). The weight $\hat{\pi}_k(x)$ is the posterior mean of the toxicity probability,

$$\hat{\pi}_k(x) = \frac{\int p_k(x; a_k) L(D|M_k(a_k)) f(a_k|M_k) \, d\alpha_k}{\int L(D|M_k(a_k)) f(a_k|M_k) \, da_k},$$

where $f(a_k|M_k)$ is the prior distribution of a_k under model M_k and $L(D|M_k(a_k))$ is the likelihood function under model $M_k(a_k)$.

For a bivariate model that models the toxicity and efficacy data of a compound, the joint distribution function can be constructed using a copula (see Chap. 6) that combines the two marginal distributions $p_e(x)$ for efficacy and $p_t(x)$ for toxicity (Nelsen 1999),

$$p_{et}(x) = 1 - \left\{ (1 - p_e^a(x))^{-c} + (1 - p_t^b(x))^{-c} - 1 \right\}^{-1/c},$$

where the association parameter $c > 0$ characterizes the correlation between efficacy and toxicity, and a and b are constants.

Copulas can also be used for studying drug combinations. In such cases, the association parameter $c > 0$ characterizes the drug-drug interactions.

Alternative to the multivariate approach, we can combine the response variables to form a composite response variable (e.g., in the efficacy-toxicity model, we can construct a univariate model based on the efficacy-toxicity trade-off). However, because the response pattern of the composite variables may not be a simple function, a Bayesian averaging model may be very helpful in this regard.

10.2.3 Safety Signal Detection

For the purpose of analysis, it is helpful to classify adverse drug events (AEs) into tiers. According to Mehrotra and Heyse (2004), Tier 1 AEs are those thought to be caused by the drug or AEs of special interest (AESI). Tier 1 AEs are predefined in the clinical trial protocol, and, if the rate is not very low, this hypothesis may be predefined and tested using the trial data. Tier 2 AEs are any AEs other than Tier 1 that are routinely collected in clinical trials. The analysis of those AEs is descriptive in nature; confidence intervals and p-values for comparison between treatment arms may be reported, but no criteria for rejecting hypotheses are prespecified. Tier 3 AEs are those from postmarketing or are spontaneous. Here we focus on Tier 2 AEs. As stated by Chi et al. (2002), from a regulatory perspective, "Safety assessment is one area where frequentist strategies have been less applicable. Perhaps Bayesian approaches in this area have more promise." Berry and Berry (2004) proposed a three-level hierarchical Bayesian model for analyzing the Tier 2 AEs according to the hierarchical structure of MedDRA (the Medical Dictionary for Regulatory Activities Terminology). MedDRA is a controlled vocabulary widely used as a medical coding scheme. It is a clinically validated international medical terminology used by regulatory authorities and the pharmaceutical industry. The terminology is used throughout the entire regulatory process, from premarketing to postmarketing, and for data entry, retrieval, evaluation, and presentation.

The MedDRA hierarchical structure includes about 25 System Organ Classes (SOCs), 350 high-level group terms, 1,700 high-level terms, 11,000 preferred terms (PTs), and 46,000 lowest-level terms. The hierarchical model will be able to synergize the information within and across SOCs and will allow early detection of safety signals and alert medical reviewers to focus on the right safety issues.

Let A_{bj} be the jth AEs in the SOC, which are assumed exchangeable within the SOC in the following three-level hierarchical mixed model. The probabilities of experiencing A_{bj} are c_{bj} and t_{bj} for subjects in the control and treatment groups, respectively. A commonly used risk measure is the log odds ratio θ_{bj}, which is a logistic transformation of the AE probabilities:

$$\begin{cases} \gamma_{bj} = \ln\left(\dfrac{c_{bj}}{1-c_{bj}}\right), \\[2mm] \theta_{bj} = \ln\left(\dfrac{t_{bj}}{1-t_{bj}}\right) - \gamma_{bj}. \end{cases} \tag{10.63}$$

When $\theta_{bj} = 0$, the probability that a patient experiences A_{bj} is the same for the control and treatment; that is, $c_{bj} = t_{bj}$.

For a level 1 model,

$$\begin{cases} \gamma_{bj} \sim N\left(\mu_{\gamma b}, \sigma_\gamma^2\right), \\[2mm] \theta_{bj} \sim \pi_b I\left(\theta_{bj} = 0\right) + (1-\pi_b) N\left(\mu_{\theta b}, \sigma_{\theta b}^2\right), \end{cases} \tag{10.64}$$

where function $I[x] = 1$ if x is true and 0 otherwise.

For a level 2 model,

$$\begin{cases} \mu_{\gamma b} \sim N\left(\mu_{\gamma 0}, \tau_{\gamma 0}^2\right), \ \sigma_\gamma^2 \sim IG\left(\alpha_{\sigma\gamma}, \beta_{\sigma\gamma}\right), \\[2mm] \pi_b \sim Beta\left(\alpha_\pi, \beta_\pi\right), \\[2mm] \mu_{\theta b} \sim N\left(\mu_{\theta 0}, \tau_{\theta 0}^2\right), \ \sigma_{\theta b}^2 \sim IG\left(\alpha_\theta, \beta_\theta\right), \end{cases} \tag{10.65}$$

where $IG(\cdot, \cdot)$ is the inverse-Gaussian distribution, and $\alpha_{\alpha\gamma}$ and $\beta_{\sigma\gamma}$ are fixed constants.

For a level 3 model,

$$\begin{cases} \mu_{\gamma 0} \sim N\left(\mu_{\gamma 00}, \tau_{\gamma 00}^2\right), \ \tau_{\gamma 0}^2 \sim IG\left(\alpha_{\tau\gamma}, \beta_{\tau\gamma}\right), \\[2mm] \alpha_\pi \sim \dfrac{\lambda_\alpha \exp(-\alpha\lambda_\alpha)}{\exp(-\lambda_\alpha)} I\,(\alpha > 1), \ \beta_\pi \sim \dfrac{\lambda_\beta \exp\left(-\alpha\lambda_\beta\right)}{\exp\left(-\lambda_\beta\right)} I\,(\beta > 1), \\[2mm] \mu_{\theta 0} \sim N\left(\mu_{\theta 00}, \tau_{\theta 00}^2\right), \ \tau_{\theta 0} \sim IG\left(\alpha_{\theta 0}, \beta_{\theta 0}\right). \end{cases} \tag{10.66}$$

The hyperparameters $\mu_{\gamma 00}$, $\tau_{\gamma 00}^2$, $\alpha_{\tau\gamma}$, and $\beta_{\tau\gamma}$ are fixed constants. Here, the function $I[x]$ is used to restrict both parameters in the beta-distribution to be greater than 1 so that the posterior density of π will not become too heavily concentrated at one of its edges.

Berry and Berry (2004) use the parameter values $\mu_{\theta 00} = 0$, $\tau_{\theta 00}^2 = 10$, $\alpha_\theta = 3$, $\beta_\theta = 1$, $\alpha_{\theta 0} = 3$, $\beta_{\theta 0} = 1$, $\alpha_{\tau\theta} = 3$, $\beta_{\tau\theta} = 1$, $\alpha_{\sigma\theta} = 3$, $\beta_{\sigma\gamma} = 1$, and $\lambda_\alpha = \lambda_\beta = 1$ in their simulations, with 10,000 observations from the posterior after a burn-in of 1,000 observations. The posterior distributions and the details of the MCMC methods are available in their paper.

10.2.4 Missing-Data Handling

Missing data are common in practice. Missing data can reduce the power of analysis and cause bias and imprecise estimation. We use Bayesian bootstrapping to illustrate the Bayesian method in handling missing-data issues.

From the Bayes Theorem, the joint posterior distribution of y_{mis} and θ is

$$\varphi\left(\theta, y_{mis}\right) \propto f\left(y_{mis}, y_{obs}|\theta\right) \pi\left(\theta\right), \tag{10.67}$$

where $\pi\left(\theta\right)$ is the prior. The marginal posterior of θ is given by

$$\pi\left(\theta|y_{obs}\right) = \int \varphi\left(\theta, y_{mis}\right) \mathrm{d}y_{mis}. \tag{10.68}$$

We can draw random samples $(\theta^{(1)}, y_{mis}^{(1)}), \ldots, (\theta^{(m)}, y_{mis}^{(m)})$ from $\varphi(\theta, y_{mis})$ to form an empirical distribution to approximate $\pi(\theta|y_{obs})$. This empirical distribution can be used for estimation and inference. For example, given the function $h(\cdot)$, we can have

$$E\left\{h\left(\theta|y_{obs}\right)\right\} \simeq \frac{1}{m}\left[h\left(\theta^{(1)}\right) + \ldots + h\left(\theta^{(m)}\right)\right]. \tag{10.69}$$

In the case that there is no analytical form available, we can easily obtain the marginal distributions $p(y_{mis}|\theta^{(t)}, y_{obs})$ and $p(\theta|y_{mis}^{(t+1)}, y_{obs})$ from the joint distribution $\varphi(\theta, y_{mis})$. The computer algorithms to obtain the posterior distribution of θ are available elsewhere (Chang 2010).

10.2.5 Meta-Analysis

As we discussed in Chap. 7, meta-analysis is a statistical technique for performing integrated analyses by combining results of several independent studies to answer specific questions. Let θ_i and $\sigma_{\theta_i}^2$ be the treatment effect and its variance for the ith clinical trial, $(i = 1, 2, \ldots, K)$.

We can propose a Bayesian hierarchical model,

$$\begin{cases} \hat{\theta}_i|\theta_i, \sigma_{\theta_i} \overset{ind}{\sim} N\left(\theta_i, \sigma_{\theta_i}^2\right), \\ \theta_i = N\left(\theta, \tau_i^2\right), \\ \tau_i^2 \sim \pi\left(\tau^2\right). \end{cases} \tag{10.70}$$

A frequentist estimate for the overall parameter is given by (see Chap. 7)

$$\hat{\theta} = \frac{\sum_{i=1}^{K} w_i^2\left(\tau\right) \hat{\theta}_i}{\sum_{i=1}^{K} w_i^2\left(\tau\right)}, \tag{10.71}$$

where τ can be estimated using a frequentist approach. However, the frequentist estimate $\hat{\tau}$ is inaccurate when the number of meta-analyses is small and $\hat{\theta}$ is sensitive to $\hat{\tau}$. This sensitivity issue can be overcome by using a Bayesian prior for τ^2. Accordingly, w_i in (10.71) is replaced by

$$w_i(\tau) = \int \frac{\pi(\tau^2)}{\sigma_{\theta_i}^2 + \tau^2} d\tau^2. \tag{10.72}$$

Particularly, for the flat prior $\pi(\hat{\tau}^2) = \frac{1}{\tau_{max}^2 - \tau_{min}^2}$,

$$w_i = \frac{1}{\tau_{max}^2 - \tau_{min}^2} \int \frac{1}{\sigma_{\theta_i}^2 + \tau^2} d\tau^2 = \frac{1}{\tau_{max}^2 - \tau_{min}^2} \ln \frac{\sigma_{\theta_i}^2 + \tau_{max}^2}{\sigma_{\theta_i}^2 + \tau_{min}^2}. \tag{10.73}$$

10.2.6 Noninferiority Design

Noninferiority trials are intended to show that the effect of a new medical treatment is not worse than that of an active-control by more than a specified margin, called the noninferiority margin.

The hypothesis test for noninferiority is given by

$$H_o : \theta_T - \theta_C \leq -\delta_{NI} \text{ versus } H_a : \bar{H}_o, \tag{10.74}$$

where θ_T and θ_C are treatment effects for the test and control groups, respectively. Here $\delta_{NI} > 0$ is the noninferiority margin, which is determined based on clinical and statistical considerations.

NI trials are also utilized in the so-called bridging studies. A bridging study (defined by The International Conference on Harmonization E5) is usually conducted in the new region only after the test product has been approved for commercial marketing in the original region due to its proven efficacy and safety. If the foreign clinical data contained in the complete clinical data package (CCDP) cannot provide sufficient bridging evidence, ICH E5 suggests that a bridging study should be conducted in the new region to generate additional information to bridge the foreign clinical data. The ICH E5 therefore defines a bridging study as a supplementary study conducted in the new region to provide pharmacodynamic or clinical data on efficacy, safety, dosage, and dose regimen to allow extrapolation of the foreign clinical data to the population of the new region.

Following Simon (1999), Liu et al. (2004) proposed the model

$$Y = \mu_P(1 - X) + \{\mu_{NT}Z + \mu_{OT}(1 - Z)\} X + \varepsilon, \tag{10.75}$$

where μ_P is the common placebo effect for both new and original regions, μ_{NT} (μ_{OT}) is the treatment mean for the new (original) region, the dummy variable $X = 1$ for the test group and 0 for the placebo group, $Z = 1$ for the new region and 0 for the original region, and $\varepsilon \overset{iid}{\sim} N(0, \sigma^2)$.

Given the data from the bridging study and prior information (μ_P, μ_{NT}, μ_{OT}) formulated from the CCDP, the efficacy observed in the bridging study of the new region is similar if the posterior probability of similarity using the concept of noninferiority is at least $1 - \alpha$; that is,

$$P_{SI} = P\{\mu_{NT} - \mu_{OT} + \delta_{NI} \geq 0|\text{bridging data, prior}\} \geq 1 - \alpha. \qquad (10.76)$$

For the proportional margin $\delta_{NI} = \lambda(\mu_{OT} - \mu_P)$, where $0 < \lambda < 1$, (10.76) becomes

$$P_{SI} = P\{\mu_{NT} - (1 - \lambda)\mu_{OT} - \lambda\mu_P \geq 0|\text{bridging data, prior}\} \geq 1 - \alpha. \qquad (10.77)$$

Based on the n clinical responses from the bridging study, the least-squares mean estimators for μ_{NT} and μ_P are given as (Liu et al. 2004)

$$\begin{pmatrix} Y_{NT} \\ Y_{NP} \end{pmatrix} = \begin{pmatrix} \sum \dfrac{XY}{N_{NT}} \\ \sum \dfrac{1-X}{N_{NP}} \end{pmatrix} \sim N\left(\begin{pmatrix} \mu_{NT} \\ \mu_P \end{pmatrix}, \begin{pmatrix} \dfrac{\sigma^2}{N_{NT}} & 0 \\ 0 & \dfrac{\sigma^2}{N_{NP}} \end{pmatrix} \right), \qquad (10.78)$$

where N_{NT} and N_{NP} are the sample sizes for the test and placebo groups, respectively, in the bridging study.

Assume the prior distribution of the parameter vector $(\mu_P, \mu_{OT}, \mu_{NT})'$ with mean $(\theta_P, \theta_{OT}, \theta_{NT})'$ and diagonal covariance matrix with diagonal elements σ_P^2, σ_{OT}^2, and σ_{NT}^2, respectively. Using the normal prior distribution, the posterior distribution is normal with mean $(\eta_P, \eta_{OT}, \eta_{NT})'$ and a diagonal covariance matrix with diagonal elements τ_P^2, τ_{OT}^2, and τ_{NT}^2, where

$$\begin{cases} \eta_P = \left[\dfrac{\theta_P}{\sigma_P^2} + \dfrac{Y_{NP}}{v_P^2} \right] \tau_P^2, \\[2ex] \tau_P^2 = \left[\dfrac{1}{\sigma_P^2} + \dfrac{1}{v_P^2} \right]^{-1}, \\[2ex] \eta_{OT} = \theta_{OT}, \\[1ex] \tau_{OT}^2 = \sigma_{OT}^2, \\[2ex] \eta_{NT} = \left[\dfrac{\theta_{NT}}{\sigma_{NT}^2} + \dfrac{Y_{NT}}{v_{NT}^2} \right] \tau_{NT}^2, \\[2ex] \tau_{NT}^2 = \left[\dfrac{1}{\sigma_{NT}^2} + \dfrac{1}{v_{NT}^2} \right]^{-1}. \end{cases} \qquad (10.79)$$

It follows that the posterior distribution of the quantity $\mu_{NT} - (1-\lambda)\mu_{OT} - \lambda\mu_P$ is normal with mean ξ and variance ω^2, where

$$\begin{cases} \xi = \eta_{NT} - (1-\lambda)\,\eta_{OT} - \lambda\eta_P, \\ \omega^2 = \tau_{NT}^2 - (1-\lambda)^2\,\tau_{OT}^2 - \lambda^2\tau_P^2. \end{cases} \tag{10.80}$$

With posterior (10.80) and similarity criterion (10.77), it is straightforward to determine the efficacy of the drug in the new region.

10.2.7 Disease Mapping

Hierarchical models can be used in epidemiological studies such as disease mapping. The goal of disease mapping is to provide a geographical distribution of a disease displaying some index such as the relative risk of the disease. Let O_i and E_i $(i = 1, \ldots, N)$ be the observed and expected number of cases of a disease in the ith region. Ghosh et al. (2006) used a multivariate normal distribution for log-relative risks $\ln \theta_i$ in their hierarchical model:

$$\begin{cases} O_i | \theta_i \sim \text{Poisson}\,(E_i\theta_i), \\ \text{where link function } \ln \theta_i = x_i'\boldsymbol{\beta} + \phi_i. \end{cases} \tag{10.81}$$

Let $\boldsymbol{\phi} = \{\phi_1, \ldots, \phi_N\}$. Assuming the conditional autoregressive model for the correlation among the ϕ_is, we can obtain the prior

$$\boldsymbol{\phi} \sim N\,(0, \Sigma), \tag{10.82}$$

where $\Sigma = \lambda\,(D_w - \alpha W)^{-1}$. Here $0 < \alpha < 1$, which ensures the prior spatial correlation, and the proximity matrix W satisfies $\Sigma_{i=1}^{N} w_{ij} = 1$. The element w_{ij} spatially connects regions i and j in a certain manner. $D_w = \text{Diag}(\sigma_1^2, \ldots, \sigma_N^2)$.

Ghosh et al. (2006) used a constant α and a vague prior for β in their example for modeling cancer rates in 56 countries. There are many other applications of the Bayesian approach in the medical and life sciences. More examples can be found in Gelman et al. (2004), Simon (1999), and Spiegelhalter et al. (2004).

10.3 Controversies and Debates

There is a long history of debate between frequentists and Bayesians. Since the nineteenth century, frequentists have dominated the field of statistics. However, there is an apparent trend that Bayesianism is starting to gain momentum. One of the distinctions between frequentist and Bayesianism is that a parameter is considered a fixed unknown in frequentism but an unknown quantity with a distribution in Bayesianism. However, with the development of random-effect modeling in the frequentist approach, this distinction is not that clear anymore. The purpose of statistical modeling and analysis is to guide our decisions. We make our decisions (or take actions) based on our knowledge or perceptions about the truth and not the truth itself. Knowledge virtually always involves uncertainty. This justifies why we consider the distributions of parameters even though the true parameters are fixed.

10.3.1 Internal Consistency

As we mentioned in the beginning of the chapter, Bayesianism and frequentism reflect different beliefs. It is usually acceptable for two controversial mathematical axiom systems to coexist as long as each of them is internally consistent and complete. We are going to discuss consistency within frequentist and Bayesian statistics.

Two fundamental principles are the sufficiency and conditionality principles.

Definition 10.6. When $x \sim f(x|\theta)$, a function T of x (also called a statistic) is said to be *sufficient* if the distribution of x conditionally on $T(x)$ does not depend on θ.

A sufficient statistic $T(x)$ contains the whole information brought by x about the distribution of θ.

When the model allows for a minimal sufficient statistic (i.e., for a sufficient statistic that a function of all the other sufficient statistics), we only have to consider the procedures depending on this statistic.

10.3.1.1 Sufficiency Principle

Two observations, x and y, factorizing through the same value of a sufficient statistic T (i.e., such that $T(x) = T(y)$) must lead to the same inference on θ.

10.3.1.2 Conditionality Principle

If m experiments $(\breve{E}_1, \ldots, \breve{E}_m)$ on the parameter θ are available with equal probability of being selected, the resulting inference on θ should only depend on the selected experiment.

The sufficiency and conditionality principles are so intuitively appealing that no proofs are required, i.e., they are considered axioms.

We now examine the same hypothesis test based on two different experiments.

Example 10.6. Paradox: Binomial or Negative Binomial? Suppose we are interested in the hypothesis test of a binary endpoint

$$H_o : p = 0.5 \text{ vs: } H_a : p > 0.5. \tag{10.83}$$

The experiment is finished with 3 responses out of 12 patients. However, this information is not sufficient for rejecting or accepting the null hypothesis.

Scenario 1: If the total number of patients, $N = 12$, is predetermined, the number of responses X follows the binomial distribution $B(n; p)$ and the frequentist p-value of the test is given by

$$\Pr\left(X \geq 9 | H_o\right) = \sum_{x=9}^{12} \binom{12}{x} 0.5^x 0.5^{12-x} = 0.073.$$

The null cannot be rejected at a one-sided level $\alpha = 0.05$. The likelihood in this case is given by

$$l_1\left(x | p\right) = \binom{12}{9} p^9 \left(1 - p\right)^3 = 220 p^9 \left(1 - p\right)^3.$$

Scenario 2: If the number of responses, $n = 3$, is predetermined and the experiment continues until three responses are observed, then X follows the negative binomial $NB(3; 1 - p)$, and the frequentist p-value of the test is given by

$$\Pr\left(X \geq 9 | H_o\right) = \sum_{x=9}^{\infty} \binom{3 + x - 1}{2} 0.5^x 0.5^3 = 0.0327.$$

Therefore, the null is rejected at a one-sided level, $\alpha = 0.05$. The likelihood in this case is given by

$$l_2\left(x | p\right) = \binom{3 + 9 - 1}{2} p^9 \left(1 - p\right)^3 = 55 p^9 \left(1 - p\right)^3.$$

These two different conclusions are not surprising to any frequentist statistician because it is a routine hypothesis that is based on the control of the type-I error rate α. However, we want to look at the problem a little more closely.

We can show that the conjunction of the sufficiency and conditionality principles leads to the likelihood principle (Robert 1997), which says that the two scenarios above should lead to the same conclusion.

10.3.1.3 Likelihood Principle

The information contained in an observation x about θ is entirely contained in the likelihood function $l(\theta | x)$. Moreover, if x_1 and x_2 are two observations depending on the same parameter θ, such that there exists a constant c satisfying

$$l_1\left(\theta | x\right) = c l_2\left(\theta | x_2\right), \tag{10.84}$$

for every θ, then l_1 and l_2 contain the same information about θ and must lead to identical inferences.

In fact, the likelihood principle is intuitively appealing, too. Since $l_1(x|p) = \frac{220}{55}l_2(x|p)$ in Example 10.5, we can, according to the likelihood principle, conclude that all information is included in $l(p) = p^9(1 - p)^3$, and the two scenarios should not lead to different conclusions (rejection or nonrejection).

Note that the likelihood principle is only valid when (1) the inference is about the same parameter θ and (2) θ includes every unknown factor of the model. The likelihood and sufficiency principles are naturally followed by the Bayesian paradigm. On the other hand, the Bayesian approach rejects other principles, such as the notion of unbiasedness. This notion was once a cornerstone of classical statistics and restricted the choice of estimators to those that are, on average, correct (Lehmann 1983).

10.3.2 Subjectivity

Subjectivity is nothing but a pretext for all kinds of abductions, including the particular choice of research subjects, experiment designs, and model selection processes. Subjectivity exists in every scientific discipline. On the other hand, subjectivity is a reflection of individual experiences; some of those experiences are closely related to the current study, and many others are remotely related. Because these relationships to the current study are unclear or difficult to specify, we call this aggregation of knowledge (evidence) a "subjective prior." However, without this subjective prior, everyone would act no more mature than a newborn baby.

Subjectivity does raise concerns in practice when a decision is required to be made jointly by stockholders who have different priors and when the decision made will have different impacts on them. The statistical criterion for NDA (new drug application) approval is an example. The current regulatory criterion is p-value $\leq$ $\alpha = 5\%$, which we all know is not a good scientific criterion. However, if we use a Bayesian criterion, which prior should be used? Should the prior be different for different drug candidates? Does it sound practical and scientific to get mutual agreement on the prior before we obtain the clinical trial results? If not, poststudy disputes could lead to a disaster.

10.4 Exercises

10.1. Divide the class into teams and perform debates between Bayesian and frequentist paradigms.

10.2. What are the differences in utilization of prior knowledge between Bayesian and frequentist approaches?

10.3. In Example 10.2, suppose $X \sim N(\theta, \sigma^2/n)$ and $\theta \sim N(\mu, \sigma_0^2/n_0)$. Derive the posterior distribution.

10.4. Suppose that in Example 10.2 the prior has just a single observation x_0 from a normal distribution. Derive the posterior distribution.

10.5. If in Example 10.5 we lose the information about how the design was conducted (i.e., we don't know whether the distribution is binomial or negative binomial, but we do know 3 responses out of 12 subjects), how do you use the information to make a conclusion for the hypothesis test?

10.6. Study the relationship between the frequentist p-value and the Bayesian p-value under a normal distribution.

10.7. Discuss the differences between Bayesian hierarchical modeling and frequentist random-effect modeling.

10.8. Discuss the importance of the exchangeability in Bayesian and frequentist paradigms, and study the exchangeability of observations from sequential trial designs.

10.9. Justify the Bayesian decision approach in general.

Further Readings and References

Berger, J.: Statistical Decision Theory and Bayesian Analysis. Springer, New York (1985)
Berger, J.: Bayesian Adjustment for Multiplicity. Subjective Bayes 2009. Duke University Statistical and Applied Mathematical Sciences Institute. December 14–16 (2009)
Berry, S.M., Berry, D.A.: Accounting for multiplicities in assessing drug safety: A three-level hierarchical mixture model. Biometrics **60**, 418–426 (2004)
Braun, T.M.: The bivariate continual reassessment method: Extending the CRM to phase I trials of two competing outcomes. Control. Clin. Trials **23**, 240–256 (2002)
Braun, T.M., Thall, P.F., Nguyen, H., de Lima, M.: Simultaneously optimizing dose and schedule of a new cytotoxic agent. Clin. Trials **4**, 113–124 (2007)
Chang, M.: Adaptive Design Theory and Implementation Using SAS and R. Chapman and Hall/CRC, Boca Raton (2007a)
Chang, M.: Multiple-arm superiority and noninferiority designs with various endpoints. Pharm. Stat. **6**, 43–52 (2007b)
Chang, M.: Classical and Adaptive Designs Using ExpDesign Studio. Wiley, New York (2008)
Chang, M.: Monte Carlo Simulation for the Pharmaceutical Industry. Chapman and Hall/CRC, Boca Raton (2010)
Chang, M., Boral, A.: Current opinion: ABC of Bayesian approach for clinical trials. J. Pharm. Med. **22**(3), 141–150 (2008)
Chang, M., Chow, S.C.: A hybrid Bayesian adaptive design for dose response trials. J. Biopharm. Stat. **15**, 667–691 (2005)
Chang, M., Chow, S.C.: Power and sample size for dose response studies. In: Ting, N. (ed.) Dose Finding in Drug Development. Springer, New York (2006)
Chen, M.H., Shao, Q.M., Ibrahim, J.G.: Monte Carlo Methods in Bayesian Computation. Springer, New York (2000)

Chi, G., Hung, H.M.J., O'Neill, R.: Some comments on "Adaptive Trials and Bayesian Statistics in Drug Development" by Don Berry. Pharm. Rep. **9**, 1–11 (2002)

Carvalho, C.M., Scott, J.G.: Objective Bayesian model selection in Gaussian graphical models. Biometrika **96**(3), 497–512 (2009)

Gelman, A., Carlin, B.J., Stern, H.S., Rubin, D.B.: Bayesain Data Analysis, 2nd edn. Chapman and Hall/CRC, Boca Raton (2004)

Ghosh, G.K., Delampady, M., Samanta, T.: An Introduction to Bayesian Analysis: Theory and Methods. Springer, New York (2006)

Lehmann, E.L.: The Theory of Point Estimation. Wiley, New York (1983)

Liu, J.P., Hsueh, H., Hsiao, C.F.: A Bayesian noninferiority approach to evaluation of bridging studies. J. Biopharm. Stat. **14**, 291–300 (2004)

Mehrotra, D.V., Heyse, J.F.: Multiplicity considerations in clinical safety analyses. Stat. Meth. Med. Res. **13**, 227–238 (2004)

Nelsen, R.B.: An Introduction to Copulas. Springer, New York (1999)

Robert, C.P.: The Bayesian Choice. Springer, New York (1997)

Scott, J.G., Berger, J.O.: Bayes and Empirical-Bayes multiplicity adjustment in the variable-selection problem. Ann. Stat. **38**, 2587–2619 (2010)

Simon, R.: Bayesian design and analysis of active control trials. Biometrics **55**, 484–487 (1999)

Spiegelhalter, D.J., Abrams, K.R., Myles, K.J.: Bayesian Approaches to Clinical Trials and Health-Care Evaluation. Wiley, Southern Chichester (2004)

Thall, P.F., Cook, J.: Dose-finding based on toxicity-efficacy trade-offs. Biometrics **60**, 684–693 (2004)

Thall, P.F., Millikan, R.E., MÄuller, P., Lee, S.-J.: Dose-finding with two agents in phase I oncology trials. Biometrics **59**, 487–496 (2003)

Wang, K., Ivanova, A.: Two-dimensional dose-finding in discrete dose space. Biometrics **61**, 217–222 (2005)

Yuan, Z., Chappell, R., Bailey, H.: The continual reassessment method for multiple toxicity grades: A Bayesian quasi-likelihood approach. Biometrics **63**, 173–179 (2007)

Yin, G., Li, Y., Ji, Y.: Bayesian dose-finding in phase I/II clinical trials using toxicity and efficacy odds ratios. Biometrics **62**, 777–784 (2006)

Yin, G., Yuan, Y.: Bayesian model averaging continual reassessment method in phase I clinical trials. J. Am. Stat. Assoc. **104**, 954–968 (2009a)

Yin, G., Yuan, Y.: Bayesian dose–finding in oncology for drug combinations by copula regression. J. R. Stat. Soc. C **58**, 211–224 (2009b)

Index

M. Chang, *Modern Issues and Methods in Biostatistics*, Statistics for Biology and Health,   291
DOI 10.1007/978-1-4419-9842-2, © Springer Science+Business Media, LLC 2011

Antihypertensive, 13
Apoptosis, 252
Approximate likelihood model, 187–188, 190
Apriori, 206
Arbitrage, 51
Area under the curve (AUC), 254
Arteriosclerotic, 68
Artificial, 117, 200, 206, 213–215, 256, 271
Artificial intelligence (AI) agents, 228
Artificial neural network (ANN), 213–215,
    256–258
Ascending, 10, 240, 242
Ascertained, 141
Assay(s), 61, 79–81, 84, 199, 242, 243
Associated kernel, 188
Asymmetric, 197–199
Asymptotic, 23, 64, 74, 110, 125, 126, 196,
    265
    variance, 125
Augmented, 124, 138
Augmented inverse-probability weighting
    (AIPW) estimator, 124
Authority, 49, 50, 139, 207
Autoimmune diseases, 38
Automata, 217–218
Automated control, 30–31
Automatic signaling methods, 223
Autonomous, 228
Autoregressive (AR), 121, 128, 284
Auxiliary variable, 123, 133, 137
Aversion, 39–40
Axioms, 261, 283, 285

B

Back propagation, 215, 257, 258
Backward(s), 46
    induction, 34, 46, 52, 56
Bacterial, 218
Bagging, 212, 213, 227
Baseline, 27, 111, 120, 134, 142, 151, 182,
    188, 190, 221
    functions, 147
Bate, A., 224
Bayes
    action, 269
    exchangeable variable inclusion, 271, 272
    formula, 262
Bayesian
    approach to multiplicity, 1, 261, 269–272
    computation, 272–275
    decision-making, 268–269
    false positive rate (FPR), 225
    inference, 126, 137, 261–265

method, 126, 224, 261–288
multiplicity, 269–272
Occam's Razor effect, 272
paradigm, 261–275, 287, 288
significance, 265
Bayesian confidence propagation (BCPNN),
    223
Bayesianism, 261, 284, 285
Bayesian network (BN), 245
BC, 171, 176, 224, 245
BCPNN. *See* Bayesian confidence propagation
BDS. *See* Blessed dementia scale
Bellman equations, 33, 34, 37, 38, 41–42, 56
Bellman's optimality principle, 33–34
Bernoulli, 129, 191, 270–271
Best/worst case imputation, 120
Beta, 79, 262, 263, 272, 275, 280
Between-study variation, 179, 190, 195
Bias, 23, 80, 100, 101, 117, 119, 120, 123,
    137, 139, 140, 151, 172, 175, 190,
    197–100, 209, 281
Bin, 192, 262, 263
Binding, 92, 243, 245–248, 255
    free, 247
Binomial, 36, 263, 285, 286, 288
Bioactive, 246
Biochemical screening assays, 242
Biocreep, 61, 81, 84
Bioerodible, 218
Bioinformaticians, 227
Bioinformatics, 205
Biologic, 219
Biological, 2, 149, 213, 218, 227, 229, 243,
    249–251, 256, 258
    organisms, 145
    pathway simulation, 248–252
    processes, 156, 217, 228, 248
Biology, 145, 217, 227, 248, 250
Biomarker, 40, 45, 78, 79, 149, 153, 157–159,
    171, 172
Biopharmaceutical, 31
Biostatistics, 233, 261
Biotech, 39, 45, 50
Bit(s), 244
Bivariate, 157, 159, 273, 274
    model, 278
    survival function, 148, 153
Blanchard-Roquain procedure, 22–23
Blessed dementia scale (BDS), 182, 201
Blind, 87, 106, 140, 229, 238, 242
Bloodstream, 68, 252
BN. *See* Bayesian network
Boltzmann probability, 246
Bonds, 243